IT'S TIME TO ASK QUESTIONS...
WHEN YOUR DOCTOR SUGGESTS THAT:

- Your child should be on Ritalin
- You need antibiotics to get rid of your winter cold
- You should be on hormone therapy after menopause
- Asthma inhalers are all safe and effective
- Steroids are a quick solution to many minor problems
- Someone in your family should undergo bypass surgery

Find out more about the dangers of many commonly used medicines and treatments in

WHAT DOCTORS DON'T TELL YOU

WHAT DOCTORS DON'T TELL YOU

THE TRUTH ABOUT THE DANGERS OF MODERN MEDICINE

LYNNE McTAGGART

AN AVON BOOK

Every illness and every patient are unique. This book is intended as a source of information only. Readers are urged to work in partnership with a qualified, experienced healthcare practitioner before undertaking (or refraining from) any treatments listed in this book.

Some of the names of individuals whose medical experiences are recounted in this book have been changed to protect their privacy.

AVON BOOKS
An Imprint of HarperCollins*Publishers*
10 East 53rd Street
New York, New York 10022-5299

Copyright © 1996, 1998 by Lynne McTaggart
Interior design by Kellan Peck
Published by arrangement with the author
Library of Congress Catalog Card Number: 98-92431
ISBN: 0-380-80761-0
www.avonbooks.com/wholecare

First Wholecare Printing: August 1999
First Avon Books Trade Printing: May 1998

Wholecare Trademark Reg. U.S. Pat. Off. and in Other Countries, Marca Registrada, Hecho en U.S.A.
HarperCollins® is a trademark of HarperCollins Publishers Inc.

Printed in the U.S.A.

WCD 10 9 8 7 6 5 4 3 2

FOR BRYAN

CONTENTS

ACKNOWLEDGMENTS

In 1988, my husband, Bryan, also a journalist, mentioned one day that he thought we should launch a newsletter called *What Doctors Don't Tell You*. We both shared a conviction that modern medicine was unproven and sometimes dangerous, and a passion to share this information with the public. I am sorry to admit this, considering how closely I am now identified with this title, but at the time I told him, quite emphatically, that the idea wouldn't fly. Also, I am sorrier to admit, I thought that title wasn't any good. So Bryan, who knew who he was dealing with, asked if I knew another good editor who might want the job. I snatched the baited hook and all these years later, here I am.

Although many books result from the silent collaboration of many parties, this one is smudged with the fingerprints of most of the people who have been involved with *What Doctors Don't Tell You,* the newsletter. Much of the information contained in this book has been published, in another form, in our newsletter over the years, and this is an attempt to pull it together into a central statement about medicine.

Although not all of our collaborators shared our intense interest in medical matters, all shared our commitment to working as a team. In a sense, this book is the product of every person who contributed in some way to the complicated business of starting a publication—and publishing company—from scratch.

I am grateful, first, to all the support teams we've had since those early days, who have willingly involved themselves with every aspect of our company, when that largely entailed packing envelopes from the top floor of our house: Amanda Hibbs, Danielle Howard, and Vera Chatz, for helping to launch us; Jan Green, Kerry and Jacquie, Jackie Goddard, and Marlene Schwertzel for early admin work; Diane Wray for persisting with a complex subscription system; Beverly Males for her good work with accounts. I am particularly grateful to our present team, the best that anyone could ever hope for: Theresa Harvey, Karen Terkelsen-Shaw, Jim McDonald, Lesley Palmer, Lisa Lathwell, and Andrew Boughton. Of equal importance were my personal support: Dorothy Rothermel, Niomi Klinck, and Marnie Clarke, whose assistance enabled me to juggle home life and work.

Thanks and acknowledgment are due to the many writers whose work in our newsletter has influenced mine: Fiona Bawdon, Deanne Pearson, Pat Thomas, and Clive Couldwell, in particular. And to our wonderful designers: Sue Buchanan, Steve Palmer, Dave Humphries, and Peter Costello.

I am indebted to a number of doctors and practitioners for their help with research and ideas, most particularly Patrick Kingsley, Ellen Grant, Harris Coulter, J. Anthony Morris, John Mansfield, Tony Newbury, Jack Levenson, Melvyn Werbach, Annemarie Colbin, Michel Odent, and Leo Galland. Our family has been privileged to be cared for by a number of special healers in both alternative and orthodox medicine, whose knowledge helped to inform my views. I am also grateful for the twenty-five panel members of *What Doctors Don't Tell You,* particularly the many doctors among them who had the faith in us to put their name to a controversial project before they'd seen one word of it.

I owe a special debt of gratitude to Harald Gaier, for his encyclopedic knowledge of the scientific evidence in alternative medicine and his generosity in sharing it.

All of the case histories mentioned in this book come from real letters we've received from our readers. With the exception of several cases that have been well publicized, the names of all such patients have been changed or shortened to protect their identities. For all their confidence in allowing me access to their private stories and pain, I am especially grateful.

I am also indebted to all our other wonderful subscribers in America and Britain for supporting us through the years and for wanting to read what we had to say.

The entire staff of Avon have my deep gratitude for their enthusiasm and courage in backing this project, most particularly Ann McKay Thoroman. Alistair Pepper of Carter-Ruck took a special interest in this book and spent many arduous hours offering wise counsel, legal and otherwise.

I also owe a special debt to my agent, Russ Galen, who is always there batting for me when I need him. And to all at Agora for their work on our newsletter in the United States.

A special mention must be made of my daughters, Caitlin and Anya, who continue to teach me more about life and health than a roomful of pediatricians ever could.

Three others stand out as particularly vital to the undertaking of this project. As a young journalist, I was privileged to edit the work of Dr. Robert Mendelsohn, whose staggeringly prescient views about medicine have largely informed mine. Dr. Stephen Davies, a nutritional pioneer, not only contributed to my own good health but provided me with a new way of looking at health and disease.

This book and my work owes its largest debt to my husband, Bryan Hubbard, whose thoughts and words are so entwined with mine that this is virtually a work of coauthorship. For his love, for his knowing what I was made to be doing before I did, for the daily joy he gives me in living and working side by side, I am forever grateful.

INTRODUCTION

This book was born from a grand passion I once had: a passion to get better.

In the early eighties, after an extraordinary patch of bad choices, I underwent a prolonged bout of stress. In every profoundly important area of my life, green lights I'd always taken for granted suddenly began turning red. If I had taken one of those little tests you find in women's magazines that add up your stress quotient—with death, marriage, divorce and moving the most stressful situations—my sums would have leapt off the chart.

In rapid succession I'd struggled under an impossible book deadline, married Mr. Wrong, divorced Mr. Wrong, bought the wrong apartment, accepted the wrong job, suffered the death of a close friend, incurred several large debts, and spent a prolonged period of intense isolation in a foreign country. I couldn't, in those days, even get a good haircut.

Shortly after emerging from the eye of this personal squall, I began to experience strange symptoms, at first your workaday "female problems"—everything from ferocious premenstrual tension and irregular periods to cystitis and almost constant vaginal infections.

As time wore on, my symptoms multiplied: eczema, hives, and allergies to a load of food and chemicals; diarrhea and an irritable bowel; insomnia and night sweats; and severe depression.

I had felt powerless for so long that my body seemed to be reacting in parallel, caving in under any sort of microbial onslaught.

For nearly all of the three years that I was ill, I made the rounds of medical circles—first the standard ones, then the periphery, with nutritionists and homeopaths, and finally the very outer rim, from breathing specialists to Bioenergeticists. By the autumn of 1986 I was hacking my way though the dense thicket of New Age therapies. I tried breathing from the abdomen. I had the negative emotions Rolfed out of me. Somebody tried to diagnose me by subjecting my hair sample to radio waves. I ploughed through autogenic training, colonic irrigation, and even a form of psychotherapy—a mixture of Wilhelm Reich and what felt like being tickled on the face. I learned something about my relationship with my mother. But I did not, at any point, get better.

By the summer of 1987 a sense of hopelessness descended over me. The worst part of being chronically unwell without a diagnosis legitimatizing it is that a lot of people don't believe you, or view your symptoms as imaginary—as a puerile sort of attention-getter. And in this land of stoics, if your illness isn't hard-core, like cancer or leprosy, you're supposed to learn to live with it, to dysfunction quietly, without complaint.

At some point it began to dawn on me that there was no miracle remedy out there that was going to turn my health around. If I was going to get better, I was going to have to take charge of the entire process myself—from diagnosis to, possibly, even the cure. Somehow I would have to figure out what was going wrong with my body and find whatever tools were necessary to cure myself. It began to make sense that I should take control of my health, since no one else would care about its outcome so passionately.

I began reading up on allergies and female problems, and one day came upon a newly discovered illness whose symptoms matched almost every one of mine. When a specialist I consulted wasn't familiar with it, I searched out a renowned doctor specializing in allergies and nutritional medicine, whose battery of tests and diagnostic sensitivity confirmed my own suspicions, and rooted out other contributory problems besides.

What I seemed to have inside me was, essentially, thrush of the body, or polystemic chronic candidiasis. *Candida albicans* is a yeast that lives in the upper bowel of most of us without doing good or harm, kept in line by our immune systems and the friendly bacteria that coexist with it. But, according to current theories (and that's all they are at the moment), when the immune system is weakened and the good-guy bacteria fall in numbers, these yeast can start multiplying out of control, sending out toxins that eventually interfere with a range of bodily functions.

Whether or not candida was the main cause of my illness, the root of the problem appeared to be an immune system that wasn't functioning at full throttle. Prolonged severe stress tends to have a depressant effect on the immune system. That, and a bunch of long-dormant allergies, including an allergy to wheat, which probably came to the fore as a result of stress, meant that I was poisoning my body every day with substances it could no longer tolerate. I'd also become sloppy about my diet, and was low in a large number of nutrients.

My treatment consisted of taking large doses of a well-tolerated drug for a time, plus a batch of specially tailored doses of supplements and a restrictive healing diet of fresh, unrefined food. A month after I'd started, my dry cleaner asked me if I'd had a face-lift.

However good these initial results, I soon realized that getting better wasn't going to be an overnight affair. For a year healing became, in effect, my career. Fortunately I had teamed up with an extraordinary doctor, and we worked together as a partnership in recovering my health, and with it, my sense of control. That year was heady and instructive, with plenty of opportunities to meditate on the science and art of healing, as well as the nature of the doctor-patient relationship. It seemed to me that patients were more likely to get better, so long as they were in charge of the decision making about their care. True healing could only begin if there existed a dialogue between doctor and patient, a democracy of shared responsibility. I also experienced firsthand that people can get well without drugs and surgery, just by altering what they eat and how they live. Healing isn't simply a matter of finding the right drug or right operation, but a complex process of accepting responsibility for your own life.

This personal experience stirred up dormant memories that had affected me deeply early in my career. As a young journalist in New York, I had headed the editorial department of the *Chicago Tribune—New York News* Syndicate. There I'd met the late Dr. Robert Mendelsohn and helped to launch his syndicated column "The People's Doctor" in the mid-seventies. As former medical director of a national program for underprivileged children, and chairman of a state licensing committee for doctors, Mendelsohn had been entrenched in the very heart of the medical establishment. Nevertheless, here was this kindly, mild-mannered man, your prototypical Jewish grandfather, blowing the whistle on all his peers by denouncing medicine as excessive and unproven. Every week his column would savage yet another medical sacred cow. Most famously, it was Bob who likened medicine to the new religion. "Medicine," he wrote, "is not based on science—it's based on faith."

Bob sent tremors through the very foundation of my belief system. I had been a product of the postwar baby boom, the Kennedy New Frontier, brought up to regard science and technology as the saviors of mankind. As a teenager I had believed in the principles of Lyndon Johnson's American dream. Most of the big problems of mankind—racism, poverty, illness—could be eliminated by social engineering and science, here in the best country in the world.

In my own journalism, when I began examining some of the social "goods" that medical science engages in—such as "breakthroughs" like the Pill—I came to realize that at times they amounted to a great deal of dangerous meddling. But it wasn't until I began to investigate my own health problems that the prescience of Mendelsohn's views really came home.

Once I got better (which took, all told, a year), I became drawn in my freelance work to medicine. I began studying the professional literature in medical libraries and learned how to read medical studies. I followed around exhausted interns working a standard eighty-four-hour shift in a special baby unit, to get a taste for the extreme conditions that young doctors had to endure (and the kind of questionable care their patients would receive under these conditions).

In time I began to feel I'd walked through the looking glass. Nothing in my university training prepared me for the peculiar, often tortured logic of medical studies. Treatments had been adopted with little or no scientific basis in fact. Studies that cast doubt on a drug's effectiveness were nevertheless applauded as evidence of success. Many of the gravest, sloppy mistakes in study design had been overlooked. Studies clearly showed that certain drugs cause cancer, yet here were top scientists dancing all around the numbers to avoid acknowledging the obvious. Medicine's own scientific literature offered overwhelming evidence that some of it not only didn't work, but was highly dangerous. This was not a "science." This was a belief system so fixed, so inherent, that any truth to the contrary was dismissed as virtual blasphemy.

Fired by the missionary zeal of the newly converted, at some point I became extremely boring on the subject. Probably out of desperation, my then-new partner (now my husband), Bryan, suggested that I start a newsletter about the true risks of medical practices—so I didn't have to tell him anymore, but could tell the world.

At the time, we didn't expect that this newsletter, which we planned to call *What Doctors Don't Tell You,* would be much more than a hobby. I was pregnant by that time, and we thought it might be a way for me to stay home with our first child and make a modest living.

From the outset, after our launch at the 1989 Here's Health show, people showed keen interest in subscribing. By then I had assembled an advisory panel of twenty-five top doctors, chosen because they themselves had blown the whistle on unproven medical practice or pioneered less invasive medical procedures. Although we rarely advertised during the first year, the newsletter seemed propelled forward by its own steam and the zealous faith of our initial subscribers; by the end of that first year we had somehow managed to accumulate 1,000 readers, and now, only a few years after that, many thousands of loyal subscribers in Britain, the United States, and all over the world.

Outrage is now the passion that powers the newsletter—as well as this book. I am livid every time I open my mail. Each morning I wade through piles of letters containing heartrending stories of personal catastrophe—children who have been killed, or husbands and wives mutilated or incapacitated through medicine. Whenever we study their cases we usually discover that the dangers of the treatments given to them were well known. Their doctors just hadn't bothered communicating this vital information to them.

The problem is, by the time they write to us, it is too late.

I have written this book because I don't want you to be another statistic in my morning mail. I do not promise you a comfortable read. Many of the facts in this book are likely to unsettle you. You may learn that much of what your doctor tells you isn't true. But that is my intention. I want to help you to become a more informed medical consumer by determining when you actually need your doctor and when his advice is best ignored. I want to save you from unnecessary treatments and dangerous cures, from "preventive just-in-case medicine" that will leave you damaged even before you've actually become ill. Besides being alerted to the hazards of many accepted practices, you'll also find many proven, safe alternatives for diagnosing, preventing, or treating many illnesses. I want to help you to learn not to be a "good" patient. Good patients, the kind who blindly follow orders instead of demanding answers, sometimes die.

The following pages will open up to you the trade secrets of what has been largely a closed shop. You'll have a chance to listen to the private conversation that medicine conducts with itself. And, once you discover just how much hokum resides in your doctor's medicine cupboard, just how much medicine relies on blind faith, received wisdom, and selective facts, not reason, science, or common sense, you can grab the power away from this false shaman and begin to take back control of your health.

MEDICINE'S FALSE SCIENCE

ONE

The Un-Science of Modern Medicine

It's comforting in life to have certainties. One of the coziest of certainties we've grown up with is that modern medicine works miracles and doctors cure diseases. In the stories we tell ourselves, Dr. Kildare and Marcus Welby, clad in symbolically pure white, engage in the business, all day, every day, of saving lives. And even though more people die in our modern-day equivalents like *ER* and *St. Elsewhere,* those doctors in the emergency room still have gadgets capable of raising the dead.

Our greatest certainty about medicine is that it is a lofty and reputable science, arrived at by scientists in laboratories by exhaustive testing and review. We proudly point to the fact that science has progressed and triumphed over chaos and darkness, over the time when doctors didn't even know that they had to wash their hands.

Since the Second World War, and the discovery of the two great miracle drugs of this century—penicillin and cortisone—medicine has indeed worked miracles. People who would have died from hormone-related deficiencies such as Addison's disease, and life-threatening infections such as pneumonia or meningitis, can now recover easily and return to normal lives. Most of the

3

great medical discoveries—painless surgery, antiseptic hospital environments, X rays—only discovered in the last century, have given us in the West the best emergency medicine in the world. If you have an unforeseen heart attack, an operable brain tumor, a near-fatal car accident, an emergency in childbirth, then Western medicine, with its array of space-age gadgetry, is without parallel for sorting you out. If a building ever falls on me, I'd like all the very latest in Western gee-whiz technology to put me back together. Indeed, if it hadn't been for twentieth-century drugs, my mother would have died in her early twenties and I never would have been born.

It was also these discoveries during the Second World War, ending abruptly with the ultimate scientific discovery, the atomic bomb, which left us with a great expectancy about science. The aftermath of victory was also the dawning of the scientific age of medicine. Science had helped us to conquer our human enemies. Now it would do battle with our microscopic ones. We were beginning to conquer space; it wouldn't be very long, as *Life* magazine promised my generation, before we conquered disease.

Doctors and medical authorities contribute to this view of infallible medical science. Whenever discussing its own track record, especially against that of alternative treatments, medicine stakes out the moral high ground, flying the territorial flag of established scientific fact. In 1980, in mounting an attack on alternative medicine, a *British Medical Journal* editorial self-congratulatingly trumpeted medicine's "record of objective evaluation of claims."[1]

By the same token, orthodox medicine denounces alternative medicine as not following suit. In 1995, one national medical association denounced alternative treatments for allergies as unscientific, warning that "until the methods have been evaluated by reputable, randomized, double-blind, placebo-controlled trials they cannot be accepted into routine clinical practice."[2]

Our faith in medical science is so ingrained that it has become woven into the warp and woof of our daily routine. In any average day in America, a family may place its entire future in the hands of medical advance. For a pregnant mother, the result of prenatal tests may determine whether she carries her pregnancy to term. Her child may be given his vaccine and her husband his blood-pressure-lowering drugs on the premise that this medicine will prevent them from getting future disease. Medical tests determine whether we can have children, continue working, have operations, are eligible for insurance, require cesareans, or, as with an HIV test that comes back positive, are shunned as pariahs. It is doctors with their miracle treatments, we believe, who will deliver us from evil, which, these days, is not temptation so much as the frightening randomness of disease.

But much as we cling to the notion of science as a force of redemption, our faith is misplaced. The truth of it is that medical science actually isn't working too well. The United States is losing the "War on Cancer."[3] Despite state-of-the-art mammogram screening equipment and surgical techniques, breast cancer mortality rates stubbornly refuse to fall. Despite hundreds of thousands of prescriptions of cholesterol drugs and the hundreds of thousands of eggs avoided on low-cholesterol diets, heart attack rates in the West basically remain unchanged. With all the fancy chemicals and computerized testing equipment we have at hand, asthma, arthritis, diabetes, cancer—virtually all the chronic degenerative diseases known to mankind—are thriving, and medicine hasn't affected their incidence one tiny bit.

One glance at the statistics shows that, except in the case of getting run over or needing an emergency cesarean, orthodox Western medicine not only won't cure you but may leave you worse off than you were before. In fact, these days, scientific medicine itself is responsible for a good percentage of disease. If you're in the hospital, there's a one in six chance that you landed there because of some modern medical treatment gone wrong.[4] Once you get there, your chances are one in six of dying in the hospital or suffering some injury while you're there. Since half this risk is caused by a doctor's or hospital's error, you've got an 8 percent chance of being killed or injured by the staff.[5] If we extrapolate the results of a 1984 study, over one million Americans are being injured in the hospital every year, and 180,000 die as a result.[6] To put the magnitude of the problem in perspective, if you live in the United States, where about 40,000 people are shot dead every year, you are nevertheless three times more likely to be killed by a doctor than by a gun.[7]

This appalling track record has nothing to do with incompetence or lack of dedication. Most doctors are extremely well intended, and probably a majority are highly competent in what they've been taught.

The problem isn't the carpenter, but his tools. The fact is that medicine is *not* a science, or even an art. Many of your doctor's arsenal of treatments don't work—indeed, have never been proven to work, let alone to be safe. It is a false science, built upon conjuring tricks, supposition, and blind preconception, whose so-called scientific method is a vast amount of stumbling in the dark.

Many of the treatments we take for granted—for breast cancer or heart surgery, even treatments for chronic conditions such as arthritis or asthma—have been adopted and widely used *without one single valid study demonstrating that they are effective and safe.* The so-called "gold standard" respected by medical scientists as the only scientific proof of the true worth of a drug or treatment is the randomized, double-blind, placebo-controlled trial—that is, a study in which patients are randomly assigned to receive either a drug or a sugar pill, with neither researchers nor participants aware of who is getting what. Nevertheless, despite the fact that thousands of studies are conducted every year, very few of the treatments considered to be at the very cornerstone of modern medicine have been put to this most basic of tests—or, indeed, to any test at all.

For all the science-speak in medicine about risk factors and painstakingly controlled data, the stringent government regulation, the meticulous peer review in professional literature—for all the attempts to cloak medicine in the weighty mantle of science—*a good deal of what we regard as standard medical practice today amounts to little more than twentieth-century voodoo.*

In their own literature, medical authorities openly acknowledge this fact. The prestigious British magazine *New Scientist* recently announced on the cover of one issue that 80 percent of medical procedures used today have never been properly tested.[8] John Garrow, chairman of HealthWatch, a group of self-appointed guardians of honesty in medicine, recently stated that ". . . more than half the forms of care offered in pregnancy and childbirth were judged to have 'unknown effects' or need to be 'abandoned.' There is no reason to suppose that care in other branches of medicine has been more thoroughly validated."[9]

Medicine as it is practiced today is largely a conspiracy of faith. Probably because of the miracle of drugs such as antibiotics, doctors have come to believe that their little black bag ought to be filled, in effect, with magic. The late Dr. Robert Mendelsohn was one of the first to liken modern medicine to a church, with doctors its high priests following the teachings with blind faith: "Modern Medicine is neither an art nor a science. It's a religion," he wrote in his book, *Confessions of a Medical Heretic* (Contemporary Books), "just ask *why?* enough times and sooner or later you'll reach the Chasm of Faith. Your doctor will retreat into the fact that you have no way of knowing or understanding all the wonders he has at his command. *Just trust me.*"[10]

Doctors believe so fervently in the power of their tools that they are willing to suspend all reasonable skepticism about current and new medical treatments—so long as these treatments fit in with orthodox medical practice. Most doctors and researchers operate on the assumption of *a priori* benefit, whether or not a given remedy has actually been proven: *we know what we're doing is right.* Enthusiasm for HRT is so great, for instance, that doctors are willing to ignore the grossest of scientific lapses in safety testing in order to promote what is looked upon *prima facie* as a good thing. *We know what we're doing is right.*

Even if studies have been done demonstrating that a treatment is ineffective or even downright dangerous, so powerful is this faith that these results often get ignored. Virtually every good study of fetal monitoring—devices employing ultrasound testing supposedly to measure the condition of the fetus during labor and birth—all show that this procedure produces a *worse* outcome for mother and child.[11] This information appears well known to many senior obstetricians—the former head of the prestigious

Perinatal Unit in Oxford, Great Britain, repeatedly has written widely about this fact—yet fetal monitors continue to be employed in every delivery room in the land. *We know what we're doing is right.*

This is probably why doctors make such rotten logicians. Many in medicine get tied into logical knots, attempting to justify apparent contradictions with the most arcane Alice-in-Wonderland reasoning. Medical critic Robert Mendelsohn used to say that his favorite line spouted by doctors was: "Breast-feeding is best, but bottlefeeding is just as good."

"High serum cholesterol levels are an important risk factor for coronary disease," wrote noted heart researcher Dr. Meir J. Stampfer of the Harvard School of Public Health, repeating the prevailing view. In the next breath, however, he added, parenthetically: "*but most patients with [heart attacks] have normal cholesterol levels*" (my italics).[12]

The faith in the infallibility of their tools allows doctors to adopt as the "gold standard" what are usually little more than experimental treatments, and employ these on millions before their effects are fully understood or the procedure has stood the test of time. The favorite line of doctors, when steamrolling ahead without proof, is that if they had always waited until they had proper evidence, Lord knows how many advances in medicine would have been held up (and how many millions of people would have died). That argument does not, of course, take into account the vast number of people who *have* died taking unproven treatments later found to be dangerous. Asthma beta-agonist inhalers, found to be linked with deaths after years of being on the market, are only one of many chilling examples of a drug whose potentially fatal side effects appear to have slipped through the regulatory nets unnoticed.[13] Still others, such as amalgam in dental silver fillings and the radical mastectomy, are treatments devised a century ago and never properly tested or reviewed to determine whether they are as safe or effective as has always been presumed.

Medicine as it is now practiced relies entirely on numbers. When judging the worth of any treatment, researchers must weigh the risks of the drugs or treatments (and all treatments in orthodox medicine carry some risks) against their likely benefits and against the risk of the illness being treated. A drug known to be effective but with serious side effects might be worth taking if you have a life-threatening illness, but not if your medical problem is a hangnail.

Medical science is, in the main, a triumph of statistics over common sense. When bumping up against unpalatable truths in the study, medical scientists, who again always assume a medical treatment to be beneficial, are inclined to put the best face on the whole exercise, or cut and paste, refine and edit, to fit the premise or explain away an undesirable result.

Recently, a large study from the Netherlands Cancer Institute showed that all women taking the Pill, no matter what their age, had an increased risk of breast cancer. Most worryingly, 97 percent of women under age thirty-six who contracted breast cancer had taken the Pill, for any length of time.[14] For thirty years doctors have been touting the Pill as the safest drug ever developed. The Dutch study, now the fifth and possibly most damning to show a link between the Pill and cancer, was a colossal embarrassment to an entire industry devoted to contraception at all costs.

However, once they trumpeted the negative findings in the beginning of their article, the Dutch researchers began back-pedaling, by qualifying the overall implications of their findings. They emphasized that the increased risk mainly occurred among certain subgroups. Because the numbers supposedly showed no increased risk of breast cancer after long-term use among women in their later thirties, their study was, in effect, *good* news: "Our findings accord with the mass of evidence that [oral contraceptive use] by women in the middle of their fertile years [twenty-five to thirty-nine years] has *no adverse effect* on breast cancer risk" (my italics).

Doctors can often minimize the risks of drugs by magnifying the risk of not using them. Most studies have been able to justify that the Pill is safe by turning pregnancy into a dangerous disease. This risk-benefit equation works only if you believe it is better to risk breast cancer, cervical cancer, a stroke, or thrombosis—all known risks associated with the Pill—than to have an unwanted baby or to use a condom instead.

A spokeswoman from the Family Planning Association, which has probably handed out its fair share of Pills to teenagers, dismissed any breast cancer risk out of hand, arguing that this theoretical risk had to be weighed against the "evidence that the Pill protects against endometrial and ovarian cancer."[15] This is a typical example of medical reasoning. This drug is beneficial because it may "protect" you against one kind of fatal cancer (a highly questionable conclusion, in any event), even though it may give you another potentially fatal cancer.

And because they live and breathe medicine by numbers, and believe in the infallibility of their tools, doctors are willing to hand out dangerous medication on the confident assumption that new tests will pick up any side effects that they cause, and yet other drugs will be able to treat these new problems. Hence the reason why family planning enthusiasts will usually patiently explain that, even though the Pill may cause cervical cancer, cervical smears should pick up early changes, at which stage things are mainly treatable. Like many in medicine, they make the fatal error of requiring medicine to be infallible. This reasoning works *if* a test that can be wrong more than half the time picks up the cancer early, and *if* medicine can always cure cancer, which thus far it has singularly failed to do.

This kind of tortuous logic was used to minimize new evidence showing a definite, indisputable link between vasectomy and the development of prostate cancer. The two studies, which examined over 74,000 men who had had vasectomies, showed that vasectomy increases the prostate cancer risk by 56 to 66 percent.[16] Those patients who'd had their operation done twenty years ago faced a whopping increase in risk of between 85 and 89 percent. In other words, having a vasectomy twenty years ago nearly doubles your risk of getting cancer.

Pretty damning evidence, one would have thought. Nevertheless, after it was published, some professional magazines encouraged doctors to tell their patients that the risk of prostate cancer following a vasectomy was minimal. The article attempted to claim that, compared to other methods of birth control (*the condom? natural family planning?*), vasectomy is "still one of the safest." A Family Planning Association spokesperson concurred: "These studies *do not tell us* that vasectomy causes prostate cancer" (again, my italics).

Doctors and medical researchers have been known to hype up the risks of a disease compared with the risks of the drug used to treat it. Dangerous drugs look good if you turn an ordinarily benign problem into a killer disease. In 1992, the U.K. Department of Health (DoH) announced the hasty withdrawal of two of the three brands of the combined measles, mumps, and rubella (MMR) vaccines. The official line circulated to the press about why these drugs were withdrawn, after having been jabbed into millions of fifteen-month-olds, were allegedly the results of a study showing that the two withdrawn brands had a "negligible" (1 in 11,000) risk of causing a "transient" and "mild" (all DoH words, these) case of meningitis. The third brand, made from a different strain of the mumps virus, supposedly did not pose this risk.

In 1989, when I first interviewed Dr. Norman Begg of the U.K.'s Public Health Laboratory Service, which recommended the vaccine in Britain, he assured me that mumps on its own was a very mild illness in children. Mumps, he said, "very rarely" leads to long-term permanent complications such as orchitis (where the disease hits the testicles of adult males, very occasionally causing sterility). The mumps component had only been added, he said, to give "extra value" to the jab.[17]

By 1992, however, when the two versions of the MMR were withdrawn, the British government painted a very different picture, announcing that mumps leads to meningitis in 1 in 400 cases. Hence, even though the old vaccine was dangerous (and it must have been pretty dangerous to get hauled off the market virtually overnight), *it was not as dangerous as catching mumps*.

But of course, two-thirds of medical practices don't have any proof at all. There is no such regulatory agency like the Food and Drug Administration to monitor surgery, screening, or diagnostic tests—nothing but peer review through national medical associations. Run by doctors for doctors, these organizations tend to rule by consensus, and by a peculiarly circular logic: If a practice is universally employed, it must be safe, even when many studies point otherwise.

In the case of surgery, most treatments get the nod without any kind of clinical trial (partly because it is very difficult to have either a randomized or double-blind trial or to reverse an operation with an unfavorable result). Consequently, some new techniques get adopted with very little in the way of proof to show they are doing any good or even not doing drastic harm.

Medicine as it is currently practiced is a private conversation by doctors, for doctors. There's no doubt that medicine maintains a double standard. Doctors often privately voice their doubts, disappointments, and fears about particular treatments in their own literature, yet fail to disclose this in any discussion with patients or the press. Recently, an alarming piece of information came to light about vaccines. The Centers for Disease Control and Prevention in Atlanta, Georgia, discovered that children receiving the triple jabs for diphtheria/tetanus/whooping cough or for measles/mumps/rubella were three times more likely to suffer seizures. Nevertheless, this information was announced to only nine scientists and was never otherwise publicized.

Another prime example of this double standard surrounded the issue of treatment for breast cancer. An editorial in the prestigious medical journal The Lancet published a scathing attack on the failure of mammography as a technology to halt the rising breast cancer death rates, and organized a conference to talk over new solutions[18]—at the same time that various government bodies were calling for increasing the frequency of mammograms.

The greatest reason that medical research is tainted is that the majority of it is funded by the very companies who stand to gain by certain results. These drug companies not only pay the salaries of researchers, but they can often decide where—indeed, whether—they get published. It's wise to keep in mind that this industry, in a sense, has a vested interest in ill health: If drug companies found cures, rather than lifelong "maintenance" therapies, they'd soon be out of business.

The constant exposure of medicine to the pharmaceutical industry, and the reliance of future medical research on these companies, has bred a climate in which much of mainstream medicine refuses to consider any other treatment options besides drugs and surgery, even when copious scientific evidence exists to support those options. Many conventional doctors are especially vituperative in their dismissal of important work by innovators, while uncritically embracing many surgical or drug-based solutions that are little more than modern-day snake oil. This has bred a climate into which healers are polarized into "alternative" and "orthodox" camps, rather than into one common group approving of anything that has a solid basis in science or clinical practice. Dr. Peter Duesberg, a leading University of California professor in molecular biology, has been publicly vilified for suggesting, with a well-reasoned argument backed up by a seventy-five-page published paper, that HIV is not the cause of AIDS.

To give you some idea how medicine handles heretics, witness how it reacted to scientific evidence supporting alternative medicine. A recent study, conducted scientifically with all the usual gold standard double-blind, placebo-controlled checks and balances that medicine prides itself on, showed that homeopathy for asthma actually works. Scientists now had some proof: *homeopathy works*. In fact it was the third study carried out by the same man since 1985 to show exactly the same result.

Nevertheless, in his published report the leader of the trial distanced himself from his results, pointing out in his conclusion that tests such as these just might end up producing false-positive, or wrong, results.[19] Despite the scientific design of the trial, an editorial in *The Lancet* flatly refused to accept the results: "What could be more absurd than the notion that a substance is therapeutically active in dilutions so great that the patient is unlikely to receive a single molecule of it? . . . Yes, the dilution principle of homeopathy is absurd; so the reason for any therapeutic effect presumably lies elsewhere."[20] In other words, the scientific method works only when it applies to things we have faith in, but not, it seems, with anything we don't understand or agree with.

The problem with this dogmatic adherence to preconception and dismissal of dissension or doubt, as far as you and I are concerned, is that it covers up the fact that much of standard medical practice may not work very well. It makes dangerous drugs look safe and effective. It makes it seem like people who don't need drugs should take them. It justifies a lot of useless surgery that may very well kill you, and certainly isn't going to make you better. It explains away many promising treatments that don't require dangerous drugs or surgery. Despite the very best of intentions, it sometimes causes untold pain and suffering, rather than contributing to your health. In fact, you are in grave danger from the moment you walk into your doctor's office, particularly at the point when he tells you he'd like to take a few tests.

— II —

DIAGNOSIS

TWO

Diagnostic Excess

Your modern-day doctor has at his disposal an array of high-tech gadgetry that allows him to monitor and measure virtually every nook and cranny of your body. He and his fellow doctors are now completely reliant upon these tests to diagnose disease. As patients, we trust tests so implicitly to provide us with a definitive view of our state of health, even to predict when we're going to get ill at some distant point in the future, that most of our children begin having tests as soon as they've been conceived.

At last count, there were more than 1,400 of these, ranging from the simple blood-pressure cuff to the most sophisticated computerized nuclear magnetic imaging devices. Back in the relatively dark ages of 1987, some 19 billion tests were performed on Americans that year alone, which works out to be eighty tests for each man, woman, and child.[1]

Despite the kind of gadgetry that would put NASA to shame, the problem is that the technology doesn't really work very well. Most tests are grossly unreliable, giving wrong readings a good deal of the time. A false-positive test sets in motion the juggernaut of aggressive treatments at your doctor's disposal, with all *their* attendant risks. But the tests themselves can be as risky as some of the most dangerous drugs and surgery, risks that are magnified because so many of these tests are patently unnecessary. In many cases, doctors protect themselves against potential lawsuits by ordering every test they can. In fact, many orders for tests are motivated by a doctor's own self-interest, since so many physicians either own or have substantial shareholdings in the facilities to which they refer their own patients.

Another problem is that, these days, technology has replaced the fine art of diagnostics—of examining a patient's clinical history and having a good look at his eyes and the state of his tongue. The problem often comes down to trainee doctors, who often order tests under the mistaken notion that their superiors desire such "just-in-case" medicine. But in many cases residents do flog their interns if they fail to request particular tests, engendering the view that more is better and that massive test taking is what constitutes good doctoring.[2]

Tests also make the fundamental error of assuming not only that all people are alike, but that people (and their measurements) always stay the same.

The other problem is that, unless your doctor has a particular feeling for taking apart computers in his spare time, he often doesn't know how to use a good deal of this gee-whiz technology. A recent study found that virtually all doctors and nurses don't know how to work a pulse oximeter, a monitoring system which is vital for monitoring patients recovering from anesthesia and recording potential life-threatening situations.[3] Consequently, they make serious errors in evaluating readings. The medics reported not being "particularly worried" when patients had levels indicating that they were seriously deprived of oxygen and needed immediate attention if they were to live.[4]

BLOOD-PRESSURE READINGS

Your problems can start even when your doctor brandishes his blood-pressure cuff to record your blood pressure. Professor William White, chief of Hypertension and Vascular Diseases at the University of Connecticut, refers to this gizmo, known in medicalese as the "sphygmomanometer," as "medicine's crudest investigation." Blood pressure, he says, can vary tremendously—as much as 30 mm Hg over the course of any day.[5] In fact, the time it's most likely to rise is in your doctor's office, when you're waiting to have the test—a phenomenon known as "white-coat hypertension."

These days, your doctor is more likely to strap you up with a portable electronic device that will measure your blood pressure at preset intervals over twenty-four hours. This is now thought to be the more accurate way of assessing your average blood pressure, although there is still a great deal of evidence that this system, called "ambulatory monitoring," likewise doesn't provide accurate enough information for doctors to decide whether a patient needs treatment for high blood pressure.[6] Even the World Health Organization now recommends that ambulatory monitoring is best conducted with multiple readings over six months. But because no one has yet bothered to do proper large-scale scientific studies, no one can agree over how long you should go on doing the ambulatory monitoring before making a diagnosis, or what actually constitutes high blood pressure over this period, or even how much blood pressure should be lowered to make it "normal."[7]

Even the variation between the arms influences a blood pressure reading. One doctor from City General Hospital in Staffordshire, England, discovered a variation of more than 8 mm Hg in systolic blood pressure between the two arms of nearly a quarter of his patients. In one case, the difference was 20 mm Hg.[8]

Things are just as confusing for pregnant women and children. Doctors and nurses can't even agree over how to record the second beat of blood pressure (called the diastole), which measures when blood fills up the heart,[9] or whether certain sounds accurately reflect diastolic pressure. This was even the subject of a heated debate at a world congress of hypertension in pregnancy in Italy in 1990, calling for an "international consensus" on how to record blood pressure in pregnant women. In fact, recently

some researchers have claimed that doctors have been using the
wrong type of blood-pressure test on pregnant women: Obstetricians and midwives prefer the blood-pressure gauge called Korot-
koff phase 4, but new research shows that phase 5 testing is far
more reliable—the reverse of the prevailing view. In one test,
virtually nobody agreed on the reading from a K4 test, while
everyone was in agreement on the K5 test.[10]

This potential for different interpretations in readings can cause
problems for you if your blood pressure is being monitored by
several people who may have had different training in how to
read the cuffs.

ECG READINGS

Besides blood pressure, your doctor's next favorite activity is
listening to the state of your heartbeat. However, these days, the
all-purpose stethoscope (never proved to have any advantages
over the naked ear) has been replaced by a number of space-age
gadgets, all designed to record the most minute changes in your
heart's ability to do its job.[11] The stalwart of any cardiac specialist
is the electrocardiogram (ECG), even though studies demonstrate
enormous potential for error in recording or interpreting correct
results. One study showed that computers, often used to interpret
ECG readings, were right only two-thirds of the time, and
missed 15 percent of cases of enlargement of the right ventricle.
Nevertheless, human beings didn't fare much better; even trained
heart specialists misinterpreted one out of every four readings.[12]
This is largely because, as with blood pressure, readings can be
affected as much as 20 percent by recent activity, time of day,
and even factors such as fear of the cardiologist's findings! The
late Dr. Robert Mendelsohn wrote of a study in which electro-
cardiography detected only a quarter of proven cases of heart
attack, and another study in which the tests found gross abnormalities in more than half of perfectly healthy people.[13] As Stephen Fulder, author of *How to Be a Healthy Patient* (Hodder &
Stoughton), notes, an incorrect ECG has led to "vague diagnoses

of organic brain disease in healthy but unruly children, turning them into medical cases."[14]

More state-of-the-art these days than the ECG is the *echo*cardiography—a diagnostic test on the heart, often using a mixture of contrast agents and soundwaves. The procedure, which involves the use of two drugs—dobutamine and atropine—had been gaining acceptance for its safety and accuracy. However, as with much "perfectly safe" new technology, doctors have only recently realized that it is more dangerous than had been thought, possibly leading to life-and-death complications.

The first major study into the procedure discovered that it can be life-threatening in one in 210 cases, requiring special treatment or a stay in the hospital; two people of the 3,000 studied suffered a heart attack after the procedure had been completed.[15]

ANGIOGRAPHY

If your doctor suspects that something is awry, he may trot you off for angiography, an X-ray test supposed to examine the state of your arteries via a contrast dye. Nevertheless, there is plenty of evidence that this test also has a poor batting average, wrongfully setting in motion one of a number of potentially lethal heart operations. In one test in Boston, half of the 171 patients recommended to have a coronary angioplasty (the operation where clogged veins are opened by tiny inflated balloons) on the basis of their angiograph were found not to need the operation. In the end, only 4 percent of the patients advised to have the angiograph really needed one.[16] Angiographs are also especially open to misinterpretation. In another study in which the pathology reports of deceased patients were compared with prior angiographs, two-thirds were found to be wrong.[17]

X RAYS

X rays are the most common procedure you're likely to be exposed to at least once in your lifetime. Ionizing radiation is actually very high frequency waves, which pass through living tissue. Depending on how dense the tissues are, the body retains some of this radiation. These absorbed rays are what gets recorded on the film as white or gray; the ones that pass completely through hit a plate of photographic film and show up as dark gray or black. Besides mammograms, bone X rays, and dental X rays, the newest kind of X rays include CAT scans, in which a moving beam of X rays creates a three-dimensional picture, usually of the brain, and fluoroscopy, which sends the X ray shadow picture onto a television screen. Occasionally contrast mediums like dyes or barium are used to provide a clearer picture.

Although the newest equipment uses lower and more precisely targeted doses, there is still no such thing as safe X rays (that goes for dental X rays, too). In all of medicine there is virtually no disagreement that ionizing radiation is damaging—and those risks are multiplying as our understanding of the medium grows. "Medical irradiation is by far the largest man-made contribution to the radiation burden of the population of developed countries," R. Wootton, professor and director of Medical Physics at Hammersmith Hospital in London, England, wrote in a textbook on the subject. In the United Kingdom, he says, X rays ordered by doctors account for over 90 percent of the total radiation exposure of our population.[18]

X rays harm people in three ways. First, they can damage individual cells (although the harm caused by the lower doses is usually quickly repaired). Rarely (but depending on exposure), this damage can convert the cell to a cancer cell. Although we don't know exactly how this works, it has been proposed that, since a cell is 75 percent water, most of the radiation will be absorbed by the water, forming free radicals, which are known to be carcinogenic.[19]

Second, if a woman is pregnant, it can injure the developing fetus, causing death or malformations.

Finally, X rays can damage the sperm or ovaries of children or adults, causing abnormalities in future generations. We also know that X-ray exposure is cumulative; the danger of something going wrong may increase every time you get another one.

We're still coming to grips with exactly how dangerous X rays are, however. Unnecessary radiation from X rays may be responsible for perhaps 1,000 cancer deaths per year in the United States, and between 100 and 250 of the 160,000 cancer deaths in the United Kingdom every year.[20] But these figures may still be conservative. A 1991 national science committee reviewed the usual assumptions that X rays were responsible for 1 percent of all leukemias and 1 to 2 percent of all other cancers, and concluded that the real risk could be as much as four times higher[21]—a conclusion also reached that same year by the International Commission on Radiological Protection.[22] Recently, multiple X rays have even been linked with multiple myeloma— a form of bone cancer. Those who'd had the most exposure had a four times increased risk, the National Cancer Institute found.[23]

As far back as the 1950s, medicine discovered a link between leukemia and prenatal X rays. X-raying pregnant woman used to be routine, on the ludicrous notion that X rays could tell a doctor whether her pelvis was "wide enough" for the fetus to fit through during birth. We now know that if children are exposed to X rays *in utero* their risk of all cancers is increased by 40 percent, of leukemias by 70 percent, and of tumors of the nervous system by 50 percent.[24] There also may not be a safe "dose threshold"; single babies who'd received five to six times less radiation than twins who'd been X rayed more frequently had the same incidence of cancer.[25] To put these numbers in perspective, for every million babies exposed in the womb to even a single rad of X rays—the equivalent of a single picture of the stomach and intestines—between 600 and 6,000 could develop leukemia.[26]

Besides cancer and genetic deformities, X rays of the brain can lead to abnormal hormonal function, possibly causing underactive thyroid and infertility, or resulting in subtle changes in the adrenal glands.[27] The Food and Drug Administration has also lately received a number of reports of patients suffering skin burns after radiation, so severe in some instances that the skin has died. The problem is complicated by the fact that these injuries don't show up for weeks after exposure. Even typical doses of fluoroscopy can result in skin injury after less than an hour.[28]

Although X-ray exposure and risk are cumulative over a lifetime, even single shots are not innocuous. According to the Health Research Group, a consumer group that reports on risks in medicine, topping the list are X rays of the upper intestine, which give an equivalent dose to the entire body of 400–800 millirads; the next highest (apart from the risk associated with X-raying the other organs) is the spine (100–500 millirads); stomach, breast, and pelvis (100–200 each); skull or shoulder (25–75); chest (20–60); with whole mouth dental X rays taking up the rear at 10–30 millirads.[29]

To put these numbers in context, in case you are feeling complacent about that low dosage from dental X rays, a single bitewing dental X ray is equivalent to smoking half a cigarette every day for a year. The Academy of Sciences figures that one barium meal shot of the intestines carries the same risk as smoking up to a pack of cigarettes a day for a year.[30]

Even if everyone in medicine knows that X rays are dangerous—possibly dazzled by another of their "miracles," the ability to "see" through living tissue, Superman style—doctors blithely downplay the dangers and make few efforts to minimize exposure when ordering up a set, even on your teeth. Most internists and orthopedists have a knee-jerk approach to ordering X rays. Even the prestigious medical journal *The Lancet* admitted that most chest X rays routinely performed on patients awaiting surgery other than on their heart or lungs were of so little benefit that over a million pounds' worth of X rays would have to be done to end up saving a single life.[31]

The Food and Drug Administration reckons that a third of all radiation is unnecessary.[32] In Britain, up to one fifth of X-ray exams are unnecessary or downright useless.[33] In one examination of patients given X rays of the lower back, more than half were absolutely unnecessary.[34]

The most common unnecessary X rays are those of the chest, limbs, and joints. America and France top the list of countries with aggressive X-ray policies;[35] in the United States, seven out of every ten people get subjected to at least one X ray every year.[36] In Canada the figures are even worse: Virtually everyone gets an annual X ray of some sort.[37] (On the other hand, British doctors order twice the number of certain types of X rays—barium meal and enema—as their American counterparts.[38])

Doctors are also cavalier about taking pictures that have already been taken before. In a 1991 survey of a representative sample of 2,229 adults, in only half of the cases of X rays being taken were people asked if the relevant part of their body had been X rayed before.

The decision of whether you need an X ray or not also depends on the whim of the individual doctor. An audit of nearly a million outpatients and hospital patients has shown that referrals for X ray varied by thirteen-fold in general and up to twenty-five-fold for chest X rays, depending on which specialist was in charge.[39]

Because the reproductive organs are susceptible to radiation damage, they should always be protected from exposure during X ray by a lead shield. Nevertheless, in one survey, in 40 percent of cases the men surveyed had not had their testes shielded, and women were unprotected two-thirds of the time.[40] (In a third of cases, no attempt was made to find out if the women were pregnant.) In another study of children, three-quarters of the time the lead shields used to protect the reproductive organs hadn't been used or placed properly.[41] And although X-raying of pregnant women dropped off sharply immediately after a study in Oxford first made links between fetal X rays and childhood cancer, this decrease lasted only for a decade. By the 1970s, doctors resumed X-raying pregnant women at a rate similar to that undertaken in the fifties—about a third of the time.[42]

Obviously there are times when X rays are invaluable—particularly when limbs are first broken (though many doctors insist on constant new shots to check the progress of healing). However, even if your doctor is responsible about "dose constraints"—the new buzzword among radiologists for the least amount of radiation necessary for individual snapshots—you still could be getting more radiation than necessary, largely from aging equipment. In 1990, one study reported that patients in some hospitals were receiving doses twenty to thirty times higher than necessary for obtaining diagnoses from machines that were, in some cases, fifteen years old.[43] "Two years ago, physicists were saying that old X ray equipment was giving out doses bigger than Chernobyl," said Liz Francis, information officer at the British National Radiological Protection Board.[44]

Even dental X rays can subject you to unnecessary risks, since they are often performed by untrained staff who can't use the equipment properly and who may either need to repeat the exercise or will set the dosage unnecessarily high.

As with most tests, there is a strong likelihood of human error in interpreting the results. One study of Harvard radiologists found they disagreed on the interpretation of chest X rays half of the time. There were significant errors in 41 percent of their reports.[45]

Myelograms and X-ray Dyes

The other danger with X rays is the contrast agents often used to highlight soft tissue of the body. These dyes have been associated with anaphylactic shock, cardiac instability, and poisoning of the kidneys, particularly among diabetics. In one study, of 319 patients with abnormal kidney function after being given "high osmolality contrast agents," nearly one in ten required kidney dialysis.[46]

Many hundreds of thousands of cases of chronic, debilitating back pain have been caused by spinal X rays, called myelograms. This diagnostic tool involves the use of a contrast medium or dye injected into the canal space and trickled into and around all the discs and nerve roots in the back, which is then X-rayed. Mounting evidence shows that a number of myelogram patients will develop a condition called arachnoiditis, causing permanent, unrelenting pain and rendering many virtually unable to move.

Arachnoiditis is a little-understood condition in which the middle membrane protecting the spinal cord becomes scarred. Nerves atrophy and become enmeshed in dense scar tissue, which presses constantly on the spine. Orthopedic surgeon Dr. Charles Burton of the Institute for Low Back Care in Minneapolis, Minnesota, one of the few doctors to make a study of lumbar sacral adhesive arachnoiditis (LSAA), estimates that it accounts for 11 percent of patients with "failed back surgery syndrome"—where surgery has left them worse off than before.

Although LSAA results from a number of different causes, in Dr. Burton's view it is mainly caused by the introduction of foreign substances into the human subarachnoid space. The foreign body most often identified in victims, he says, is iophendylate (Pantopaque), the oil-based dye used for myelograms. In LSAA, he says, iophendylate is often found in a cyst within the scar tissue mass.

An estimated one million people worldwide suffer from arachnoiditis caused by this dye, and even this figure could be conservative. Until the 1980s, nearly half a million myelograms were being performed in the United States every year.

This is exactly what happened to Brian from Massachusetts. In 1980, after a staphylococcus blood infection causing paralysis, fever, and pain, Brian had to undergo back surgery. Before his operation, a myelogram was performed on him, which left residual dye in Brian's coccyx.

In 1993, after spraining his back, he developed severe muscle spasticity, which caused pain in his legs and lower back. Each night now, the pain forces him out of bed every one or two hours. An MRI scan and X ray finally revealed that Brian had arachnoiditis and that the myelogram he'd had left residual dye in his coccyx. "Eighteen months, and several doctors later, with muscle relaxants, physical therapy, epidermal injections, chiropractic, and even seizure drugs like Dilantin, nothing seems to work," he says.

Pantopaque was introduced in the United States in 1944 after the medical profession was convinced that it was safe. This was despite animal studies showing that Pantopaque caused arachnoiditis (the Swedes banned the product from use in humans in 1948).[47] Even though the product was discontinued by Glaxo with the onset of water-based dyes and imaging techniques, iophendylate continued to be used around the world until supplies ran out, and many back specialists continued to maintain that the dye was safe.

The Food and Drug Administration and the British government also have made no moves to ban oil-based myelograms. "Despite the fact that iophendylate was identified as being causally related to the production of arachnoiditis from the time of its introduction, its use in the United States has never been restricted by industry, government, or the medical profession," says Dr. Charles Burton.[48]

It took patients with myelogram-induced LSAA bringing legal suits against the manufacturers before anyone else took notice. In the United Kingdom, the Arachnoiditis Society has some 1,000 members, and a class action suit was taken against Glaxo. After detailed negotiations, Glaxo reached a settlement with the 426 plaintiffs of £7 million, without admission of liability.

The water-based dyes now being used instead are not without risk. One woman being investigated for sciatic pain (back-caused leg pain) with iopamidol (Niopam 200), a water-soluble contrast medium, was immediately rendered paraplegic,[49] as was another middle-aged woman given a myelogram with itohexol (Omnipaque), another water-soluble dye.[50] Dr. Burton says that some new mediums have caused such pain that the X rays have had to be performed under general anesthesia. "The medical profession has not yet succeeded in finding a benign, effective myelographic medium," he says.[51]

BONE SCANS

Besides looking for broken bones, X rays are now being used to screen for osteoporosis. That might be a good idea—if we had a test that could be relied upon to deliver an accurate result. The problem is, as many medical experts agree, that even the latest techniques in bone scanning should be interpreted with caution, since changes in bone mass may not signify anything.[52]

The instruments are imprecise, multiple measurements may be

wrong, even the assumptions upon which we scan bone are open to question—for example, the very notions that bones have a density that can be measured or that we can treat it and effectively reverse bone loss.

The latest souped-up bone scan is the "dual energy X ray absorptiometry"—a fancy sort of X ray. But an accurate reading in this technique can easily be knocked off. "A walk around the room causes the measurement to change by up to 6 percent (at the hip), which corresponds to six years of bone lost at the usual rate," says Susan M. Ott, associate professor in the Division of Metabolism, University of Washington in Seattle.[53] Poor machine quality control and a high percentage of operator error also throw off results.

The favored technique, measuring many different areas of the body at the same time—one shot of the top of the leg produces five separate measurements, for instance—also increases the risk of a false-positive reading.

"Apparently dramatic changes can be taken as indicating improvement or dramatic bone loss but may simply be due to the precision of the measurement and poor repositioning technique," wrote David M. Reid, a rheumatologist at City Hospital in Aberdeen, Scotland, and his colleagues.[54]

In fact, the entire exercise of measuring bone mass may be useless, because bone mass doesn't necessarily have anything to do with bone strength. For instance, fluoride causes bone mass to increase dramatically, but decreases its strength. This is why elderly populations in highly fluoridated communities show an increase in osteoporosis. Similarly, some drugs may increase bone mass by 5 percent, but because bone structure has been damaged, it isn't strengthened with the drug. New research shows that only half the people considered to be at most danger from a fracture because of their reduced bone density will actually suffer one.[55]

It's important to understand that bone in healthy individuals is a dynamic entity, constantly undergoing interior remodeling. Two sets of cells are responsible: osteoclasts—the construction workers—which rip down the worn-out bone; and osteoblasts—

the architects—which utilize calcium, magnesium, boron, and other minerals to build up healthy new tissue. This process is called "resorption." All that the usual drugs for osteoporosis such as estrogen, calcitonin, or etidronate (called "antiresorbing drugs") do is to lower this process of turnover and renewal, preventing the hard-hat osteoclasts from doing their job. Eventually, there is no further bone formation.

Some researchers argue that the presence or absence of low bone density is a meaningless indicator of risk of fractures or osteoporosis.[56] In one nine-year study of 1,000 middle-aged women, the group considered at *high* risk of osteoporosis actually had fewer fractures than the group not considered at risk. Bone density screening has never been shown to be effective in preventing fractures, according to a large review of published work on bone density screening.[57]

Bone scans may have a one-time use to help in diagnosing women suspected clinically of osteoporosis, but appear to be too variable to be relied upon as a general screening test for women without symptoms.

CAT SCANS

As with most other industries, the advent of the computer has taken the medical X-ray business to a new level. In the 1970s, computed axial tomography, now usually known as CAT, or CT, scans, revolutionized diagnosis, particularly of soft tissue of the body, offering pictures with up to twenty times the detail of ordinary X rays. CAT scans take a 360-degree series of cross-sectional X-ray images from multiple angles—up to thirty shots—by passing a pencil-thin beam through a particular portion of the body, sometimes with the use of a contrast agent. This information is then passed through a computer, which reconstructs the image on a video screen, allowing the operator to see this portion of the body from any angle. It is also stored so that the doctor can take photographs of the video screen or call up the information in the future.

Your problem is that now that your doctor has computerized diagnostic toys at his disposal, he's more likely to want to play with them. Although doctors have attempted to claim that CT scanning reduces the need for other tests such as brain scans, arteriography, or exploratory surgery, this may be a false saving. While no doubt CAT scanning represents the height of twentieth-century technology, it also poses far more risks than most other tests, blasting you with far higher doses of radiation. In 1991, one study in Britain showed that CAT scans accounted for only 2 percent of the total X-ray examinations but 20 percent of the overall collective dose, and so were the largest single source of exposure from X rays.[58] This risk is magnified if you don't stay stock still during the half minute or so of the test and it has to be repeated. In Japan nearly one-eighth of the population was getting CT-scanned as far back as 1979.[59]

Furthermore, although all the early studies showed that CAT scans reduced diagnosis time, helped doctors to understand their diagnosis, reassured doctors about their diagnosis or treatment plans, and avoided the need for other tests, very few demonstrated that this knowledge in any way reduced illness, shortened hospital stay, or prevented death.[60] There are also questions of accuracy. Despite the dangers of high-dose radiation in children, particularly of their sexual organs, it is often used to diagnose cerebral (brain) hernia after lumbar puncture for meningitis. Nevertheless, one study found that one-third of children with hernias were misdiagnosed as normal.[61]

Despite any real demonstration of value, other than as a diagnostic toy, use of CAT scanning has moved briskly apace. Patients who have a seizure are scanned, even before a clinical history is taken, to rule out alcohol withdrawal.[62] So beloved is this gadgetry that it has even been used to research the cause of the common cold, the researchers concluding that their study patients had (wait for this) swelling of the mucous membranes.[63] Besides megadoses of radiation, CAT scans (indeed all X rays) have long been known to cause cataracts and other lens opacities, such as nuclear sclerosis,[64] and could affect thyroid function.[65]

MRI Scans

The dangers of CAT scans and the use of computers led to the development of nuclear magnetic resonance, which developed into magnetic resonance imaging (MRI). This relatively new screening procedure has been hailed as a promising alternative to X rays for providing detailed pictures of soft body tissue, particularly the brain and spinal cord.

Although it was originally believed that the good "pictures" afforded by MRI would eliminate the need for injectable dyes, this hasn't proved so. Contrast agents are needed to detect brain tumors, for example. Unlike the contrast materials used for CAT scans, which contain iodine, those used for MRI are magnetically active substances.

Currently, the only MRI contrast materials approved by the Food and Drug Administration are chelates, containing a rare earth element called gadolinium. When injected into a patient's veins, this works similarly to iodine contrast agents, but is supposed to be far safer, with severe reactions occurring in about one in 350,000 patients.

MRI is mainly used to view the nervous system, for suspected strokes, brain tumors, multiple sclerosis, brain infections such as meningitis, epilepsy, developmental disorders of the brain such as hydrocephalus, and problems of the spinal cord or vertebrae. Its advantages over CAT scans are that it shows better tissue contrast, enables you to get images in multiple planes, has no radiation and a safer contrast medium, and enables you to view veins and the top and front joining of the skull. The big drawback is that you must undergo a much longer scanning time, and results can be flawed if you move at any time during the procedure.

MRI is supposed to be fairly accurate for detecting multiple sclerosis; one study of MS patients showed a 95 to 99 percent accuracy in detecting the disease.[66]

But, again, there are large question marks about its accuracy. According to a medical textbook on CAT and MRI, many initial reports that MRI gave more detailed images than CAT were "overly optimistic." All the initial fanfare, which came from individual cases of patients, could not be confirmed by subsequent larger studies using full scientific methods. The earlier studies turned out to be not well controlled.[67]

Lately, MRI has shown to be less than accurate in detecting early prostate cancer[68] or coronary artery disease.[69] It is now thought that MRI is better than CAT for the brain and spine, because of its ability to take shots of the top of the head and front of the skull and to detect subtle tissue changes, but CT is better for studying any sort of trauma—such as blows to a body part—or the bones or calcium.

In MRI, you are placed inside a massive cylindrical magnet weighing up to 500 tons—large enough to envelope the entire body. While you are inside the magnet a quick pulse is applied, creating a magnetic field some 50,000 times stronger than that of the earth.[70] The effect of this is to excite the nuclei of atoms within body cells. These hyped-up nuclei produce radiofrequency echoes, which get translated into images on a computer.

The problem is that no one yet knows the likely long-term effects of subjecting the body to a magnetic field powerful enough to send magnetic objects flying across the room.

Microbiologist Wendell Winter and colleagues at the University of Texas Health Center at San Antonio stated that exposure to electromagnetic fields may not be totally harmless. They subjected a number of living things to a range of electromagnetic fields and found that they stimulated the growth rate of cancer cells.[71]

Research on chick embryos has demonstrated that they are at risk with the increased temperatures; female mice chronically exposed showed changes in their white blood cell count. Other animal studies show that MRI can cause birth defects in the eyes[72] and damage to the ears.[73] Several patients with pacemakers have died when the magnetic forces altered them.[74]

One of the big problems with MRI scannings is claustrophobia. Up to one-third of patients given MRI scans have felt so claustrophobic that the tests had to be abandoned.[75] "After an

MRI scan for my neck, I had appalling claustrophobia (during it), with memory loss," writes Jill. "I kept crying, shaking, couldn't write, stammered, had nightmares for two weeks afterward. It was fifty-five minutes of hell—worse than the two previous CAT scans. It must affect the brain cells with all that magnetism."

Perhaps the most unsuspected problem caused by radiofrequency fields of MRI is localized heating, a risk that is magnified among babies or patients who are anesthetized.[76] For instance, in one poll of ten American departments of radiology, the overwhelming majority of serious injuries relating to MR imaging were burns.[77] This heating can also cause future fertility problems in men, since sperm are rendered sterile if heated up to body temperature. One study found that average scrotal skin temperature was significantly raised by an average of 2°C, with the highest change 4°C.[78] Four separate studies support Jill's contention that the technique causes memory loss.[79]

If you are pregnant, have a pacemaker, have a metal prosthesis such as an artificial hip, or have retained shrapnel or cochlear, carbon-fiber implants, you should avoid MRI. Implants in particular can either move or become foci for the heating effect of MRI, causing discomfort and local tissue damage. Besides the dangers of metal inside your body, every metallic object in the scanning room becomes a potentially lethal missile once the MRI device is turned on. The most serious reported injury with MRI occurred when an oxygen tank near the magnet started flying and struck a patient's face.[80]

If your doctor wants you to undergo the procedure you should make sure he first takes your full medical history, since the protocol for using MRI differs depending on what you are investigating. According to multiple sclerosis specialist Dr. Patrick Kingsley, when diagnostic toys like MRI weren't available, any reasonably experienced neurologist could make a confident diagnosis of MS based on a patient's symptoms and history. The only reason perhaps to proceed with an MRI scan is if the neurologist wishes to rule out a brain tumor that might be amenable to surgery.

LAB TESTS

Besides X rays, laboratory tests of all persuasions are subject to the grossest sort of error. The Centers for Disease Control and Prevention in Atlanta, Georgia, studied a representative sampling of laboratories all over the United States and found that about a quarter of all tests had incorrect results.[81]

Even an editorial in *The Lancet* maintained that many routine laboratory diagnostic tests are a waste of time and money.[82] This includes blood counts and biochemical screening when you're admitted to the hospital. One study, it said, showed that the illnesses of only six out of 630 patients were diagnosed from routine blood and urine tests. In another study of over 1,000 patients in an adult psychiatric unit, routine blood and urine tests contributed to less than 1 percent of diagnoses; nearly three-quarters of diagnoses were made on the basis of the patient's medical history or a physical examination.[83]

Doctors can't even agree on blood sugar levels in diabetics. A Scottish study found marked differences in the results between the two tests—one which measures carbohydrates in the blood, the other, just glucose—used to assess control of blood sugar levels and whether good blood sugar control has been achieved.[84]

The HIV Test

The most shameful instance of an unreliable lab test used for diagnostic purposes is the AIDS test. The enzyme-linked immunosorbent assay (ELISA) test is most frequently used to test your HIV status, and is usually considered proof positive that you are infected with HIV. A test called Western Blot is often used as a confirmation. For the ELISA test, a sample of the patient's blood is added to a mixture of proteins. It is assumed that if HIV antibodies are present in the blood, they will react to the HIV proteins in the test.

The proof that HIV causes AIDS hinges entirely on the idea that detection of an antibody response to the virus is proof of its actual presence. Doctors assume that if your body has made antibodies specific to HIV, it must mean that a protein of the virus—and so the virus itself—is present. In other words, the so-called AIDS tests cannot test for the presence of HIV, just the presence of antibodies to it—the usual sign that the body has fought off infection and won.

With the Western Blot, these HIV proteins are isolated in bands; when mixed with a blood sample, each protein band will show up if it has bound to an antibody.

Besides being unable actually to detect HIV, these tests are notoriously unreliable; in Russia, in 1990, out of 20,000 positive ELISA tests, only 112 could be confirmed using the Western Blot, according to Australian biophysicist Eleni Papadopulos-Eleopulos, who has studied both tests in depth.[85] The French government considers these tests so unreliable that it recently withdrew nine of the thirty HIV tests that were available.

The other problem is that neither test is specific to HIV; both react to many other proteins caused by other diseases. For example, the protein p24, generally accepted to be proof of the existence of HIV, is found in all retroviruses that live in the body and do no harm. This means that p24 is not unique to HIV, as Dr. Robert Gallo, codiscoverer of the HIV virus, has stated repeatedly. Hepatitis B and C, malaria, papillomavirus warts, glandular fever, tuberculosis, syphilis, and leprosy are just a few of the conditions that are capable of producing biological false positives in ELISA tests.[86]

In one study, antibodies to p24 were detected in 13 percent of patients with generalized papilloma virus warts, 24 percent of patients with skin cancer, and 41 percent of patients with multiple sclerosis.[87] In one study conducted in 1991, half the patients with a positive p24 test later tested negatively.[88]

Western Blot, supposed to be the more accurate of the two, has proven no better than ELISA. Dr. Max Essex of Harvard University's School of Public Health, a highly respected AIDS expert, found that the Western Blot gave a positive result to some 85 percent of African patients later found to be HIV-negative. Eventually, he and his researchers discovered that proteins from the leprosy germ—which infects millions of Africans—

can show up as a false positive on both ELISA and Western Blot, as can malaria.[89] In one study of Venezuelan malaria patients, the rate of false positives with Western Blot was 25 to 41 percent.[90]

This poor track record is disturbing when you consider that the main AIDS "risk" groups—gay men, drug users, and hemophiliacs—are exposed to many foreign substances such as semen, drugs, blood transfusions and blood components, hepatitis, Epstein-Barr virus, and many other factors or diseases known to cause false positives in HIV tests. Other populations exposed to a greater than normal amount of disease—such as Africans and drug users—also make many more antibodies than the rest of us and therefore are likely to end up with a false reading.

Blood transfusions can also bring up a false-positive HIV test result. In one study, the amount of HIV antibody detected in ELISA tests was greatest immediately after blood transfusion, and thereafter decreased.[91] One volunteer was given six injections of donated HIV-negative blood at four-day intervals. After the first injection his HIV test was negative, but the HIV-positive antibody response increased with each subsequent transfusion.[92]

Of course, the greatest problem with an HIV test is that a positive test labels you HIV positive for life. Being HIV positive can bar you from insurance, employment, marriage, or even entry into another country. The HIV test can also launch many healthy patients on the inexorable road to "just-in-case" AIDS treatment with drugs whose considerable, even life-threatening side effects bear uncanny resemblance to the list of symptoms doctors describe in HIV infection or full-blown AIDS.

"OSCOPY" TESTS

Most other tests you're likely to encounter are more invasive, requiring that your doctor inject or penetrate your body with something. These can include tests such as endoscopy or laparoscopy, where an optic tube or "scope" is passed through a bodily orifice in order to inspect the inside of the appropriate body cavity—the stomach, lungs, colon, or uterus.

One big problem, which has recently come to light, is that endoscopy is killing one in 2,000 patients. This poor batting average came to light only because a special audit was carried out to look into the long-term effects of the technique.[93] The study discovered that patients were dying up to thirty days after having the test, usually from heart or respiratory complications. Complications are occurring because the test requires the patient to be sedated, which means the patient can still respond but cannot feel any pain. Nevertheless, patients who are sedated must be carefully monitored; inadequate monitoring is the cause of 20 percent of all deaths related to anesthesia.

Another recurrent problem with "oscopy" tests, such as endoscopy and bronchoscopy, are outbreaks of infection occurring in hospitals caused by inadequately sterilized flexible fiber-optic endoscopes and bronchoscopes. Endoscopy have also been implicated in more serious cases of infection, such as hepatitis B.[94]

The devices are cleaned and disinfected either manually, which is time-consuming for a busy hospital, or, increasingly, by automated machines. After investigating an outbreak of *Pseudomonas aeruginosa,* causing infection of the gallbladder, which occurred in one hospital, the Centers for Disease Control found the culprit to be a thick film of *P. aeruginosa* that had formed in the detergent holding tank, water hose, and air vents of the automated disinfecting machine. Attempts to disinfect the machine according to the manufacturer's instructions using commercial preparations of glutaraldehyde were unsuccessful.

After the second outbreak, the Food and Drug Administration requested that one of the manufacturers send out a safety alert to all hospitals with its products, recommending that a stringent rinsing program be adopted for the cleaning of the machines. The FDA has also suspended the further sale of any of the machines until the contamination problem is resolved.

The other types of tests include those in which tissue or fluids are withdrawn for examination, such as biopsies, bone marrow aspiration, or spinal tap (also called lumbar puncture). About one-fifth of lumbar punctures lead to injury. Although it had always been assumed that injuries occurred when a junior doctor carried out the procedure, new evidence now finds that mistakes occur across the board, even with very experienced practitioners.[95]

Spinal taps have also been used to diagnose children with bacterial meningitis, the disease's most dangerous form. But research now shows that, with spinal taps, children are thirty times more likely to develop herniation, a catastrophic complication of bacterial meningitis, with a high risk of death or damage.[96]

As for biopsy, when a sample tissue is being removed to help diagnose suspected cancer, doctors are now beginning to realize that, unless the tumor is entirely removed at the same time, such tampering may cause the cancer to spread. "Such a biopsy on a secondary tumor, which was diagnosed after a 'local' needle biopsy, I consider responsible for the death of my beloved wife, Geena, at the age of fifty" writes Matthew. "Geena was then radiant, playing sports and active in the garden. She was also into alternative therapies and fighting her cancer magnificently." He goes on:

> However, she was pressurized into that surgical biopsy by arrogant dismissals of our expressed fears, and assurances that such a test carried no risk; the doctors stressed the need to locate the primary tumor immediately so that "urgent treatment" could start.
>
> Tragically, medical dogmatism prevailed over our instincts and better judgment, and the biopsy took place. That biopsy caused the tumor (in her neck) to spread rapidly.
>
> It was agonizing to witness. Just two months later, radium had to be prescribed to reduce its growth. From day two of the "treatment," Geena experienced abdominal pain. After its conclusion in September, her decline was precipitous.
>
> A few weeks later, an emergency hysterectomy had to be performed to treat what was finally diagnosed as cancer of the ovaries.
>
> Surgery could not extract all the cancer; what remained spread like wildfire. "Last-ditch" chemotherapy was powerless to prevent it. Geena died on November 23rd.
>
> Twelve years ago, my father died within two weeks of a "routine" biopsy test on his lung.

With this great potential for error and danger, it is vital that you forego any test—even the most seemingly gentle—unless it is truly vital. Also insist on a thorough verbal and physical exam before you get a test. Oftentimes, taking a good clinical history will give your doctor enough information to preempt a routine test. Finally, think twice about annual checkups when you are feeling perfectly healthy.

TESTING THE TEST

Before you agree to the simplest test, including one for your blood pressure, ask your doctor some of the following questions:

- **Do I really need this test?** Is there another, safer way of determining the same thing (such as a thorough interview and physical exam by an experienced doctor)?

- **What will you advise me to do if the tests are normal/ abnormal?** If your doctor cannot do anything about any abnormal findings, why take the test?

- **What are the risks of this test? Of the treatment?** Again, you may have to do your homework, contacting the medical journals and even the manufacturers of the test (*see pages 231–33 for more suggestions about how to do your own research*).

- **What are the qualifications of the operators (and how many hours are they likely to have been on duty when you take the test)?** If the operators are interns at the end of a seventy-two-hour stint, you would be wise to insist on more experienced—and rested—parties to handle the equipment.

- **When was the equipment last checked for safety/ accuracy?**

- **What dosage (of radiation or ultrasound, say) will I receive? Are there any protective devices (shields, in the case of radiation) that I can wear?** A protective apron worn when you receive dental X rays can prevent the rest of your body from getting "zapped" at the same time.

- **Is it possible to use earlier test results so that I am not exposed to further risk?** Insist that your dentist keep your X rays permanently on file. And if you move, insist that they be transferred to your new dentist.

- **What is the real risk of my developing the condition you're investigating?** If the doctor suggests a mammogram to investigate a breast lump and you're fifteen and have never been exposed to hormones, the risk of your developing breast cancer at your age may be far less than the risk of the test.

All this test taking presumes that you have symptoms, which is why you went to your doctor in the first place. These days, you're more than likely to get screened for diseases even *before* there's anything wrong with you—and never more so than from the first moment you are "diagnosed" as being pregnant.

THREE

Prenatal Testing: Dead Certainty

The moment you first miss a period, medical science informs you that you will not be able to give birth unless you are subjected to a large round of prenatal tests, all supposedly designed to "put your mind at rest." In reality, these tests have the opposite effect. According to medical science, for instance, my oldest daughter, Caitlin, could have had Down's syndrome. If I had listened to the experts I might have aborted her or lost her through a high-tech, test-induced miscarriage. The very thought sends a chill down my spine.

When I got pregnant, I firmly resisted all recommendations to have ultrasound monitoring and amniocentesis despite being a reasonably elderly primigravida (thirty-seven) at conception, because of my fears about their known and unknown risks.

Nevertheless, when I was sixteen weeks pregnant my doctor, who respected my wish to avoid amniocentesis, suggested that I take a routine prenatal alpha-fetoprotein (AFP) test. The test measures the level of AFP produced by the fetus and present in the mother's bloodstream.

It was designed to detect babies with rare neural tube defects such as spina bifida, as evidenced by a "high" reading. Although the test wasn't designed for it, low readings are now thought to be associated with an increased risk of Down's syndrome.

"Just to put your mind at rest," my doctor cajoled.

Since it only involved taking a blood sample from my upper arm rather than invading the uterus as all other prenatal tests do, I let myself be talked into it. After all, I was having a fantastic pregnancy. I was convinced my baby was perfectly healthy. Now I'd know for sure. What was there to lose?

A week or so later, my doctor's secretary rang and asked me to phone him. "What for? Did the test come back?" I asked apprehensively.

"That's what he wants to discuss with you."

For an agonizing half hour I stayed on the phone waiting for him to get on the line. When he did, it was to report the words I'd never even thought to consider: "The results of the AFP test are borderline low."

I burst out in hysterical sobbing, and only after five minutes had calmed down sufficiently to ask what I already knew that meant.

"There's a slight possibility of Down's syndrome."

I don't remember much of the rest of the conversation. My doctor tried a few gentle reassurances—we could find out for sure through a combination of amniocentesis and ultrasound; this combination of tests had a high degree of accuracy; the other borderline situations he'd investigated had turned out all right.

Finally I managed to say that I would call him back. I had some secretary drag my husband out of a meeting to tell him the news, and after he rushed home we considered our options. We could run through the battery of tests with ultrasound and amniocentesis, and risk miscarrying a perfectly healthy baby or damaging it through the test—both known risks of the procedure. We then discussed the ramifications of a test result confirming that I was carrying a handicapped child.

We would be faced with the decision of aborting a five-month-old fetus—not some lima-bean-sized tadpole, but a perfectly formed, nearly viable human being. It meant going through labor and giving birth to a dead baby or, if he wasn't expelled in that manner, having the body removed, piece by piece.

I looked down at my bump. For me, that simply was not a possibility I could contemplate, no matter how deformed this child might be, which made the entire AFP exercise an utter waste of time. If you are not prepared to abort a handicapped fetus, there is no point in going through with the tests.

I hated medicine at that moment for creating a situation that could be resolved only through the high-tech measures I had so wished to avoid. If I had never had the AFP test, I thought, I would never have had to consider subjecting my baby to a battery of possibly damaging tests just to bury the doubts raised by the first test result.

In the end, to our minds, there was only one reasonable path: to ignore the test and to listen to our hearts, which told us that the baby was fine.

This is what we chose to do. I called my doctor to tell him, and my husband and I never spoke about the test again. Sure enough, it turned out that we had been traumatized for nothing. The test was wrong. At the end of my term, out came our perfectly normal, healthy baby.

Despite the murmurs from your obstetrician about the very best in medical technology, most prenatal testing is little more than ritualistic nonsense.

ULTRASOUND SCANS

The ultrasound scan is the most likely test you'll be given, following hard at the heels of your urine test confirming pregnancy in the first place. Most women these days can show off pictures of their babies in the uterus when they are not much past the tadpole stage. First developed during the Second World War to track down enemy submarines, ultrasound scanning began to be used in the 1970s for diagnostic testing and eventually for pregnancy.

In the radiology industries ultrasound is known as the biggest growth area, with equipment manufacturers enjoying a 20 percent growth in sales over the next few years and some 60 to 90 million investigative tests of all sorts performed every year.[1] Although originally planned to be used for aiding high-risk pregnancies, the exam is now presently looked upon, as New York's Columbia University Professor Harold E. Fox once put it, as the equivalent of a "physical exam of the fetus *in utero*,"[2] with a good reading the tacit assurance of a healthy baby.

In the United States, pregnant women are generally told by their doctors that ultrasound is as safe as a television set. Obstetricians take the airy position that there are 50 million people walking around today who were scanned *in utero,* and with no laboratory evidence to indicate that it is a hazard, they must be all right.[3] And it is true that the very short pulses of sound that produce echoes and ultimately the pictures you see on the screen when they hit soft tissue—1,000 pulses to a second, each lasting one millionth of a second—have never been definitely shown to cause heating or bubbles in the tissues of human babies.[4]

Nevertheless, this position ignores a growing body of medical evidence to the contrary, so much so that all of the pertinent regulatory bodies urge obstetricians not to use ultrasound routinely.

The enthusiastic and uncritical embracing of this new technology reminds many of what happened in the United States with diethylstilbestrol (DES), the wonder drug of the fifties that was supposed to cure miscarriage. The side effects of the drug are only now showing up in adult offspring some thirty years later, in the form of reproductive problems and cancer.

The fact is, any woman who has had a fetal ultrasound scan is participating in one of the biggest laboratory experiments in medical history. American regulatory bodies approved the use of ultrasound without any long-term studies being done, leading the public to assume that the procedures are safe.

"*No well controlled study has yet proved that routine scanning of prenatal patients will improve the outcome of pregnancy*." That was the official statement put forward by the American College of Obstetrics and Gynecology (ACOG) in 1984.[5] At a 1988 meeting in London jointly held by the Royal Society of Medicine and the ACOG, several top obstetricians, as well as the executive director of the ACOG, disclosed that of eight major studies attempting to evaluate the effectiveness of ultrasound, "none has shown [that] routine use improves either maternal or infant outcome over that achieved when diagnostic ultrasound was used only when medically indicated."[6]

A number of American governmental bodies now concur, including the National Institute of Child Health and Human Development study group, the assistant director of Congress' Office of Technology Assessment of Congress, and a top epidemiologist for the Centers for Disease Control, America's most important epidemiological center.

As studies into the effects of ultrasound began to be done in the late eighties and nineties, they confirmed earlier suspicions. Two researchers in Switzerland did an analysis of all the scientific (that is, randomized, controlled) studies of ultrasound scanning to evaluate its effect on the outcome of pregnancy. Their conclusion: Ultrasound doesn't make one bit of difference to the ultimate health of the baby. This means it doesn't improve the live birth rate or help to produce fewer problem babies.[7] One reason it makes no difference in terms of live births is that the babies who are usually aborted after a scan shows up a severe malformation are usually those who would have died during pregnancy or shortly after birth, anyway.

The only good reason to use ultrasound, the researchers concluded, is to screen for gross congenital malformations—not to ensure your baby is "all right," the usual vague rationale offered to most pregnant woman with no suspicious symptoms.

Another study of 15,000 American women also found "no significant differences in the rate of adverse perinatal outcome (fetal or neonatal death or substantial neonatal morbidity)" between those scanned and those in the control group. The number of premature babies was identical in the two groups, as were the outcomes of multiple births, late-term pregnancies, and small-for-dates babies.[8] As Dr. Richard Berkowitz of New York's Mount Sinai Medical Center concluded: "None of the studies published to date demonstrates an effect on the outcome of pregnancy in most low-risk women."[9]

In fact, some studies show that, with ultrasound, you are more likely to lose your baby. A study from Queen Charlotte's and Chelsea Hospital in London found that women having doppler ultrasound were more likely to lose their babies than those who received only standard neonatal care (seventeen deaths to seven).[10]

The evidence is fairly conclusive that ultrasound doesn't do any good in normal pregnancies. But does subjecting an embryo to ultrasound at a delicate stage of development do any lasting harm? New studies have emerged showing that ultrasound scanning may indeed cause subtle brain damage. According to a Norwegian study of 2,000 babies, performed by the National Centre for Foetal Medicine in Trondheim, those subjected to routine ultrasound scanning were 30 percent more likely to be left-handed than those who weren't scanned.[11] Evidence from Australia demonstrates that frequent scans increased the proportion of growth-restricted babies by a third, resulting in a higher number of small babies.[12] Exposure to ultrasound also caused delayed speech, according to Canadian research. Professor James Campbell, an ear, nose, and throat surgeon in Alberta, Canada, compared a group of seventy-two children who had speech problems with a similar group with no such difficulties. He found that most of those with delayed speech had been exposed to ultrasound *in utero,* whereas most of those with normal speech had not. "The possibility of subtle microscopic changes in developing neural tissue exposed to ultrasound waves has to be considered," he concluded.[13]

These findings are particularly alarming given that the women in the study had only one scan apiece. Most pregnancies in North America involve at least two scans, and others many more, whether or not there is even a whiff of a problem.

At the conclusion of the Australian study, the authors warned that it might be "prudent to limit such examinations to circumstances in which the information is likely to be useful."[14]

Animals have exhibited delayed neuromuscular development, altered emotional behavior, and lowered birth weight with exposure at the equivalent of current diagnostic levels.[15] Rodents exposed to high-intensity ultrasound have also had low birth weights and nerve damage.[16]

Children who'd been exposed to ultrasound *in utero* had a higher incidence of dyslexia, according to one study.[17] Mothers whose babies were scanned show a 90 percent increase in fetal activity,[18] the effect of which on their future development is anyone's guess.

Work performed in the laboratory may provide some clues as to how scanning could cause damage. We know that sonography produces biological effects in two ways: heat and cavitation (the production of bubbles that expand and contract with the sound waves). We also know that ultrasound causes shock waves in liquid, but we don't know if it does so in human tissue—or for that matter, amniotic fluid. Finally, we don't know whether the effects are cumulative—that is, if they increase with multiple exposure or duration. This is an important issue now that doctors routinely order multiple scans. It also may have a bearing on electronic fetal monitoring, which employs ultrasound (although at one-thousandth of a scan's peak intensity) to monitor the baby's heartbeat during labor and delivery, often by being aimed at one spot for twenty-four hours.

An analysis of *in vitro* studies shows that ultrasound has produced cell damage and changes in DNA. The most widely quoted studies are those of radiologist Doreen Liebeskind at New York's Albert Einstein College of Medicine. After exposing cells in suspension to low-intensity pulsed ultrasound for thirty seconds, she observed changes in cell appearances and motility, DNA, abnormal cell growth, and chromosomes, some of which were passed on to succeeding cell generations. In a documentary made of Dr. Liebeskind's results, the film showed normal cells with rounded edges more or less moving in tandem. After exposure to ultrasound, the cells became "frenetic and distorted," and entangled with one another, wrote Doris Haire, president of the Foundation of Maternal and Child Health, one of America's best-briefed and most vociferous critics of routine ultrasound use.[19] Robert Bases, chief of Radiology at Albert Einstein College, reviewing what he termed the "bewildering array of ultrasound bioeffects described in over 700 publications since 1950," said Dr. Liebeskind's results had been confirmed by four independent laboratories.[20]

Dr. Liebeskind herself theorizes that these cell changes may affect the developing brain. "There may be some subtle or delayed effect on neuron interconnection or some type of effect that is not readily apparent until later," she says.[21] Dr. Liebeskind and others believe the *in vitro* studies can help to pinpoint the subtle effects on humans that epidemiologists should be looking for. "I'd look for possible behavioral changes—in reflexes, IQ, attention span," she wrote.[22]

The International Childbirth Education Association (ICEA) has maintained that ultrasound is most likely to affect development (behavioral and neurological), blood cells, the immune system, and a child's genetic makeup—a view that has been borne out by the recent evidence about weight and development in exposed children.[23]

Ultrasound has also been shown to affect many parts of the mother's body. A British study demonstrated that ovarian ultrasound can trigger premature ovulation in the mother.[24] There also have been published reports showing ultrasound's potential to damage maternal erythrocytes (mature red blood cells) and raise chorionic gonadotropin levels (the hormone that helps to maintain the pregnancy).[25] Again, we're not really sure what this means, and whether a woman is more likely to miscarry after ultrasound exposure.

Despite the assurances of your obstetrician about the safety of scans, every major American government agency has insisted that ultrasound not be used routinely on pregnant women. The FDA, the American Medical Association, the ACOG, and the Bureau of Radiological Health have all cautioned doctors to use ultrasound only when indicated (say, to investigate unexplained vaginal bleeding)—a caution that has got thrown to the winds. They also specify that there is no research proving this diagnostic test is safe. The Bureau of Radiological Health, for instance, has stated: "Although the body of current evidence does not indicate that diagnostic ultrasound represents an acute risk to human health, it is insufficient to justify an unqualified acceptance of safety."[26]

Besides the safety issue, there are considerable questions about accuracy. There is a significant chance that your scan will indicate a problem when there isn't one, or fail to pick up a problem actually there. One study found a "high rate" of false positives; 17 percent of the pregnant women scanned were shown to have small-for-dates babies, when only 6 percent actually did—an error rate of nearly one out of three.[27] Another study from Harvard showed that among 3,100 scans, eighteen babies were erroneously labeled abnormal, and seventeen fetuses with problems were missed.[28]

Yet a third Swiss study pooling the results of all ultrasound studies concluded that 2.4 per 1,000 women will be given a false diagnosis of a malformed fetus. This high error rate has chilling repercussions for families who decide to opt for late-term abortions after a scan shows that their child has spina bifida.[29] In fact, the Swiss researchers concluded that the negligible benefits of ultrasound scanning (which don't improve the outcome of pregnancy) are not worth exposing pregnant women to the "risk of false diagnosis" of malformations.

Not long ago, the British press was filled with stories of women who may have aborted healthy babies due to inaccurate scans. In one, Jacqui James of Brierley Hill in the West Midlands, a twenty-four-year-old mother of two, was told scans done at Birmingham Maternity Hospital during her twenty-seventh week of pregnancy showed that her third baby was not growing properly and likely to have brain damage. After a family discussion, she decided she had no choice but to have an abortion. Because she was more than six months pregnant, the "abortion" was done by cesarean section. However, the baby girl, which survived the operation for forty-five minutes, was later found to be perfectly healthy.[30]

Ultrasound may be useful very late in pregnancy to help confirm suspicions of such conditions as placenta previa (potentially fatal low-lying placenta in late pregnancy) or the position of twins. Otherwise, the only rationale for scanning most uneventful pregnancies is to satisfy our curiosity, to try to get a little closer to the mystery of life.

Besides the inherent risk of the technology, you also risk having an untrained operator who will give you an inaccurate reading. "Modern sonography is plagued by a growing number of untrained practitioners, many of whom use such self-conferred credentials as 'level 1 examiner' to excuse their ignorance," said an article in *Radiology,* a medical journal specifically aimed at X-ray and sonograph technicians.[31] In nearly one-third of offices examined in one study, the operator had no training other than that acquired from the doctor.[32] This utterly flouts the recommendation of the ACOG that technologists complete an accredited training program and doctors receive three months' formal training followed by two months' practical experience before offering their diagnostic services.

FETAL MONITORING DURING LABOR

The *New England Journal of Medicine* reluctantly concluded, after examining seven major studies, that this form of ultrasound provides no benefits to newborns, even premature ones. In reviewing the data, the *Journal* accepted that the study was the final proof that fetal monitoring is ineffective in decreasing the chances of a stillbirth, a low Apgar score, or neurological problems in high-risk infants. It only increases the chances of a woman having a cesarean section.[33] This conclusion was reached following a study, carried out in several medical centers in the state of Washington, which tested the widely held view that high-risk babies who were electronically monitored died less frequently and had better outcomes than low-risk babies monitored by simple auscultation (trumpet stethoscopes or other sonic aids). The study, which looked at premature infants in several hospitals, found that those babies monitored had no better chance of being born live than those monitored by ordinary auscultation. The final death knell was sounded when a major California study found that the test's false-positive level—reporting a problem where there is none—is an alarming 99.8 percent, resulting in thousands of unnecessary cesareans.[34]

Even the former head of the Oxford Perinatal Unit, Iain Chalmers, has gone on record to say that the major, properly conducted studies show that the mortality rate among technologically monitored babies was higher than that among controls.[35]

"A review of this evidence was first published eight years ago," wrote Chalmers,[36] "and the lack of evidence to support the use of this widely adopted form of obstetric technology has been reiterated at intervals since then.[37] For obvious reasons, it is the kind of evidence that some obstetricians would rather overlook."

Unless you are suspected of having twins or a low-lying placenta, you might be wise to avoid knee-jerk ultrasound testing, particularly before your twentieth week of pregnancy when the baby is still forming.

AFP TESTS

Most of the rest of the new prenatal tests are designed to detect Down's syndrome, and new ones are devised as fast as some of the older ones seem to get discredited—this despite the fact that none of these screening tests seems to be making much difference. Despite 30,000 amniocenteses and 3,000 chorionic villus tests performed each year in the United Kingdom, less than 20 percent of Down's syndrome babies are detected. This may have something to do with the fact that 70 percent are born to younger mothers who don't have the tests—a fact that tends to pour cold water on the idea that Down's syndrome is solely a result of the "tired eggs" of relatively elderly mothers.

In fact, despite medicine's attempts to protect mothers from having Down's babies, the incidence of the condition is going up. This could either be because the tests—usually amniocentesis or alpha-fetoprotein—are not detecting the condition, or because parents are choosing to continue with pregnancies of the babies diagnosed as suffering from the condition.

The most substantial risks you face of deformed or retarded children may result from the diagnostic tests themselves.

AFP Test

Before you go in for amnio or CVS, you're likely to have, as I did, an AFP test or a "triple test," developed by the University of Leeds in Britain to replace advancing maternal age as the only risk factor for giving birth to a Down's syndrome baby.

There is no doubt that the batting average on the alpha-feto-protein tests is appalling. After my own experience, I heard of at least three friends or acquaintances with false-positive AFP readings. Doctors accept there is a 3 to 4 percent error rate of abnormally high readings on first screening, according to writer Helen Klein Ross. "This means that of every 2,000 women tested," she says, "100 will have an abnormal reading, but *only 1 or 2* will be carrying a fetus with this congenital defect."[38]

Even this estimate of inaccuracy could be conservative. One study done in 1982 estimated a failure rate of 20 per cent.[39]

According to the late Dr. Robert Mendelsohn, one of the first to call attention to the problems of this test in his American column *The People's Doctor,* the test has false negatives, too, as evidenced in an article in *The Lancet* concerning two babies born with spinal defects whose mothers nevertheless had normal AFP readings.[40]

According to Helen Ross, the AFP test "misses about 40 percent of spina bifida cases, 10 percent of anencephaly cases, and 80 percent of fetuses with Down's syndrome. All of which makes a negative result by no means reassuring."[41]

Twins or a miscalculation about the date of conception are two common ways that test results are thrown off. In my case, we were sure about the dates, but my daughter Caitlin turned out to be a full ten-month pregnancy, born twenty-eight days past her estimated due date (first babies who are not induced are very often late, and my obstetrician doesn't induce labor if there is no evidence that anything is awry). As a slow grower, she probably deviated sufficiently from the norm to show up as "abnormal."

In other words, what this test mostly produces is a good deal of needless anxiety, which can be dispelled only by subjecting your baby to amniocentesis or ultrasound, two procedures with their own potential risks. Indeed, for anyone younger than about thirty-nine, the risk of losing a healthy baby through amniocentesis (about 1 in 100) may be greater than the risk of having a baby with Down's syndrome—if indeed age has anything to do with it.

The Triple Test

This test analyzes three substances in the mother's blood as markers for Down's syndrome. These measured levels, plus the mother's age and genetic history, are thrown into some mathematical stew in order to determine her personal odds of having a Down's baby. The test is supposed to be a better marker than age alone for determining whether a woman should go on to have amniocentesis, which more accurately determines whether a child has Down's syndrome. At best, the test detects 70 percent of Down's babies in women over thirty-five, and only 50 percent in women younger than this.[42]

All those who receive a positive triple test result must wait five or six anguished weeks before receiving the results of the recommended amniocentesis to confirm or deny the suspicious results of the first test. If you are one of the unlucky ones who receives a false positive, you will needlessly undergo amniocentesis, which increases the risk of miscarriage from 3 to 4 percent. In other words, one out of every one hundred women with a false-positive triple test opting for amniocentesis may abort a normal baby.

CHORIONIC VILLUS SAMPLING

Chorionic villus sampling (CVS) was supposed to be the answer to every older mother-to-be's prayers. Although amniocentesis is well established as a test to detect Down's syndrome, you have to wait to have the test until your sixteenth week of pregnancy, then wait two or three weeks more before results are available. If the test shows an abnormality, and you do not wish to continue, you must undergo a second-trimester abortion, which entails, in effect, giving birth to a dead twenty-week-old fetus, with all the physical and psychological ramifications that entails.

Then in the early seventies some medics from Sweden and the Far East figured out that you could take a tiny sample of the tissue of the "villi," the hairlike projections of the chorion (the sac containing the embryo in the uterus, which becomes the placenta) between the ninth and twelfth week of pregnancy and it would tell you the genetic typing of the fetus.

This could help to screen for Down's syndrome, as well as sickle cell anemia, muscular dystrophy, and sex-linked abnormalities. The villus sample is taken with a needle inserted transabdominally (through the walls of the abdomen) or transcervically (through the vagina).

Lately, a number of concerns about chorionic villus sampling have finally been confirmed by several large-scale studies. The latest, conducted by Britain's Medical Research Council, of over 3,000 women from seven different European countries, examined the results of pregnancies of women who'd had CVS against those who'd had amniocentesis.[43]

Compared with women undergoing amniocentesis, those who elected CVS were more likely to lose their babies. Only 86 percent of the women in the CVS group had successful pregnancies, compared to 91 percent in the amniocentesis group. This was due to a greater number of fetal deaths before twenty-eight weeks, a higher number of terminations of supposed abnormalities, and a higher number of neonatal deaths, largely due to a higher number of premature babies born before thirty-two weeks.

CVS can cause massive loss of blood from the uterus, which may lead to the death of the fetus. This discovery from the Erasmus University in Bilthoven, the Netherlands, counters an earlier view that the fetus could survive such a loss of blood.[44]

"The results of this trial suggest that the policy of chorionic villus sampling in the first trimester reduces the chances of a successful pregnancy outcome by 4.6 percent," concluded the MRC report.[45]

The study couldn't tell for sure how many of the CVS tests were false positives because not all aborted or miscarried fetuses were tested. However, the researchers did find three false positives, one in the CVS sample and two in the amniocentesis group, and one false negative with CVS. Two other cases in the CVS group were thought to be false positives.

False positives and negatives are potentially common because the genetic material found in the chorionic villus may not be identical to that of the fetus. In the MRC study and elsewhere, samples of the chorionic villus were found to contain abnormal chromosomes, but the babies resulting were nevertheless normal. Two doctors from Copenhagen reported such an instance; the woman went ahead and terminated what turned out to be a normal baby.[46]

In another case in Brest, France, CVS carried out on a fetus showed the chromosome linked to cystic fibrosis was present. Despite the test results, the parents decided to proceed with the pregnancy and the mother gave birth to a healthy baby girl. The doctor who reported the case estimates the chances of such a false positive are one in six.[47]

What this means, of course, is that the chorionic membrane itself could have a defect not shared by the fetus, possibly resulting from a twin that has died and been reabsorbed. Or, it could mean that abnormal placental tissue in these early stages doesn't mean anything in the long term (the placenta of the Copenhagen case showed normal cultures on biopsy after the abortion). In other words, the entire theory upon which CVS rests—that chorionic villus will tell you about the state of the fetus—could be wrong.

Reports are now flooding in of limb abnormalities among babies whose mothers had CVS. At the Churchill Hospital in Oxford in Britain, five cases of limb-reduction defects (where arms or legs are abnormally short) occurred among nearly 300 pregnancies that had been investigated by CVS at fifty-five to sixty-six days of pregnancy.[48]

Italian researchers from Catholic University in Rome found that four of the 118 cases of "transverse" limb reductions born between 1988 and 1990 in Italy occurred among babies born to mothers who'd had CVS.[49]

From their own data, they reckoned the risk of these deformities occurring for mothers given CVS at any point in the pregnancy was 1 in 200. This compares with an ordinary risk of 1 in 3,100 among the population at large. The risk of deformities from CVS would be even greater if other malformations besides limb reductions were considered. In one study of mothers given CVS, all seventy-five had produced a baby with some birth defect, from lost limbs to damaged nails.[50]

Far from being less invasive, the earlier the CVS was given, the more severe the abnormality. The greatest deformities occur among fetuses given CVS fifty-six days after conception.[51]

It's believed that vascular disruption or puncture of the amniotic sac might have something to do with producing the deformities. Whatever the damage results from, it's clear that the tiny villi aren't quite as dispensable as medicine believed.

The Centers for Disease Control and Prevention now recommend that doctors warn parents of the risk of CVS causing limb defects to their babies at least up to seventy-six days' (nearly eleven weeks') gestation. The CDC also warns that testing can be dangerous in fetuses older than nine weeks—assumed in the past to be the safest period. The Centers' views go against the recent World Health Organization's pronouncement that there is no risk of limb defects if CVS is carried out after the ninth week. One theory for the discrepancy in the two findings may be due to the inexperience of obstetricians at some centers, who may unwittingly be causing damage during the test.

Because of the questionable accuracy of CVS, you might have to have amniocentesis to confirm its results, thus subjecting your baby to two major insults and multiplying your risk of miscarriage. The risk of losing a baby through CVS has now been put at nearly 5 percent. When you add amniocentesis on top of that, you start moving up to a very substantial miscarriage risk of one in sixteen.

AMNIOCENTESIS

Amniocentesis is by far the preferred test for Down's syndrome and other genetic abnormalities. The procedure involves having a needle (guided by ultrasound) inserted into your abdomen and uterus and drawing out amniotic fluid. These cells are then cultured for two or three weeks and the chromosomes of the cells examined, which explains the three-week delay between the test and its results.

The risks of miscarriage are assumed to be 1 to 1.5 per 100 pregnancies, largely from damage caused by the needle or the possibility of introducing infections to the uterus. In 1978, the Medical Research Council also reported a 3 percent increase in neonatal respiratory distress and a 2.4 percent increase in congenital dislocations of the hip and club feet. The high miscarriage rate is worth keeping in mind if you are a woman who has delayed childbearing until you are over thirty-five and now are carrying a much-wanted baby.

Because of the specter of a late-term abortion should the test prove positive, many women are opting for early amniocentesis. However, the latest information is that early amniocentesis greatly increases your risk of miscarriage. It is also slightly more likely to cause cases of club foot than does CVS, according to research at the King's College Medical School in London.[52]

Early amniocentesis has proven to be so dangerous that Dutch researchers may abandon their trials into the procedure because they do not consider it ethically justified to continue. At the time of writing, since the Dutch started their tests eight women have miscarried after having an early amniocentesis, similar to the losses noted in another trial of 120 women given the test. Dr. F. Vandenbussche and his colleagues from the Leiden University Hospital have warned other doctors that "there certainly seems no justification for the continuing unqualified advocacy of early amniocentesis on the basis of beliefs and uncontrolled observations."[53] Another study showed that children whose mothers undergo amniocentesis reported "significantly higher" levels of hemolytic diseases (related to red blood cell levels) than children who didn't have the test.[54]

There are also plenty of false positives, even with this supposedly highly accurate test (there were more false results with amniocentesis than CVS in the MRC study). Anyone doubting that it can't happen to them should read the letter sent to the *Spectator* congratulating Dominic Lawson, after his bold refusal to have amniocentesis and even bolder defenses of the joys of having the resulting Down's baby. "You have a human being in your hands," wrote the letter writer, "and that is what really matters." He goes on:

> *This time last year my wife was pregnant, at the age of forty-two. The hospital called us to explain the possibility of a Down's syndrome baby at her age. Foolishly and arrogantly, we agreed to have the test. We were told that the risk of a resulting miscarriage was 1 in 200, which I considered remote.*
>
> *The long and short of it all is that we lost a healthy baby, and on September 20, 1994 at 10:45 I had the task of carrying the tiny coffin for burial. It is a day I will never forget, and I will forever blame myself for the decision to have the test.*
>
> *Please be pleased with yourself and have no regrets. Today we wish we had a Down's syndrome baby to care for and love. However, we are grateful that we have two surviving children. There must be many others who made the mistake of having the test, lost the baby, and have nothing now but regrets.*[55]

Radiation and Down's Syndrome

Amid this massive effort to prevent Down's syndrome, no one is asking whether they are looking in the right place. Robert Mendelsohn, who belittled the entire notion of "tired eggs" based on age, was one of the first to warn mothers than their chances of Down's syndrome increased with the amount of accumulated exposure to X rays, not their age per se. "Despite overwhelming evidence that this is the case, doctors continue to tell all older women that they shouldn't have babies because their eggs may be weary, rather than determining how much radiation exposure they have had."[56]

Mendelsohn's farsighted view about the connection between Down's syndrome and radiation was recently validated. Researchers from the Freie University in Berlin discovered a direct link between Down's syndrome—which suddenly increased six-fold in the city in January 1987—and the Chernobyl nuclear reactor accident, which happened nine months earlier.[57]

These women were breathing in high levels of radiation—especially iodine-131—for two weeks after the accident, during which time they conceived.

The researchers were able to discount the usual theory that Down's syndrome is related to the age of the mother. The average age of the mothers with Down's babies during the year of the nuclear accident was virtually identical to the average age of mothers with Down's babies the decade before, and the percentage of women over thirty-five with Down's babies after Chernobyl was identical to the percentage over the decade before. After making the discovery, the German researchers uncovered other studies that supported their conclusions. Incidents of Down's syndrome increased dramatically in Kerala, India, and Yangjiang County, China, after women were exposed to similarly high levels of background radiation from the soil.

The study group, led by Professor Karl Sperling, accepts that its evidence "contradicts current textbook opinion." The age of the mother per se doesn't seem a reliable indicator of Down's syndrome, other than the fact that an older mother may have a high buildup of radiation in her system, from X rays. They concluded that any exposure to ionizing radiation, especially around the time of conception, should be avoided.

A similar connection was made by scientists exploring the rate of Down's births and tests at nuclear plants. They examined a community in Fylde in Lancashire, England, and discovered that the incidence of Down's births peaked in 1958 and 1962 to 1964, when there were higher levels of nuclear fallout. The pattern was also followed in 1957, when there was a fire at the nearby Windscale—now called Sellafield—nuclear power station. Women over the age of thirty-five seemed most affected, again perhaps because they had already accumulated some radiation during their lifetimes and the nuclear reaction radiation sent these levels over the top.[58]

The German and English findings add evidence to the argument that Down's syndrome is the result of environmental factors and not simply age. In fact, a major study in 1990 discovered that Down's syndrome babies had higher levels of aluminium in their brains than did normal babies.[59]

The discovery that different racial groups have a markedly different rate of Down's syndrome offers more evidence of an environmental cause. A recent study, which tracked births in seventeen states across the United States between 1983 and 1990, discovered that American blacks have fewer Down's babies than any other racial group (with 7.3 per 10,000) and Hispanics fare the worse (with 11.8 per 10,000). The Down's syndrome rate also varied markedly between states, with 5.9 per 10,000 recorded in Kansas and 12.3 per 10,000 in Colorado.[60]

In a new book, the result of over 30 years' research into Down's children, the condition appears not as daunting as medicine would have us believe. Psychologist Janet Carr has monitored a group of fifty-four Down's children since 1964 and found that they do not suffer from ill health any more than a similar group of normal children. There was no significant excess of marital stress or breakdown in parents of Down's children, and no adverse effects on siblings. In fact, virtually all the families simply loved their Down's members, and wouldn't have dreamed of ending their lives.[61]

GETTING HEALTHY BEFORE CONCEIVING

For any woman worried about producing a normal baby, it may make the most sense to get yourself healthy before conceiving, rather than relying on a batch of tests with questionable records of safety and effectiveness. There is plenty of evidence showing a relationship between deformities at birth and low zinc, magnesium, and selenium levels in the mother.[62] Foresight, the Association for Preconceptual Care, a British organization dedicated to ending fertility and birth defects through better parental nutrition prior to conception, advocates that parents follow whole-food low-allergy diets, cut down on drinking, and sort out vitamin/ mineral deficiencies and excess levels of toxic metal accumulation in the body before attempting to conceive. In a recent study, 89 percent of a group of 418 couples went on to give birth to healthy babies after following the Foresight diet and supplement program. In the study groups, no baby was born before thirty-six weeks and none was lighter than 2.4 kilograms (5 pounds 5 ounces). There were also no miscarriages, perinatal deaths, malformations, or babies requiring admission to special care. Of the 418 couples, 75 percent had either previous infertility problems, miscarriages, or stillbirths; many were over forty.

FOUR

Catching It Early

SCREENING FOR CANCER

Doctors tend to visualize many diseases as a little army that starts small, enlisting, at most, a soldier or two. If they can locate and flush out the enemy when it's only two or three strong, they figure they can get in there early with their nuclear warfare and win the war, even before it gets going. The best way to root out these errant cells, they've convinced us, is with a screening test.

Because cancers can grow before you get ill or exhibit symptoms, they have been the main target of catch-it-early warfare. For all of us who dread the frightening randomness of "silent" killers such as cancer, which are reaching epidemic proportions, this is a highly comforting notion. Doctors have managed to convince us that we can escape death just by having a simple annual screening test.

So persuasive is the catching-it-early argument that medicine has also managed to convince governments to spend millions of dollars putting into effect mass screening programs. At the moment, women are the primary targets of these annual tests, mainly for cervical and breast cancer, although there has been talk of ovarian cancer screening, and prostate and bowel cancer screening programs for men. Cervical screening and mammography have been in place for years in the United States, but European countries like Britain have only recently begun wholesale breast and cervical cancer campaigns, screening three-quarters of eligible groups.[1]

Despite all the money being poured into massive screening campaigns, no screening programs anywhere are making the slightest impact on cancer mortality. In fact, because of their inordinately high potential for false-positive readings, screening may only be increasing the number of patients mutilated through unnecessary drug treatment or surgery.

Even the respected medical journal *The Lancet* admitted in a no-holds-barred editorial that despite "all the media hype, the triumphalism of the profession in published research, and the almost weekly miracle breakthroughs trumpeted by the cancer charities," the number of women dying from breast cancer refuses to go down. "Let us stop complaining that screening ought to work if only we tried harder and ask why this approach is so disappointing."[2] One recent estimate is that mammography is ten times more likely to pick up a benign cancer—leading to unnecessary treatment and surgery—as it is to prevent one single cancer death.[3]

SMEAR TESTS

The most widespread screening test of all is the Pap smear, after a fellow named Dr. George Papanicolaou who first developed it. In 1941, Papanicolaou and a colleague published a study demonstrating that malignant changes in the cervix could be diagnosed by examining cells taken from the vagina.[4]

This simple, relatively painless test involves scraping a small sample of tissue from the neck of the uterus and sending a slide of it to a lab for analysis to see if any unusual cells are present. It was first adopted in various Western countries after publication of results from the pilot screening program in British Columbia showed that it was having an impact on lowering mortality rates. After seeing the British Columbia results, doctors began enthusing that the Pap smear would sound the death knell for cervical cancer.[5]

In the United States, with one out of every eight women developing breast cancer, women's groups are demanding action on all women's cancers, including cervical cancer. In response, the Centers for Disease Control and Prevention released the National Strategic Plan for the Early Detection and Control of Breast and Cervical Cancers (NSP), a collaborative program between the Food and Drug Administration, the National Cancer Institute, and the CDC. This promises to heat up the screening program, increasing the number of women and the frequency with which they are screened for these diseases.

Most doctors regard cervical cancer screening as part of standard good practice, recommending that all women between the ages of twenty and sixty-five repeat the test every three to five years. *The Lancet* even recently recommended that the screening be extended to women over sixty-five, now considered a high-risk group.[7]

But who would quarrel with the benefits of a simple, painless, risk-free test that promises to eradicate a common killer of women?

Nobody, if it actually worked. *The problem is there is no convincing evidence anywhere to suggest that it does.* Professor James McCormick of the Department of Public Health at Dublin's Trinity College, an expert on mass screening tests, who studied much of the available medical literature on the subject, has concluded: "There is no clear evidence that this screening is beneficial, and it may well be doing more harm than good."[8] By harm he means that many thousands of women are being subjected to risky treatments that could affect fertility for a condition they do not have or which could revert to normal.

First of all, it's hard not to think, once you examine the figures, that medicine has backed the wrong horse. Cervical cancer is not the massive killer it's often made out to be. The number of women who die from cervical cancer represents less than one-sixth of the number of women who contract breast cancer. In *The Health Scandal,* author Dr. Vernon Coleman says that cervical cancer doesn't even make the top ten causes of death among women, falling behind breast, lung, colon, stomach, ovarian, and even pancreatic cancers.[9] And only 1.6 of every 1,000 women with abnormal smears go on to develop cancer.[10]

The smear test has also never been proven to save lives in any country where it has been introduced. In fact, every study shows that it is making virtually no impact. The only area in Canada where screening has been universally adopted is British Columbia; nevertheless, the death rate of cervical cancer there matches the death rate for the rest of the country.[11] Mortality rates from cervical cancer may have fallen in British Columbia, but they also fell in other parts of Canada without organized screening programs.[12]

In many countries, the death rate from cervical cancer fell *before* the test was introduced and has stubbornly remained at a comparable figure. There is also no evidence to support the common contention that things would be worse but for the test. Dr. McCormick and his colleague, the late Petr Skrabanek, say that the blind enthusiasm for cervical screening "has produced a climate in which it has been impossible to mount controlled trials."[13] Twenty years ago, Dr. Herbert Green, a New Zealand doctor who had the temerity to dispute many dearly held assumptions about cervical cancer, was even found guilty of disgraceful misconduct for conducting a trial to see whether cancer is inevitable after an abnormal screening test.[14]

A major new British study confirms that cervical screening isn't doing any good, since death rates from cervical cancer haven't varied in two decades, despite virtually universal screening. These findings are based on monitoring nearly a quarter of a million women in Bristol over twenty years. In 1992, the death rate was similar to that of 1975, when continuous screening was introduced.[19]

If screening has managed to put a slight dent in the death rate nationally, it comes at an unacceptable cost, says Dr. McCormick. Many thousands of women are given false positives and unnecessarily treated and possibly even left infertile or with terrible side effects. During every area-wide screening in the Bristol area, 15,000 women have been told they were at risk of cancer, and more than 5,500 investigated and treated for mild abnormalities that never would have progressed to cancer.

Between 1988 and 1993, nearly 226,000 women were screened, and abnormalities were supposedly found in more than 15,000—or about one out of every fifteen women. This figure is absurdly high compared with the actual rate of cervical cancer, which kills one woman in 10,000. The Bristol level of false positives (where a "discovery" of cancer turns out to be false) demonstrates to what extent cervical screening is simply causing unnecessary worry in healthy women.[20]

The greatest problem lies with the very medical foundation on which the test is based. *Mounting evidence suggests that the smear campaign may be based on a faulty assumption: that abnormal, or "precancerous," cells on the cervix lead to cancer.* This assumption has been inferred from two facts: 1) that cervical cancer progresses slowly and, 2) if caught early enough, can be cured.

There are four categories of abnormal lesions, or "cervical interstitial neoplasia": CIN I, II, III, and cancer. What we don't know is whether the early lesions—those in the CIN I and II categories—will go on to develop cancer, or even what to do about them. In one study examining the accuracy of cytology (cell) screening, some 10 percent of women screened had cervical abnormalities, "most of which," notes Professor McCormick, "would not progress to cancer."[21]

Medicine also doesn't really understand the usual progression of this kind of cancer, a fact they have tacitly begun to admit. Some cervical cancers appear to regress if left alone, while others progress so rapidly that the three-to-five-year gap recommended by most screening programs would fail to pick them up in time. On this fragile foundation, women with an abnormal smear are frightened and stigmatized by the term "precancerous" when no one knows whether it is appropriate or not.

This very situation happened to Anna. After her smear test came up positive, the twenty-five-year-old spent months worrying that she had cancer. She also felt deeply embarrassed by the test results, as though it were a public comment on her sex life, since cervical cancer is known to occur among women who are highly promiscuous. In the end, she discovered that she had suffered all her distress for nothing. Follow-up tests some months later proved the first test was wrong.

One study in 1988 showed that nearly half of smears with mild abnormalities reverted to normal within two years. None of the patients developed invasive cancer during long-term follow-up.[22] Similar results occurred in a 1992 study in northeast Scotland, demonstrating that there is no steady progression from mild to moderate to severe abnormality of cells.[23]

A recent Canadian study showed that simple inflammation of the cervix may throw up an abnormal smear. Of 411 women examined by researchers at the Memorial University of Newfoundland, in St. John's, Newfoundland, the smear tests of nearly a third were shown to have inflammatory changes, nearly half of whom were shown to have some sort of infection. Ironically, even here the test was unreliable: half of the remaining women with normal smear tests also had an infection.[24]

Besides this confusion over the significance of various results, the test is so inaccurate as to be virtually pointless. There is no guarantee that a Pap smear will pick up the fact that you have cancer, and a fair likelihood that you will be told you have an abnormality that doesn't actually exist. In one study, the authors admit to false-negative rates of between 7 and 60 percent.[25]

In another report, one in every five cervical cancer deaths was due to poor management or misdiagnosis by doctors. In one in every seven of these cases, the smear tests had been read as normal. Reanalysis of the slides showed that early abnormalities had in fact been present, but were missed.

Interpretation of the results varies wildly, depending on who is looking at the slides. You could even get a different interpretation from the same person looking at the same slide on separate occasions. This is particularly so, says Professor McCormick, with the minor changes that give rise to most reported abnormalities.[26]

The 1992 report from the National Audit Office, "Cervical

and Breast Screening in England," found a wide disparity in interpretations of findings and a lack of benchmarks against which to compare results. The audit found that in some areas of England, nearly a fifth of all smears were classified as abnormal, compared with 3 percent in other areas.[27] This lack of any standards is responsible for many false diagnoses of cancer.

In Scotland, some 20,000 tests done over the last five years under the screening program at the Inverclyde Royal Hospital had to be reexamined after evidence that the doctor doing the analysis may have misread the results. On a preliminary reexamination, 40 out of 1,000 smears taken since 1988 were found to be "inadequate" and to require a repeat test.[28]

Large numbers of smears are also technically not up to scratch. Dr. Chandra Grubb, head of the Department of Cytology at the Royal Free and University College Hospital in London, estimates that some 10 percent of all smears sent to cytology departments are useless, and a further 40 percent are of limited usefulness because doctors haven't taken the smear correctly or have taken it from the wrong site.[29] With this kind of terrible batting average, the likelihood is that screening not only isn't going to pick up your cancer, but could set you on the road to potentially risky treatments when you don't need them.

The conventional treatment for early "precancerous" lesions employs a colposcopy (a magnifying glass with a light) and biopsy (exploratory surgery), diathermy (burning the abnormal cells) or cytotherapy (which employs a freezing probe to freeze the outlaw cells). These procedures can all cause hemorrhage or permanently damage the cervix, resulting in an "incompetent" or narrowed cervix, and thus affect a woman's chances of carrying a baby to term.

Dr. Robert Mendelsohn liked to tell the story of a colleague of his whose wife received a positive reading. She went ahead with a cone biopsy, which caused such excessive bleeding that she had to have an emergency hysterectomy, during which she almost died from the anesthesia. All because of a test that might have been wrong in the first place.[30]

One of our readers, a young woman in her early twenties,

had been diagnosed as having stage 2 to 3 abnormal cells, and was scheduled for an operation to have them frozen or burned out. At the eleventh hour, she decided to have a second smear test at another laboratory. Her new test showed that the first test was wrong; her problem turned out to be a simple infection.

Individual doctors also differ widely in their views of how to treat abnormalities. One report showed that many doctors opt for radical treatment such as cervical conization for cases of mild abnormalities, which would eventually resolve themselves without intervention.[31]

Some reports demonstrate that getting in there early and aggressively treating cervical abnormalities doesn't do any good, anyway. In one recent study, referring women with mildly abnormal smear test results for the more invasive examination produced no more favorable outcome than adopting a policy of watchful waiting. Referring women for a colposcopy exam, often with a biopsy, or simply giving them a repeat smear test after several months produced identical results: 1.6 per 1,000 cases developed into cervical cancer. This means 2,500 women were sent for colposcopy—with its inherent risks of causing infertility—to save one case of cancer.[32]

Some countries now specifically recommend that women with minor cell abnormalities—"borderline or mildly dyskaryotic smears"—adopt a path of surveillance—that is, have the smear test repeated six months later. The women should be referred for colposcopy only if the smear continues to show abnormality.

MAMMOGRAMS

Mammography—an X ray of the breast designed to pick up early malignancies—is the other screening test being stepped up sharply. Breast cancer, the overall number two cancer killer after lung cancer, claimed the lives of an estimated 46,000 American women in 1993.[33] England and Wales have the worst breast cancer death rates of fifty Western nations, with 29 per 100,000 of the population dying from the disease.

As the commonest female cancer and the main cause of death in women under fifty-five, breast cancer has become a political football, with breast cancer activists on both sides of the Atlantic demanding government action. In the United States, Congress responded to pressure from breast cancer activists by ordering that the National Institutes of Health increase spending on breast cancer research and treatment by nearly 50 percent—to some $132.7 million. Lately, the American Cancer Society has begun employing tactics such as designating October 19 "National Mammography Day" ("Be sure she makes the appointment that could save her life," read the ad in the medical literature, sponsored by the ZENECA HealthCare Foundation), even offering individually tailored letters and telephone calls.[34] In the United Kingdom, the government launched its National Breast Screening Programme in 1990, offering mammography to women aged fifty to sixty-four, and its first year exceeded its target of screening 70 percent of the million women invited to participate every three years. Nevertheless, in some quarters this isn't good enough. The American College of Obstetricians and Gynecologists has called for more frequent mammograms among women over fifty.

All this activity may comfort those who wish to see medicine doing *something* about breast cancer. However, nobody can agree on who should be screened and how often. Wide variations exist between countries (and even between different governmental bodies) as to which groups of women would most benefit. And the bottom line is that the level of breast cancer mortality remains constant, despite huge efforts to improve early detection and local treatment.

Breast cancer deaths in England and Wales fell by 12 percent between 1987 and 1994. However, health officials who ascribe this sudden drop to their extensive mammogram screening programs have no reason to be self-congratulatory. New research has discovered no evidence to link the two, although screening has helped detect more cases earlier. The British National Cancer Registration Bureau believes that the fall may be more likely associated with the increasing use of the drug tamoxifen, which slows cancer growth, than with any screening. Since nationwide screening was introduced in 1988, recorded incidence of the disease in the fifty to sixty-four-year age group rose by 25 percent.[35] Furthermore, the fall in mortality began in 1985, but the first screening units were not working until three years later, and Great Britain as a whole wasn't sufficiently covered until 1990. As Royal Marsden Hospital breast cancer specialist Michael Baum writes, claiming that any part of the drop in mortality is due to the screening program is "intellectually dishonest."[36]

Baum estimated that, based on current statistics, the British health services would have to spend close to the equivalent of $3.3 million on universal mammogram screening to benefit one woman out of 10,000 among the under-fifties.

After the publication of a Swedish meta-analysis a few years ago, which pooled results from five studies conducted over five to thirteen years on some 300,000 women, most members of the medical establishment have adopted as gospel its results: that for women fifty and over, regular screening can reduce breast cancer mortality by 30 percent.[37] It is also generally agreed that *no* studies have shown a benefit for women younger than fifty.[38]

In early 1994, the National Cancer Institute broke ranks with bodies such as the American Cancer Society by reversing its earlier recommendations that all women over forty should have routine mammograms. The new advice included only women over fifty. The reason for this reversal of policy, it reiterated, was that no studies of routine screening mammography have shown a "statistically significant reduction in mortality in women under the age of fifty."[39] This decision was followed by a similar move by the government of New Zealand.[40] Michael Baum and Ismail Jatoi, another top breast cancer specialist, wrote a special feature labeling American doctors "negligent" for giving mammograms to women under fifty, because it can often do more harm than good.[41] Nevertheless, despite all medical evidence to the contrary, the American Cancer Society and the American College of Radiology have carried on urging all women over forty—which of course includes this limbo group between the ages of forty and forty-nine—to have annual mammograms.[42]

This "30 percent risk reduction" has been adopted as a mantra by the medical profession. It has provided a justification of sorts to screen many groups, such as women under fifty, where benefits of screening have never been shown. Despite the new recommendations from the National Cancer Institute, a researcher from the University of North Carolina discovered that 89 percent of doctors in her region were still screening even though they were aware of the change in recommended procedure.[43]

As a perfect example of just how ingrained routine screening is, Minerva, the pen name of a columnist in the *British Medical Journal,* cheerily admitted that there is "little hard evidence" but "plenty of sound reasons" for believing that screening for those over sixty-five is just as important as for those in their fifties. As age is the most important risk factor for the disease, and sixty-five-year-olds may go on to live another twelve years, she added, "it's *got* to be good for them."[44]

But even among the over-fifties, there is no conclusive evidence that mammographic screening is doing any good. In the much-quoted Swedish study, the researchers came up with their figure by pooling all the results of three bands of age groups—the forty to forty-nine-year-olds, fifty to sixty-nine-year-olds and seventy to seventy-four-year-olds—into an overview. The study showed a positive benefit (29 percent reduction in mortality) among the women in their fifties, but none among the women in their forties or those in their seventies.

However, when you actually examine the science behind these statistics, this is the only study to show clear benefit, even among the fifty-year-olds. The 30 percent improved survival figure being bandied about derives from several articles that examined *all* the studies of screening and attempted to pool the results. Although most studies didn't show a clear benefit, the article concluded that those that were most scientific, or "randomized" (that is, women assigned randomly to either screening groups or controls) all proved to be of benefit.[45]

However, Dublin's Dr. McCormick and his late colleague Petr Skrabanek, both scourges of unproven medical practice, have pointed out that three of the four of those trials considered most scientific "failed to reach statistically significant benefit for women aged fifty and over."[46] These included two studies of an aggregate of 80,000 women, which were dismissed as "too small" by one set of screening proponents.[47] In other words, to reach their favorable statistics, academics have combined entirely different types of scientific studies—those that set out with several groups of women to see what happens to them over time, versus analyzing what has already happened to several groups of women—in an attempt to make the insignificant advantages of screening appear significant. In fact, two of the best breast cancer centers in the United Kingdom failed to lower deaths significantly using annual clinical exams and every-other-year mammograms.[48]

It's also wise to keep in mind what this 30 percent supposed reduction in mortality actually translates into. At best, it may prevent or postpone one cancer death for between 7,000 and 63,000 women invited for screening every year.[49]

The latest study from the University of British Columbia in Vancouver has come out with the astonishing suggestion that we junk mammograms altogether. Researchers studied all the trials since the early ones that claimed a 30 percent reduction in deaths from breast cancer in women over fifty. There has been far less publicity, the Canadian researchers point out, about all the studies that have been done since those early days, showing that mammography does no good for anyone in any age group, but does great harm through false positives and get-in-there-early intervention. The study attacked mammography after discovering that only one in fourteen women with a positive mammogram result indicating breast cancer will actually have the condition.

"Since the benefit achieved is marginal, the harm caused is substantial, and the costs incurred are enormous, we suggest that public funding for breast cancer screening in any age group is not justifiable," these epidemiologists concluded.[50]

In another Canadian study, researchers analyzed six trials into breast cancer screening, and discovered only one in fourteen women with a positive mammography result indicating breast cancer will actually have the condition. As with cervical cancer, this means that many women are going through needless worry and treatment on the basis of an inaccurate test.[51]

In fact, treating women who have had a false-positive mammography test represents a third of the cost of providing screening for all women. Swedish researchers monitored 352 women who'd been given false-positive readings. They discovered the women had made 1,112 visits to doctors, had 397 biopsies, 187 follow-up mammograms and 90 in-hospital surgical biopsies before being pronounced clear of cancer. Even after six months, only two-thirds of the women had been given a clean bill of health. All this needless medical intervention cost more than $400,000; women under fifty accounted for 41 percent of costs.[52]

The rationale for screening has always been that the earlier you catch it, the smaller the tumor will be, and hence the greater your chances of beating the disease. However, this rationale doesn't take into account that cancer doesn't always metastasize at the same rate. Breast cancer isn't a tidy disease that progresses in the same way for every woman; sometimes it spreads throughout the body, other times it advances in the breast alone. Much of our treatment doesn't influence the outcome in any case.[53]

One reason may be that mammograms actually increase mortality rates. Among the under-fifties, more women die from breast cancer among screened groups than among those not given mammograms. The Canadian National Breast Cancer Screening Trial (NBSS), published in 1993, which screened 50,000 women between the ages of forty and forty-nine, showed that more tumors were detected in the screened group, but not only were no lives saved, but a third more women died from breast cancer in the group first offered screening.[54] Similar results occurred in three Swedish studies[55] and also in those conducted in New York.[56] One of the Swedish studies, conducted in Malmo, showed nearly a *third* more cases of breast cancer in women under fifty-five given mammograms over ten years.[57] Even when you adjust results and allow that cancers among women aged fifty-one to sixty-nine—the so-called "high-risk group"—have been detected, screened women have nearly a 2 percent higher incidence of breast cancer than controls.[58]

That more younger screened women die may reflect the fact that mammography is indiscriminate, picking up many cancers that would do no harm if left alone. The scattergun nature of the technology has several implications. This ability to pick up any sort of tumor falsely increases the incidence of breast cancer by a quarter to a half.[59] Adding all these benign tumors, which of course don't lead to death, into the cancer data also has the effect of making it look like more people in the screened population survive because of early detection.

The third effect of regular mammograms is that they lead to massive, unnecessary treatment because benign tumors are often mistaken for malignant ones. In one study of over a thousand women undertaken by Harvard Medical School, only a quarter of the women whose mammograms had recorded some abnormality were actually found to have malignant tumors. Other radiology departments referring patients to the Harvard Center had an even worse batting average—getting it right only one-sixth of the time. And of course an inappropriately strong mammography report, which might include statements such as "malignancy cannot be excluded," raises the anxiety level of the patient and referring physician and often ends up with the woman on the operating table.[60]

Professor McCormick is particularly worried about the ability of mammograms to pick up ductal carcinoma in situ (DCIS). Since the advent of screening, the incidence of DCIS has skyrocketed, from 2.4 per 100,000 women in 1973 to 15.8 cases per 100,000 in 1992.[61] Although many women being diagnosed with DCIS are undergoing radical mastectomies, this form of cancer is "not a synonym for other forms of cancer," says Professor McCormick. Not only do many experts misunderstand DCIS, but most cases of this condition, says McCormick, would not do a woman any harm.[62]

Up until now, only relatively high doses of radiation have been associated with an increased risk of breast cancer. However, new evidence demonstrates that even moderate strengths of strong X rays raise the risk of breast cancer five or six times in women who carry a certain gene, occurring in about 1 percent of the population—or in at least one million American women. In 1975, Dr. C. Bailar II, editor in chief of the *Journal of the National Cancer Institute,* concluded that accumulated X-ray doses in excess of 100 rads over ten to fifteen years may induce cancer of the breast.[63] A single-view mammogram offers the average breast a dose of about 200 millirads (0.2 rad).[64]

However, women with the ataxia-telangiectasia gene, says Dr. Michael Swift, chief of medical genetics at North Carolina University, have an usual sensitivity to radiation and could develop cancer after exposure to "appallingly low" doses. He estimates that, in the United States, between 5,000 and 10,000 of the 180,000 breast cancer cases diagnosed each year could be prevented if women with the gene were not exposed to the radiation from mammograms.[65]

Besides a genetic susceptibility, the physical trauma caused by the force of mammograms could be a factor in spreading cancer. At the moment, mammograms use 200 newtons of compression, the equivalent of 44 1-pound bags of sugar per breast. Some of the modern foot-pedal operated machines are designed to exert one-third again as much force—the equivalent of your breast being squashed by 58 bags of sugar.[66] The force is thought to be necessary in order to get the best quality of image while keeping the radiation dose to a minimum.[67] A number of researchers believe that compression during mammography can rupture cysts and disseminate cancer cells.[68] This phenomenon has been observed in animal studies; if a tumor is manipulated, it can increase the rate of its spread to other parts of the body by up to 80 percent.[69]

Many biopsies to investigate a suspicious lump found on mammography have their own set of problems. In this standard procedure, a thick needle is inserted into the breast under local anesthetic to remove a small piece of tissue. This is then examined for cancerous cells. In one study of women undergoing biopsy, a quarter had problems afterward with the wound left by the needle such as infection or bleeding. Nine patients reported a new breast lump (all benign) developing under the biopsy scar between one to seven years after surgery. Eight patients continued to have pain in the area where the biopsy had been taken up to six years after the operation, and seven reported unsightly scars.[70]

Fine-needle aspiration, which can be done on an outpatient basis, has been served up as the less-invasive alternative when a lump has been found; in this instance, a fine needle with a syringe is inserted in the breast to draw out a specimen of the lump's contents. However, doctors have been known to puncture the lung during this procedure, causing pneumothorax (in which air enters the chest, causing the lung to collapse). In 74,000 fine-needle aspirations of the breast, this occurred in about 133 patients (0.18 per cent).[71]

The experience in many countries suggests that mammograms also have a high rate of inaccuracy. In Canada, during the first four years of the eight-year trial on breast cancer screening, nearly three-quarters of test results were unacceptable. Only in the last two years of the trial were more than half the tests up to the required standard.[72]

As for women under fifty, another Canadian study showed that some 87 percent of so-called cancer cases detected by mammograms were false alarms.[73]

The high level of false positives is partly due to poor standards in equipment. A third of women's clinics in the United States were not accredited, as of early 1994. The FDA admitted that many of them were inaccurately reporting mammograms and that some women were receiving doses of radiation that were far too high.[74] Just how poor the standards are was revealed by a 1989 survey of a cross-section of mammography units carried out by the Department of Health in Michigan. One-third of the units studied routinely exceeded the various standards of radiation exposure.[75]

The United States aimed to correct this problem with the Mammography Quality Standards Act, passed in October 1992, which was to establish quality-control standards and a certification system for the more than 10,000 medical facilities that perform and interpret mammograms. These quality-control standards relate to the training and education of personnel, the equipment, and the dosage used, among other criteria. Doctors would also have to have continuing education in reading mammograms and be expected to interpret an average of forty mammograms a month. As of October 1994, every facility performing mammograms had to obtain a certificate or provisional certificate to continue to operate legally.

However, although setting standards may undoubtedly improve some of the appalling mistakes made in the past, it may do nothing to improve the inherent imprecision of the technology itself. Even mammograms of the best quality can be misread by highly experienced radiologists. In one study carried out by Yale University, ten seasoned radiologists, with twelve years' experience in reading mammograms, each given the same 150 good-quality mammograms, differed in their interpretation a third of the time. In a quarter of cases they also radically disagreed over how the patients should be managed (such as whether they should have follow-up mammograms or exploratory surgery). Even among the twenty-seven patients later definitely diagnosed as having breast cancer, the radiologists varied widely in their diagnosis. Nearly a third of cancers were wrongly categorized. One radiologist did not detect a cancer that was clearly visible, while another thought it was developing on the breast opposite the one where it actually was.[76]

Even if regular screening doesn't spread or cause cancer, its dubious benefits may not be worth the pain reported by a third of women undergoing the screening.[77] Helen, now in her early fifties, has suffered with lumpy breasts and severe mastitis for twenty years. She's had several routine "horizontal" mammograms and a fine-needle aspiration of a cyst she found twelve years ago. Then, in 1991, she had another mammogram. "This time I had to stand upright and each breast was squashed vertically against the machine. The pain was excruciating. Tears welled up in my eyes and I could hardly stop myself from shrieking. The pain lasted in both breasts for three or four days before gradually subsiding," she says.

SCREENING FOR OVARIAN CANCER

These days, most gynecologists routinely screen for ovarian cancer. This widespread screening was prompted by the highly publicized death in 1989 of the actress and comedienne Gilda Radner at the age of forty-two from ovarian cancer. Screening involves ultrasound, pelvic examinations, and analysis of the blood.

However, this flurry of activity among doctors is against the express recommendations of the American government. The National Institutes of Health (NIH) recently recommended *against* routine screening, declaring that it is inaccurate and even dangerous.[78]

The NIH said that these tests are so unreliable that surgeons have unnecessarily operated on many women who don't have the disease. Even if doctors do get it right, by the time the cancer shows up it's too late. And in only a quarter of cases is ovarian cancer detected at a stage early enough for effective treatment.[79]

PROSTATE CANCER

With prostate cancer, medicine has been pushing routine screening of the over-fifties for the second major killer of older men. The three screening techniques include prostate-specific antigen (PSA), transrectal ultrasound (TRUS), and digital rectal examination (DRE). However, a new analysis by the Toronto Hospital in Ontario, Canada, concludes that high inaccuracy associated with these methods can also do more harm than good. The main risk is unnecessary surgery, which causes widespread incontinence and impotence in a third of cases.[80] Furthermore, no evidence exists to show that men given a prostatectomy will survive any longer than those left alone and undergoing "watchful waiting."

One study discovered that 366 men given the "all clear" with a PSA test went on to develop prostate cancer, while raised values—which indicate the presence of the cancer—were found in just 47 percent of men who in fact had prostate cancer.[81]

Recently it has been discovered that the PSA can give false readings if the man has ejaculated in the previous two days. Men over forty have very high PSA levels immediately after ejaculating, and though these start to fall significantly only six hours later, it takes forty-eight hours or more for the levels to normalize.[82]

SCREENING AGAINST SCREENING

So how can you protect yourself against cancer, or—perhaps more importantly—against the screening tests themselves? Unless you have various risk factors in your family or yourself, there is no good scientific reason why you should engage in regular screening of any sort if you are healthy and have no symptoms. Professor McCormick says the most important early warning for cervical cancer (early enough in most cases for treatment) may be a persistent vaginal discharge or any sort of intermenstrual bleeding, for instance, after coitus. The likelihood of cervical cancer increases with a woman's number of sexual partners, whether she smokes, takes the Pill or other prescribed hormones, whether she's had any sexually transmitted disease or began her sexual life early. If you don't fall into any of these categories, be wary of your doctor pressuring you into taking the test, particularly as he or she now stands to benefit financially from it.

If you do have to have a cervical exam, you might wish to insist on a visual examination of the cervix. In a study of 45,000 women in Delhi, India, where cytological screening is not available, visual exams picked up nearly three-quarters of the cancers found among the sample group, by means of cervical erosions that bled when touched, small growths or, in general, a suspicious-looking cervix.[83]

As for mammograms, medicine in general has downplayed the importance of regular physical examination of breasts as a diagnostic tool. An adviser to Britain's chief medical officer admitted that "more than 90 percent of breast tumors are found by the women themselves."[84] In fact, a seven-year study of 33,000 women showed that self-examination could reduce breast cancer deaths by up to one-fifth. Although some lumps detected by mammogram aren't palpable (able to be felt with the hand or fingers alone), the reverse is true as well. Indeed, one researcher believes that routine screening lulls you into a false sense of security, so that you tend to ignore warning signs such as suspicious lumps.[85]

If you don't want a mammogram, make sure to opt for a regular program of self-examination (your doctor can teach you how to do it) and breast examination by your doctor. If he or she is unwilling or has limited experience of physical examinations, you might ask to be referred to a clinic where these are routinely carried out, or find another doctor.

If you do decide to have a mammogram, shop around. Make sure the equipment is specially designed for mammography and therefore able to give the best image with the least radiation, and ask a lot of questions about the number taken each week, as well as when the machine was last inspected. (Machines should be tested at least once a year.)

If a lump is found, either through mammography or self-examination, you need to establish whether or not it is malignant. Some harmless cysts can be identified as such through a physical examination. If your doctor tells you it's a cyst but still suggests sending you for a biopsy, find out if it's really necessary. A benign lump often changes with your cycle, becoming more tender before a period; a cancerous one won't.

If you do produce a lump, you might wish to consider ultrasound, which may be safer (for all but fetal cells). Although the technology is vastly improving and will probably eventually develop into a good tool, there are still some problems with accuracy. The success of ultrasound largely depends on the skill of the operator, as images can be hard to read and are open to misinterpretation. In particular, operators worry about visualizing "artifacts"—that is, a ghosted image of something that isn't there—or mistaking something quite normal for something sinister, confusing a normal structure for an abnormality. This all adds up to the fact that you should only have a test performed with highly trained operators who are well skilled in all the latest equipment and equally well trained in artifacts and all the ghost images that ultrasound can produce.

With breast examinations, the most commonly used equipment is "real time" high resolution ultrasonography—which means you see on screen exactly what the transducer is picking up at that moment. According to one study of one hundred women with at least one breast nodule, the overall rate of accuracy of ultrasound was 74.8 percent. This, of course, means that the diagnosis was wrong in one out of four cases. In ten cases the ultrasound diagnosed benign breast cysts as cancerous, and also missed one breast cyst and one abscess altogether.[86]

According to Professor William Lees, Director of Radiology at UCL Hospitals Trust in London, the best ultrasound should have Doppler as part of the system and use the two types in tandem, which will boost an operator's confidence about the accuracy of his diagnosis.

Color Doppler ultrasound measures the flow of blood, which in malignant tumors tends to be abnormal. The overall view of this technology is conflicting, however. In one study, overall accuracy for detecting breast tumors was 82 percent.[87]

Nevertheless, the technology appears to be improving; presently the color method is used by comparing a color spectrum analysis compared with surrounding tissue; in cancerous tumors, the color is typically more intense with sharp margins. In one study among seventy patients, this method missed only a single tumor.[88]

Professor Lees believes that a skilled operator combining both methods should approach an accuracy rate of 85 percent.

To date, the most accurate diagnostic method is combining ultrasound with "high speed" punch biopsies, when lesions have been identified by ultrasound. In one facility in Germany, this technique reached an accuracy rate of close to 100 percent.[89]

At the end of the day, ultrasound seems to have a similar batting average to mammograms. In one review of eighty patients with both benign and malignant lesions, mammograms picked up five cancers missed by ultrasound, but ultrasound discovered nine cancers missed by mammograms. In yet another study, ultrasound picked up four cancers that weren't yet palpable.[90]

The most important questions you should ask concern the

expertise of the operator. Always opt for someone highly experienced, particularly in breast scans. Don't be shy about asking his accuracy rate or if there have been any serious cases he has missed. Also ask about the state of the equipment—how new it is, how accurate, and when it was last serviced.

For breast cancers, the best prevention of all is to avoid the birth control Pill, HRT, and all other prescribed hormones, which have proven cancer risks, to breast-feed your babies for as long as possible, and to eat a diet rich in fresh organic fruits and vegetables and essential fatty acids (EFAs).

As for ovarian cancer, only those women over age fifty in high-risk groups—those whose relatives have contracted ovarian cancer, have no children, are from North European stock, or have histories of breast, colon, or endometrial cancers—should be regularly monitored. However, if your test comes up positive, it's important that you have the results confirmed by other methods before consenting to surgery.

With prostate cancer, your best odds appear to be avoiding the test, unless you have symptoms. If you do get cancer, consider maintaining a watchful wait-and-see attitude and use other forms of therapy, such as hormonal treatment, rather than rushing into surgery, particularly if you are over seventy. Prostate cancer is, in the main, a slow-growing form of cancer, and you're much more likely to die with it than from it. According to autopsy studies, a third of men in the European Union have prostate cancer, but only 1 percent will die from it before something else claims their lives.[91]

— III —

PREVENTION

FIVE

Crazy about Cholesterol: Medicine's Red Herring

Despite what appears to be a reasonable track record for killing off people once they get ill, modern medicine promotes the view that doctors have enough understanding of your body to prevent illness even before it has begun. Increasingly doctors have turned their hand to what they like to call "preventive" medicine—that is, dispensing "just-in-case" medicine to you and your loved ones while you're still healthy, to stop disease before it starts. Throughout medical history, preventive medicine has been responsible for a number of alarming medical notions— such as routinely X-raying pregnant women to measure their pelvic size, which contributed to an increase in childhood leukemia, or giving them diethylstilbestrol to "prevent" miscarriage, which also caused cancer and infertility among an entire generation of children.

THE CHOLESTEROL FALLACY

Although the fashion these days is to blame most disease on genes—a bad call at birth—medicine has attempted to identify certain risk factors in lifestyle that increase a person's chances of coming down with a disease. In the 1960s doctors first hypothesized that lowering blood cholesterol levels would prevent heart attacks and strokes. This led to the belief that if we lowered cholesterol—either by drugs or by limiting fat intake—we could prevent heart attacks; this in turn has led to an entire food and medical industry devoted to screening for high blood cholesterol and lowering it through processed, low-fat foods and the avoidance of many healthy foods such as eggs. Since then, everyone in the Western world has become obsessed with fat. Young patients in the United States and the United Kingdom have been bullied onto long-term medication if screening tests show a high cholesterol level. In the United States, cholesterol drug use has increased tenfold in the last decade, with 26 million prescriptions written in the United States alone in 1992. In the United Kingdom, between 1986 and 1992, the number of prescriptions for cholesterol-lowering drugs increased sixfold.[1]

Even the burger chain McDonald's has got in on the act, boasting the low-fat content of their hamburgers in advertisements placed in prestigious medical journals, designed to convince doctors to get their patients sold on the healthy benefits of Big Macs and "Happy Meals."

Nevertheless, we have never been able to *prove* a cause-and-effect relationship between cholesterol and heart disease, only that heart attack victims are *assumed* to have high blood cholesterol levels, which in turn are *assumed* to be the cause of hardened arteries. It's also been *assumed* that a high dietary cholesterol intake causes a high blood cholesterol level, and sets off a chain of events leading to a heart attack.

In fact, cholesterol-lowering may be one of the biggest red herrings of the century. After thirty years or more of this "preventive" medicine, evidence is emerging that neither cholesterol-lowering drugs nor many of the recommended artificially low-cholesterol diets may do anything to prevent heart disease, and might actually *increase* your chances of dying. Many of the regimes recommended by medicine may, in fact, be among the main culprits in causing heart disease. Nor has any cholesterol-lowering drug been proved over time to be capable of lowering overall mortality rates; in many cases, the number of heart attacks may have dropped, but deaths from heart problems have not lowered significantly, and overall deaths caused by other factors have risen.

Recently, new scientific evidence proves that cholesterol may not even be the main cause of heart disease. One study involving nearly 20,000 men and women from Copenhagen demonstrated that only those with cholesterol blood levels in the top 5 percent were at risk of developing heart disease.[2] The amazing fact of it is, *most heart patients have normal cholesterol levels*.[3]

Although many small studies have been suggesting this for some time, the most comprehensive of heart research studies finally came out and said it, too: Cholesterol cannot be looked on as the only cause of coronary disease.

In the 1950s, the Seven Countries Study was set up to understand the causes of heart disease. But after collating their data, gleaned over twenty-five years, the researchers had to conclude that risk factors were a complex mix of factors, including cholesterol, smoking, high blood pressure and, most especially, diet. The importance of diet was suggested by the marked difference in levels of heart disease in different countries.[4]

Many populations with high levels of heart disease don't have correspondingly high levels of fat in their diets. For instance, a group of Dutch researchers traveled to Minsk (Belarus), an area unusually high in heart disease, and took fatty tissue samples from a group of men and women who'd been hospitalized for minor problems. After analyzing the fat samples, the researchers could find no evidence that the Minsk sample contained unusually high levels of saturated fats or unusually low levels of essential fatty acids (EFAs), both considered risk factors for heart disease. They concluded that dietary fat probably wasn't the major cause of heart disease in that area.[5]

Other research suggests that in blaming cholesterol, we could have fingered the wrong culprit. One study discovered that the problem was more likely to be the blood-clotting factor fibrinogen. Men with fibrinogen levels in the top fifth were four times more likely to suffer from heart disease than those with levels in the bottom fifth. Smokers, apparently, have high levels of fibrinogen, which would explain the long-held concerns about the link between smoking and heart attacks. Other research blames high levels of homocysteine, an amino acid.[6]

The latest theory is that your biggest risk factor is a low melatonin level. Doctors from the University of Vienna found that people with a heart problem tend to produce lower levels of this hormone at night. Normally, healthy people release melatonin while sleeping, which tends to stop or slow the activity of the endocrine glands. These glands affect growth and metabolism.[7]

Whether this proves to be the new "risk" factor or just the latest red herring, the fact is that cholesterol hasn't been proved a risk factor for *anything*. A major new California study discovered that neither high nor low cholesterol levels seem to have any bearing on any of the major illnesses, including heart disease and cancer. Researchers from the University of Southern California, who analyzed about 2,000 deaths among a group of 7,000 middle-aged men, all of Japanese descent, concluded that early deaths were caused by other risk factors, but never cholesterol on its own.[8]

Even in elderly patients, who would logically seem most at risk, science hasn't been able to link high cholesterol levels with heart disease. A large batch of patients over seventy were followed for four years. A high cholesterol level (over 240 milligrams per deciliter) didn't put them at a greater risk of dying from anything, including heart disease, a heart attack, or unstable angina.[9]

For women, a low-fat diet may actually increase their risk of heart disease. In one group of 15,000 Scottish women, those with higher levels of cholesterol than men were shown to be less likely to die from heart disease than men with the highest levels. Lowering a woman's cholesterol levels also seems to lower her levels of high-density lipoprotein, the good form of cholesterol that actually protects against heart disease.[10]

Regardless of sex, past evidence has suggested that the number of people likely to be helped by cholesterol-lowering drugs is small. In one study, only those "at very high initial risk of coronary heart disease" were likely to benefit; for those at medium risk, the drugs made no difference; while those at lower risk were more likely to die if they were being treated than if they weren't.[11]

Even if they do lower cholesterol levels over the short-term, cholesterol drugs may not have any long-term value in preventing arterial disease. Even after years of taking simvastatin, a cholesterol-lowering drug, patients from a number of centers in Europe were no better off in preventing their arteries from getting clogged up than if they'd never had any drug treatment.[12]

As this kind of evidence began pouring in, many doctors stepped forward to voice their concerns about the open floodgate of cholesterol lowering. Michael Oliver, director of the Wynn Institute for Metabolic Research of the National Heart and Lung Institute in London, emphasized that there was a decided lack of evidence in all the big studies performed to date that any drugs were saving lives.[13]

This growing skepticism among doctors was virtually swept aside in late 1994 by the publication of a single trial, the Scandinavian Simvastatin Survival Study, which appeared to vindicate cholesterol-lowering drugs, at least among those patients with a heart condition and high cholesterol levels. Dubbed the 4S study, it followed 4,444 patients ("four" was obviously the leitmotiv here) with a heart condition and high cholesterol levels. After five and a half years, the group given cholesterol drugs had a 42 percent lower rate of fatal heart attacks and a one-third reduction in heart disease over those given a placebo. (Women in the group did not enjoy the same improved survival statistics; although only a fifth of the study population were women, in the placebo group the mortality rate was half of what it was for men, suggesting, once again, that high cholesterol levels may be a meaningless indicator of future heart disease in women.)[14]

Within a week, the medical press was back on the cholesterol bandwagon, proclaiming, "Simvastatin saves lives."[15] Michael Brown and Joseph Goldstein, the 1985 Nobel prize winners for their work on cholesterol, broke what had been a long silence over the cholesterol controversy at a 1994 meeting of the American Heart Association in Dallas to talk of the "landmark" results and "definitive answer" provided by the Scandinavian study.

Hard at the heels of the 4S study was a Scottish study, the West of Scotland Coronary Prevention Study (WOSCOPS). This purported to show that, with men who had high levels of cholesterol but no history of heart disease, pravastatin, another "statin" cholesterol-lowering drug, could prevent heart attacks by a third.[16] Other studies, including one reviewing all the other studies, concluded that pravastatin could reduce the rate of heart attacks by at least 60 percent and could slow hardening of the arteries.[17]

Although there were many important differences between these trials, the effect on the rank and file in medicine was galvanic. The WOSCOP study was widely interpreted to mean that otherwise healthy men with high cholesterol levels could take cholesterol drugs and reduce their chances of dying of heart disease by nearly a third. All patients with higher cholesterol levels, of whatever age or sex, were being placed on cholesterol-lowering drugs for life.[18] One hospital in Dundee, Scotland, which maintained statistics about the level of cholesterol-drug prescribing before and after the publications of the 4S study, found a striking increase both in the percentage of patients whose cholesterol was being measured (by a third) and in the percentage of patients being prescribed drugs (by nearly eight times).[19] Many of those receiving the drugs were elderly or female, even though the drugs hadn't really been studied in terms of either category of patient. In fact, though the 4S study showed limited benefit of cholesterol-lowering drugs for women, and though women weren't even included in WOSCOPS, more than half of all cholesterol patients now receiving the drugs in the United States are women.[20]

Only a few brave dissidents have questioned the design of the 4S study and point out what they view as a number of basic flaws. For one thing, anyone with coronary heart disease was allowed into the study, whether his illness was caused by hardened arteries or not. In the treated group, there were thirty-eight additional people who had, by the time they entered the study, already been given bypass surgery or angioplasty and who therefore were less likely to die. And fifty-four more smokers were in the control group, which just might have had something to do with their greater mortality rate.[21]

William Stehbens of the Wellington School of Medicine in New Zealand pointed out (and, as a pathologist, he should know) that diagnosing CHD or gauging the severity of atherosclerosis is a highly inexact science—until people die. In the 4S study, the actual difference in the death rate between the two groups from all causes was only 3.3 percent. Finally, Stehbens notes, almost in an aside, that the control group took a placebo containing methylcellulose, which when given intravenously to rabbits causes tissue storage in arteries, a condition that sounds not dissimilar to the effect of atherosclerosis.

In the WOSCOP study, the deaths from heart disease in the control group (those not taking the drug) were higher in number than in the general population—closer to the average deaths in people ten years or older—suggesting that particular people chosen to represent the "average citizen" happened to be more ill than usual.[22] Furthermore, although pravastatin did reduce cholesterol levels and the number of heart attacks or death from heart attacks in the WOSCOPS, *it did not significantly save lives from other coronary disease or any other cause. A review of all the studies with pravastatin also failed to show that a reduction in heart attacks translated into a significant number of lives being saved.* Any improvements in the death rate, other than from heart attacks, were not considered "statistically significant."[23] And even if you tally in the survival statistics from heart attacks, overall survival over five years in the WOSCOPS trial was only increased from 96 to 97 percent, and in the 4S trial from 87.7 to 91.3 percent.[24] This means that many people with no history of heart attack may be put on cholesterol-lowering drugs indefinitely for an extremely minimal gain. A new study shows that pravastatin is little better than a sugar pill in protecting against a second heart attack.[25]

The other problem with a cholesterol-lowering "prescription for life" is that there is a great deal we still do not know about this category of drugs. Patients are being counseled to take statins up until the time they die, even though the benefits of these drugs have not been tested in the elderly. In fact other research shows that a higher cholesterol level is less of a risk factor (or possibly even irrelevant) after the age of fifty-five. And of course we don't know what effect these drugs have on someone who takes them over many years.[26]

Dr. Thomas Newman of the University of California at San Francisco, who has written extensively on medical policy concerning cholesterol, has examined epidemiological data suggesting that these drugs are less beneficial to women, the elderly, and younger men (in both of the big cholesterol studies, the subjects were all middle-aged men).[27] There may even be a slightly increased rate of death among women on cholesterol-lowering drugs.[28] But in any case, doctors don't agree about whether women should lower their cholesterol. Earlier evidence has shown that a woman's risk of developing a heart condition isn't lessened even if cholesterol levels are lowered through diet. There is no evidence linking high cholesterol levels in women with heart conditions in later life.[29]

Some researchers also have noted that slightly more people died from all causes in the 4S study. Although this number wasn't considered significant, we need more studies of the drugs to figure out if cholesterol-lowering drugs could be responsible for increasing deaths from other causes.[30] So far, we do know that a low blood cholesterol concentration can cause hemorrhagic stroke.[31]

Few have paused to add up the financial implications of these studies. If the WOSCOPS showed a 2.2 percent prevention in heart attack, this translates into the fact that 143 men with high cholesterol levels must be treated for five years to prevent one death from a cardiovascular cause. Pravastatin costs $100 for a month's supply, or $6,000 for each patient for those five years. That means that $858,000 worth of drugs needs to be purchased and consumed to prevent perhaps one death. Since middle-aged women have only about a fourth the incidence of heart disease as men, it may cost as much as $3.4 million to prevent the death from heart disease of one woman.[32] And if we're talking about only mildly elevated cholesterol, the number of people you need to treat to prevent a heart attack goes up even more.[33]

A Violent End

The biggest problem with cholesterol lowering is that patients on cholesterol-lowering programs are more likely to die *from other causes*. In the early nineties a number of large-scale studies began appearing which showed that patients on cholesterol diets or drugs were more likely to die from violent deaths, including suicide, than those eating what they wanted.[34] This bizarre connection was dismissed as a quirk—until it was confirmed by a number of subsequent international studies.

New research from Italy has confirmed that low cholesterol levels indeed tend to make people suicidal. Researchers from Corso studied the blood levels of 300 people who'd attempted suicide, against an identical number who hadn't ever tried to harm themselves. In virtually all cases, the suicide group had lower levels of cholesterol close to the time they tried to kill themselves.[35] Men whose cholesterol levels are lowered with drugs double their likelihood of committing suicide, according to French research.[36]

Cholesterol drugs, or even a very low-fat diet, may contribute to a decrease in serotonin, a brain hormone that normally keeps harmful impulses, such as aggressive behavior, in check. In animal studies, mice with lowered cholesterol levels also showed a decrease in the number of serotonin receptors in their brains.[37] One effect of the new class of selective serotonin reuptake inhibitor (SSRI) antidepressants, such as fluoxetine (Prozac), is to block serotonin from reaching certain cells in the nervous system. Numerous instances of violent or suicidal tendencies have been reported among patients taking these drugs.

One study in a geriatric unit in Italy found that among older people, the risk of depression was highest among those with the lowest blood cholesterol concentration.[38]

Researchers from the University of California at San Diego

have their own theory about the link between low cholesterol and violent death. The California researchers found that depression was three times more common in those with low blood cholesterol than in those with higher levels in those over seventy. What's more, they also found that the extent of depression correlated with the level of cholesterol: the lower the cholesterol, the more depressed the patient.[39] This problem may only occur in older people, since there has never been any evidence of a relationship among younger people between violence and drugs taken to control cholesterol levels. We do have some evidence that people on weight-loss programs have significantly reduced levels of tryptophan in their blood. Women also placed on very-low-fat diets have lower levels of tryptophan and a significant change in their levels of serotonin.[40] Tryptophan, an essential amino acid, is what serotonin is mainly derived from, and we get tryptophan from certain foods, mainly proteins, and dietary supplements. When the diets of several countries are compared, those with low tryptophan intake have a higher rate of suicide. We also have evidence that patients suffering from severe depression have low levels of tryptophan, and get worse if they are put on low-tryptophan diets. As their depression improves, so do their levels of tryptophan.[41]

Other evidence has shown a greater risk of suicide the higher the level of cholesterol,[42] and one overview trial failed to find an association.[43] However, the answer may lie in changes in our diet over the last century that have altered the ratio of the two classes of essential fatty acids, with a decrease in omega-3 fatty acids, such as are found in fatty fish and flaxseed oil. When this ratio is altered (as it would be for either a high- or low-fat diet), patients have been shown to have increased levels of depression.[44]

Whatever the association, it's obvious that medicine doesn't yet understand the delicate interrelation of hormonal messages that the brain receives, nor the dietary requirements necessary to sustain them. By some well-intended fiddling here and there, it could be creating a good deal more havoc than the very worst Western diet.

Unsafe and Unsatisfactory

Cholesterol drugs have been targeted as unsafe for other reasons. Many doctors have stopped prescribing clofibrate following a World Health Organization trial which revealed that it increased the mortality rate among sufferers by 44 percent, which fell back to normal once the drug was withdrawn.[45]

Questran (cholestyramine), another drug routinely prescribed to lower one's cholesterol levels, can cause constipation, flatulence, heartburn, nausea, diarrhea, stomach upsets, skin rashes, and, rarely, fat in the feces. It can also lead to vitamin K deficiency, which may cause increased bleeding due to the inability of the blood to clot properly. In animal studies, cholestyramine has been linked with intestinal cancer.[46] Cases of sexual dysfunction have been reported in patients taking gemfibrozil, another cholesterol-lowering drug. Several studies have shown that certain cholesterol drugs may increase rates of cancer by a third.[47] Lowering cholesterol levels may also increase the risk of death from stroke.[48]

Margaret was on Zocor (simvastatin) for eighteen months. She says she never would have taken it had her doctor told her about its side effects:

> When I complained to my doctor about these effects, he dismissed them. To my complaint about dry mouth, for example, he said that I did not drink enough water. Nosebleeds, which I'd never had before, brought no comment from him, other than that I should see an ear, nose, and throat surgeon to have my nose cauterized.
>
> A cardiologist helped me to get my blood pressure down, which corrected the extreme breathlessness I had been experiencing. But since starting on Zocor, increased breathlessness practically immobilized me—at the least bit of exertion! Even though I stopped taking the drug in August, my severe itching continues.
>
> Recently, I saw an advertisement about a similar cholesterol drug in a magazine. In the fine print, the ad clearly states some of the side effects that I've suffered. Why has

*my doctor never considered that Zocor could be the cause of
my problems?*

As Margaret rightly points out, dry mouth, shortness of breath,
blood–clotting problems, and itching are but a few of the host
of side effects with cholesterol-lowering drugs—including, in
some cases, the risk of a heart attack.

The latest suspicion is that cholesterol-lowering drugs may
cause cancer with long-term use. Cholesterol policy expert Dr.
Thomas Newman of the University of California at San Francisco, and his colleague Dr. Stephen Hulley, analyzed the data
published in the American drug reference bible, the *Physicians'
Desk Reference,* plus population studies of cancer and cholesterol
levels and clinical trials of cholesterol lowering to discover a
definite link between some of the popular cholesterol-lowering
drugs and a risk of cancer. Tests carried out on rodents clearly
show the carcinogenic effects of the drugs, especially if taken
over the long term. Drs. Newman and Hulley suggest that the
levels of statin cholesterol–lowering drugs being taken by humans
are close to the levels that have proved carcinogenic in these
experimental animals.[49] In Britain, gemfibrozil, marketed as
Lopid, has been linked to tumor growth in mice and rats, but
only when the animals have been given ten times the recommended dose per day. Although other drugs have been shown
to cause cancer in animals without posing a threat to humans,
Newman and Hulley argue that the human exposure to cholesterol-
lowering drugs is much closer to the dose that causes cancer in
rodents. The United Kingdom's drugs reference guide, the *ABPI
Compendium of Data Sheets and Summaries of Product Characteristics,*
reports a "significant increase" in liver cancer in rats given the
overdose. Since approval, several cholesterol-lowering drugs have
been associated with lung, thyroid, testis, and lymph node
cancers.[50]

The scientists note that the drugs were approved by the Food
and Drug Administration on the basis of less than ten years'
clinical trials. The full effects of the drugs may not become clear

for thirty years, particularly as many people are now being encouraged to take the drugs for many decades.

The carcinogenic potential of two of the drugs, lovastatin and gemfibrozil, were discussed in a drugs advisory committee meeting of the FDA. The drug manufacturer representative of lovastatin "downplayed the importance of the studies," the California researchers maintain. The data were also prepared in milligrams per kilogram of body weight, which may have confused the committee.

Even though they approved the drug, the FDA committee appears to have had reservations. Their original recommendation was that gemfibrozil should be used as a drug of last resort, only after exercise, diet, and weight control have failed to lower cholesterol levels. The popularity of the drug since then suggests it has been far more widely used than the committee wanted.

Although Newman and Hulley agree that extrapolating evidence of damage in rodents to humans is an uncertain business, they do not press for an all-out ban. Their view is that the benefits of the drugs outweigh the risk among men with very high blood cholesterol at a short-term high risk of heart attacks— so long as they take the drug for under five years. However, those not at high risk should avoid the drugs, they feel, particularly if they have a life expectancy greater than twenty years.

Although the renewed faith in cholesterol drugs has taken the focus away from diet as a preventive exercise, the old low-cholesterol diet recommended by the World Health Organization and the American Heart Association is being called into question.

Diets with high percentages of polyunsaturated fats have been demonstrated to lower cholesterol level, but without reducing the risk of heart disease or death. In fact, some theoretical studies question whether this diet doesn't actually *increase* arterial plaque formation.[51] According to Petr Skrabanek and James McCormick, some large-scale studies have examined the effects of the standard WHO recommendation of limiting fat intake to 30 percent of total dietary intake, with no more than 10 percent each of saturated, polyunsaturated, and monounsaturated fats. After 828,000 man-years of study, they wrote, there were four fewer deaths in 10,000 men per year. "Such a small difference is well within the limits of chance."[52]

There are dietary measures that have been shown to reverse heart disease, but they are more complex than those that simply lower fat. To determine whether comprehensive lifestyle changes might affect coronary atherosclerosis, a group of patients embarked on a low-fat vegetarian diet, stopped smoking, trained in stress management, and engaged in moderate exercise. They were compared with another group with similar clogged arteries who did not undergo the special lifestyle modifications. After a year, the vegetarian group's coronary arteries had widened by 3 percent, while the control group's had narrowed by 4 percent. In all, 82 percent of the experimental group had shown improvement, demonstrating that a comprehensive lifestyle change could reverse even severe coronary atherosclerosis without drugs after only one year.[53] A more recent study measuring coronary arteries with a special CT scanning showed that disease was reversed in 99 percent of patients over five years.[54]

In another study, patients given a cholesterol-lowering diet alone also were able to reverse coronary artery disease—nearly as much as those given the diet drugs.[55] And women runners were found to have higher levels of high-density lipoprotein (HDL—the "good" cholesterol needed by our bodies that appears to protect against heart disease), the more they exercised.[56] Giving up smoking, which appears to exacerbate the vascular abnormalities of people with high blood cholesterol, is possibly one of the most meaningful lifestyle changes you can make.[57]

Nevertheless, there is some question about which low-fat diets are appropriate. Some very-low-fat diets can change some of the levels of HDL cholesterol or result in low levels of essential fatty acids, which have been associated with an increased risk of heart attack.[58] Even the two heart doctors who performed the vegetarian diet studies disagree over whether patients should be strict vegetarians or have a high- or low-carbohydrate diet.[59]

Margarine and Other Plastic Food

Another problem is that patients on low-fat diets often consume specially processed low-fat foods, which may themselves contribute to disease. Most processed and low-fat foods are deficient in essential fatty acids; the usual effect of consuming them is to set up an imbalance in our bodies, which lowers the "good" cholesterol and increases the "bad" cholesterol.[60]

One of the most dangerous of these low-fat foods appears to be margarine, made from hydrogenated oils. This is performed by heating up the oil to a high temperature and sending hydrogen through it.

Hydrogenation began after 1912, so that polyunsaturated fats could compete with butter and lard. During hydrogenation, trans fatty acids are produced; these artificial unsaturated fatty acids have a different molecular structure to those found in the tissues of humans and other mammals. This production process, used in the manufacture of margarine, creates "trans isomers" of fatty acids, which resemble the chemical configuration of saturated fat.[61]

The amounts of trans fatty acids (TFAs) in processed foods can range from 5 percent to 75 percent of the total fat; U.S. law does not require manufacturers to state the amount of hydrogenated fat in a product, only whether or not it is present at all.[62] TFAs can have a "disastrous" effect on your body's ability to use essential fatty acids, says nutritional expert Dr. Leo Galland, author of *Superimmunity for Kids* (E. P. Dutton) and *Four Pillars of Healing* (Random House). They are even worse when heated, turning into something akin to the polymers in plastic.

Hydrogenated fats are in fast foods such as chips and doughnuts, and in the vegetable oils contained in shortenings and biscuits. They account for up to 10 percent of the content of some margarines.

George V. Mann, a doctor from Nashville, Tennessee, who has researched and written widely on the subject, argues that lipoprotein receptors in cells are impaired by TFAs. Since this impairment prevents the body from processing cholesterol-bearing low-density lipoproteins, the cells crank up their rate of synthesizing cholesterol, eventually leading to high levels in the blood. We know from numerous studies that blood cholesterol quickly increases in people fed TFAs.[63] Another study, this one by Harvard

Medical School, of 85,000 women over eight years found that those eating margarine had an *increased* risk of coronary heart disease.

The more TFAs you eat (and are stored in body fat), the greater your apparent risk of heart disease. One Welsh study showed a strong association between TFA content in body fat and death from heart disease.[64]

Partially hydrogenated vegetable oils have not only failed to provide the expected benefits as a substitute for highly saturated fats but have "contributed to the occurrence of coronary heart disease," the Harvard researchers concluded.[65]

Dr. Mary Enig, formerly of the Department of Chemistry and Biochemistry at the University of Maryland, who analyzed the trans fatty acid content of some 600 foods, reckons that Americans eat between eleven and twenty-eight grams of trans fatty acids a day—or one-fifth of their total intake of fat. To give you some idea of how this happens, one large portion of French fries cooked in partially hydrogenated oil contains 8 grams of trans fatty acids, as does 60 grams of imitation cheese.[66] The Harvard study reckons that TFAs could account for 6 percent of all deaths from heart disease, or 30,000 deaths a year in the United States alone. And of course heart disease rates are high in northern European countries, where consumption of TFAs is high, and low in the Mediterranean countries, where the main dietary fat is olive oil and TFA intake is low.

An epidemic of heart disease can be directly linked to the introduction of partially hydrogenated fats in food, with the first major outbreak recorded in 1920. Before the First World War, when cheese and butter were staples of the diet, death from coronary thrombosis was rare. Nonetheless, researchers consistently linked heart disease to animal fats, found in butter, giving margarine manufacturers the opportunity to claim their products were better for your heart.

The influential EURAMIC study, which covered eight European countries and Israel, suggested there is no conclusive evidence to show that margarine is linked to heart problems. But it did warn that there could be some connection in countries where there is a very high margarine intake.

The EURAMIC study based its findings on two groups of men—one with a serious heart condition and another without any history of heart problems. They discovered that both groups had similar levels of trans fatty acids in their tissues.[67]

There may also be another issue here. In Dr. George V. Mann's studies of the African Maasai, young men consistently had low cholesterol concentrations, even though their diets were high in saturated fats, mainly from milk and beef. Dr. Mann concluded that the Maasai, who got about 4 to 7 grams a day of TFAs from cow's milk, were below the threshold at which the body's ability to metabolize fat starts to be impaired. In the United States, the average daily intake of TFAs is 12 to 20 grams daily. Or it may well be that the story is even more complicated than this. The Maasai could be protected because they eat whole foods—albeit those containing saturated fats—and not the adulterated ones consumed by most people in the West.

The Trouble with Today's Food

The main reason that medicine is so befuddled about this entire cholesterol business is its insistence upon searching for—and isolating—a single, dietary risk factor. There is also great (and misplaced) interest in a piecemeal approach to nutrition—in the particular micronutrients that combat this or that disease. In taking this approach, medicine blinds itself to a couple of obvious differences between Westerners and all the more "primitive" populations with low heart disease, including cultures such as the Inuits, who thrive on a high-fat diet.

Numerous studies show that when more primitive populations begin to consume a Western diet, they start dying of heart attacks. But the main difference between what they're eating and what we're eating is not meat or fats but *whole foods*. The culprit appears to be the large-scale adulterating, or "dismembering," of everything we put in our mouths. This includes the massive addition of refined sugar, which increases blood fats and lowers the strength of the immune system.

In examining current twentieth-century Western diets, Dr. Stephen Davies, who has pioneered nutritional medicine in Britain, points out that people haven't changed much over 40,000 years—but, at least here in the West, our diet has.[68] He quotes S. Boyd Eaton and Melvin Konner, writing about paleolithic nutrition in the *New England Journal of Medicine:* "Even the development of agriculture 10,000 years ago has apparently had a minimal effect on our genes. Certain hemaglobinopathies and retention of intestinal lactase into adulthood are 'recent' genetic evolutionary trends, but few other examples are known."[69]

In other words, the business of food might be modern and industrial, but our stomachs are still in the hunting-and-gathering stage. At that time, we consumed 21 percent of our total dietary energy from fats, 34 percent from protein, and 45.7 grams of fiber (with cholesterol intake a whopping 591 milligrams, compared to the usual recommendations these days of 300 milligrams). Today, the average U.K. male takes in 14.1 percent of his dietary energy from protein and 37.6 percent from fats, with only 390 milligrams of cholesterol and 24.9 grams of fiber.

By modern-day dietary standards, cavemen should have been dropping like flies. But clearly fat is a very small part of the story. One of the results of modern agribusiness, with its domestication of animals, birds, and fish, is a substantial lowering of our consumption of essential fatty acids, which we now know are vital to a healthy immune system. "Intensive livestock farming of pigs and chickens in particular, where the animals are kept indoors in overcrowded conditions, is associated with nutrient deficiencies of these animals," writes Stephen Davies. "Food processing and refining techniques further compromise nutrient content, as do intensive farming techniques which result in soil demineralization. Agrichemicals and other environmental pollutants find their way in to the food chain, and further disrupt the nutrient value of the foods and stress our detoxification . . . mechanisms."[70]

What Stephen Davies is saying is that many degenerative illnesses such as coronary heart disease could be, in large part, the failure of our bodies to catch up with the twentieth century's virtual revolution in what constitutes "food." In other words, the culprit isn't necessarily cholesterol or any other single food, but the very means we now employ to grow, collect, sell, and prepare what appears on the table. Think of the extraordinary demands placed on each of us by the wholesale stripping of vital nutrients from our food and the inclusion of thousands of strange new elements into our diets.

Today's meat business makes liberal use of steroids, antibiotics, tranquilizers and beta-blockers. Agrichemicals currently employ pesticides, herbicides, rodenticides, fungicides, and nitrate fertilizers. Current food processing refines wheat and sugar, which reduces their trace mineral and vitamin content, as do current storage methods, food irradiation, and the addition of some 3,794 food additives, colorings, sweeteners, texture modifiers, and preservatives.

Native Nutrition

Because most dietary recommendations are faddish, your safest bet is to follow some of the basic dietary principles shared by many healthy native populations. In his book *Native Nutrition: Eating According to Ancestral Wisdom* (Healing Arts Press), naturopath Ronald F. Schmid, examines studies of native populations by Dr. Weston Price and Dr. Francis M. Pottenger: Inuits of Alaska, the Swiss of the Loetschental Valley, Native Americans, Africans, and South Sea islanders. All these populations, which lived on fresh fruits and vegetables, grains, wild game and fish or healthy, free-roaming animals, and, in some cases, fresh, unprocessed dairy products, were or are impressive for their strong, healthy bodies, straight, perfect teeth, and freedom from the degenerative diseases plaguing us nowadays in the West.

Although their diets varied enormously (the African Maasai mainly eat meat, milk, and blood, while the traditional Maori of New Zealand eat fish, kelp, and roots), they share certain basic similarities. According to American dietary expert Annemarie Colbin in her excellent book *Food and Healing* (Ballantine), all these native diets have in common food that is fresh (or preserved naturally, whether smoked, dried, or pickled); it is grown locally and organically, in season; and it is cooked by traditional methods.

Whenever possible, eat fresh whole foods and eschew packaged and processed foods, anything that has been added to, refined, enriched, or in some way interfered with. This would include most processed baked goods, canned sauces, commercial peanut butter, sweets, "cheese" foods, potato chips, and corn chips. Especially steer clear of anything such as margarines whose labels list nonfoods such as partially hydrogenated vegetable oils. There is no health reason to cut out or limit eggs (so long as they are free-range), which are an excellent source of protein. Otherwise, eat a wide variety of foods, sort out your food allergies beforehand, and cut down on animal fats as the centerpiece of your meals. In general, most European oils are less refined than those produced in the United States. In fact, the safest course is to cook with extra virgin olive oil that is still made by traditional methods.

SIX

Vaccination: Knee-Jerk Jabs

Josie McNally thought she was doing right by her baby son, William. He was a healthy, normal, happy one-year-old and she wanted to make sure to keep him that way. On December 1992, her doctor recommended that he come in for his routine measles/mumps/rubella (MMR) shot to protect against these dangerous diseases. Josie thought nothing of it; William had sailed through his infant shots and, besides, the doctor knew best.

Ten days after William's shot, something turned horribly wrong. William began convulsing, and Josie and her husband had to rush him by ambulance to the hospital. When Josie suggested her son might be reacting to the vaccination, the doctor shook his head. The fit coming after the shot could be nothing more than coincidence; it probably wouldn't recur. The senior pediatrician at the hospital agreed; the shot appeared to have nothing to do with it.

But the fits didn't stop, and before long William became gripped by seizures, sometimes forty a day. He also developed a rare immune-system reaction. Now three years old, he's diagnosed as epileptic, continues to have convulsions uncontrollable by medication, and has the developmental age of an eighteen-month-old. In her trips in and out of the hospital, Josie began meeting other mothers whose children also had similar problems, which started right after their MMR shot. And not long after he was given it, the vaccine William had was withdrawn. Nevertheless, to this day no one in the medical profession will officially acknowledge the vaccine had anything to do with it.

Most doctors fervently believe that vaccines are one of medical science's greatest success stories, responsible for wiping out many deadly infectious diseases. In fact, lurking inside most doctors is an altruist who likes to think that the eradication of disease is not only possible but just around the corner. Every so often, the World Health Organization will announce an actual date when it fully expects that diseases such as polio, measles, or diphtheria will be wiped off the planet forever.

The ardency of this faith has emboldened the profession to produce ever more shots to combat not only major killers such as polio but also a number of the mostly benign copassengers of childhood, such as measles, mumps, and chicken pox. Counting all multiple boosters in the entire suggested schedule, American children can receive some thirty vaccinations by the time they go to school, most in the first few months of life; Britain, with its tuberculosis vaccine offered at birth but no hepatitis B or chicken pox vaccine, ends up with a slightly more modest twenty-five. The U.S. government and the World Health Organization have even sponsored the development of what they imagine will turn out to be a genetically engineered, time-released "Holy Grail," a supervaccine containing the raw DNA of up to forty different diseases at one go, which will be squirted into a newborn's mouth at birth and send out booster doses at timed intervals throughout an individual's life.[1] Lately, there are vaccines being worked on for asthma, earaches and respiratory diseases, AIDS, cancer, and even to prevent pregnancy.

It is with vaccines that the brave-new-world technocrats of medicine have lost all reason about disease and its prevention. So steadfast is this faith in the rightness of their cause that it prevents doctors from acknowledging clear factual evidence demonstrating the dangers and ineffectiveness of certain vaccines, or even cases of a disease in children who have been vaccinated against it. It also turns otherwise reasonable doctors or scientists into bullies and hysterics, shouting down dissenters, using emotional blackmail to bully parents into submission and resorting to emotive appeals, rather than common sense or fact, to argue their point of view. In the United States parents are threatened with the withholding of welfare payments if they fail to give their kids the live triple measles/mumps/rubella vaccine. Chicago health authorities have tried to give vaccination a bit of street credibility by employing loudspeaker sales pitches mixed in with salsa music to encourage mothers in Hispanic neighborhoods to bring their children in to get their shots. To launch its countrywide campaign to vaccinate school-age children against measles and rubella, the British government ran stark, emotive black-and-white television ads suggesting that measles strikes fatally and at random.

In this recent U.K. campaign to inoculate all British children from five to sixteen with the measles/rubella shot, parents were given flimsy pamphlets with virtually no mention of the side effects long accepted by international governmental bodies. Doctors and health authorities badgered parents who'd decided against the shot with letters and phone calls to try to change their minds. And all sorts of medical experts were confidently announcing publicly that this campaign would undoubtedly eradicate measles from these shores for all time.

Britain's Department of Health pressed ahead with one of the most ambitious immunization campaigns ever seen in an industrialized country, informing parents that side effects to booster shots are very unlikely, having been "carefully studied by looking at large numbers of children in the United States."[2] In fact, the evidence on which this claim was based was rather more meager. Before the campaign they received a fax from the U.S. American National Immunization Program officials explaining that the only evidence that boosters were safer was based on questionnaires sent to college students receiving the shots. Medical scientists consider this type of study a highly unreliable and unscientific measure of safety and effectiveness. The real safety of reactions or boosters shots would not be known for another year, when a trial involving 1,800 children in the United States would be completed.

What's worse, the U.K.'s Public Health Laboratory Service completed a study before the campaign began, demonstrating that children given the measles/mumps/rubella shot were *three times* more likely to suffer from convulsions than those who didn't receive it. Two-thirds of the cases of seizures were due to the measles component alone. The study also found that the MMR vaccine caused five times the number of cases of a rare blood disorder over that expected. This study was never mentioned during the campaign, but was only published in the medical literature, and not until four months after the campaign was completed.[3]

Because vaccines represent the very epitome of modern medicine—the triumph of science over nature—scientific trials are most subject to medical spin-doctoring in order to paint a positive face on a negative result, ignoring any results they don't wish to hear. In America, the U.S. government requested that the National Academy of Science review all the medical literature and report fully on what were the known and proven dangers, if any, of the various childhood vaccines. In two separate reports the NAS's Institute of Medicine, which gathered together leading pediatricians and medical scientists for the task, concluded that all nine vaccines used at the time had the potential to do serious harm. Although these conclusions were eventually included in lengthy fact sheets given to parents prior to their children's vaccinations, the National Commission on Childhood Vaccines has pushed to have them edited, on the grounds that they "confuse" parents.

In Britain, the Department of Health commissioned a report on the whooping cough vaccine by Professor Gordon Stewart, formerly of the Department of Community Medicine at the University of Glasgow and now an adviser to the World Health Organization, who has long studied the vaccine. When his studies showed the risks of the vaccine outweighed the benefits, the

DHSS referred the report to the Committee on the Safety of Medicines, which chose not to act on it.[4]

In this zealous climate, amid the rush to "conquer" every possible disease, in which entire reputations rest on defending vaccination at all costs, no one is pausing to examine the possible long-term effects of pumping up to ten or more different antigens into the immature immune systems of a generation of babies under fifteen months. In all the studies done of vaccination, epidemiologists have never investigated whether there is an upper limit to the number of shots a baby can tolerate, after which all sorts of subtle damage—asthma, learning disabilities, hyperactivity, or chronic earache, for instance—come into play. *In fact, nobody has done any long-term safety studies at all.* "We only hear about the encephalitis and the deaths," says Dr. J. Anthony Morris, formerly a director of virology at the Food and Drug Administration and the National Institutes of Health. "But there is an entire spectrum of reactions between fever and death, and it's all those things in between that never get reported."[5]

At the heart of the logic behind vaccination is the theory of herd immunity—that is, if enough people get vaccinated against a certain disease, it will eventually disappear. Besides an element of wishful thinking in the face of highly complex organisms such as viruses, which constantly mutate and change, the problem with this line of reasoning, of course, is its tyrannical approach: Eliminating a disease is more important, in the eyes of medicine, than your child's health, which might be damaged from a vaccine, or your right to decide what is best for your family. Decide against vaccination for your child and you are considered not only an irresponsible parent but an irresponsible citizen of your community and even the world. In the United States, childhood shots have been given a further fillip by the Clinton Administration's Childhood Vaccine Act, which now makes it more difficult for parents to get exempted from vaccinating their children.

In many Western countries all children are obliged to be vaccinated in order to get into school—a policy, particularly in places such as the United States, that would seem to fly in the face of a number of constitutional freedoms. In this hysterical climate, the government and the medical community have made it their right to insist on administering a substance to a minor that it cannot guarantee is safe.

A BLUNT INSTRUMENT

Vaccination is a blunt and highly imperfect instrument. The main problem isn't so much that vaccines don't work, but that they work haphazardly. The premise of vaccination rests on the assumption that injecting an individual with weakened live or killed virus will "trick" his body into developing antibodies to the disease, as it does when it contracts an illness naturally. But medicine doesn't really know whether vaccines work for any length of time. All that the usual scientific studies can demonstrate (as they are only conducted over the short term) is that vaccines may create antibodies in the blood. What may happen is that a number of vaccines are capable of measurably raising antibodies to a particular infectious illness, but for only a short period of time. Or even if they do raise antibodies indefinitely, this may have nothing to do with protecting an individual from contracting the disease over the long (or even the short) term. In fact, having antibodies in the blood may not be the only way the body recognizes and defends itself from disease. For instance, large numbers of people who have had illnesses such as diphtheria never produce antibodies to the disease.

In one report, for instance, measles antibodies were found in the blood of only one of seven vaccinated children who'd gone on to develop measles—they hadn't developed antibodies from either the shot or the disease itself.[6] And lately, the U.K.'s Public Health Laboratory in London has discovered that a quarter of blood donors in Britain between twenty and twenty-nine had insufficient immunity to diphtheria, even though most would have been vaccinated as babies. This percentage doubled among the fifty-to-fifty-nine age group.[7]

MYTH NO 1: DISEASES HAVE BEEN ELIMINATED PURELY AS A RESULT OF VACCINATION

The success of vaccination is based entirely on assumption. Because the incidence and death rate of many infectious diseases have radically declined, with improved sanitation and hygiene, housing, better nutrition, and isolation procedures, at coincidentally the same time that vaccines have been introduced, medicine has assumed that vaccination is entirely responsible for the eradication of these diseases. Many medical textbooks lead off with the boast that one of medicine's great achievements is the eradication of smallpox through vaccination. However, if you actually examine the epidemiological statistics, you discover that between 1870 and 1872, eighteen years after compulsory vaccination was introduced, four years after a coercive four-year effort to vaccinate all members of the population was in place (with stiff penalties for offenders), and at the point where 97.5 percent of the population had been vaccinated, England experienced the worst smallpox epidemic of the century, which claimed more than 44,000 lives. In fact, three times as many people died from smallpox at that time as had in an earlier epidemic, when fewer people were vaccinated.

After 1871, the town of Leicester refused vaccination, largely because the high incidence of smallpox and death rates during the 1870 epidemic convinced the population it didn't work. In the next epidemic of 1892, Leicester relied solely on improved sanitation and quarantines. The town suffered only nineteen cases and 1 death per 100,000 population, compared with the town of Warrington, which had six times the number of cases and eleven times the death rate of Leicester, even though 99 percent of its population had been vaccinated.[8]

The World Health Organization has pointed out that the key to eradication of the disease in many parts of West and Central Africa was switching from mass immunization, which was not working very well, to a campaign of surveillance, containing the disease through isolation procedures.[9]

Sierra Leone's experience also demonstrates that vaccination wasn't responsible for the end of smallpox. In the late sixties, Sierra Leone had the highest rate of smallpox in the world. In January 1968 the country began its eradication campaign, and three of the four largest outbreaks were controlled by identifying and isolating cases alone, without immunization. Fifteen months later, the area recorded its last case of smallpox.[10]

Polio

More than any other, the polio vaccine is pointed to with pride by every government as definitive proof that mass vaccination programs work. The government is quick to note that during the plague years of polio, 20,000 to 30,000 cases per year occurred in America, compared to twenty to thirty cases a year today. Nevertheless, Dr. Bernard Greenberg, head of the Department of Biostatistics at the University of North Carolina School of Public Health, has gone on record to say that cases of polio *increased* by 50 percent between 1957 and 1958, and by 80 percent from 1958 to 1959, after the introduction of mass immunization.[11] In five New England states—Massachusetts, Connecticut, New Hampshire, Rhode Island, and Vermont—cases of polio roughly doubled in 1954 and 1955, after the polio vaccine was introduced.[12] Nevertheless, in the midst of the polio panic of the 1950s, with the pressure on to find a magic bullet, statistics were manipulated by health authorities to give the opposite impression.

One such way was to give the old disease a new name—"viral or aseptic meningitis" or "cocksackie virus." According to statistics from the Los Angeles County Health Index, for instance, in July 1955 there were 273 reported cases of polio and fifty cases of aseptic meningitis, compared with five cases of polio and 256 cases of aseptic meningitis a decade later.[13]

In the early part of this century, over 3,000 deaths were attributed to "chicken pox," and only some 500 to smallpox, even though authorities agree that chicken pox is only very rarely a fatal disease.[14]

Martha recently experienced this sort of fast-shuffle name change with whooping cough:

> Not long ago, after our two-year-old developed full-blown whooping cough, I took her to our doctor, prepared to face a reprimand for neglecting to have her vaccinated. However, the doctor diagnosed asthma and prescribed Ventolin. I was so unconvinced by this diagnosis that I consulted another doctor within the practice. To my amazement he insisted that whooping cough no longer exists (due to mass vaccination) and confirmed the diagnosis of asthma. I then pressed for a sputum test to prove or disprove the existence of whooping cough.
>
> I later received a patronizing phone call, following my doctor's discussion with a local microbiologist. 'They do not test for whooping cough because it does not exist,' I was told. I then asked, should the condition clear up in a few weeks, presumably asthma would have been an unlikely diagnosis? To which he replied: 'We now have a new condition called viral asthma which is similar to whooping cough.' He said they see many children with this condition. He added, "Since they stopped testing for whooping cough there have been no recorded cases in our area."

Diseases such as polio operate cyclically. The great polio epidemics occurred in the 1910s, the 1930s and the 1950s; then cases sharply dropped off down to nearly zero. But at the height of the fifties epidemics, after the vaccine was introduced, as author Welene James says, quoting another writer, "The vaccine took the credit instead of nature."[15] The late medical critic Dr. Robert Mendelsohn once noted: "Diseases are like fashion, they come and go."[16] Many vaccine programs claim the credit for what is simply the tendency of illnesses to wax and wane. Far from science having anything to do with finally stamping out polio or tuberculosis, both diseases decided, a number of years ago, to take a breather and are now making a comeback—tuberculosis in many Western countries, polio in many parts of Canada, and diphtheria in Russia and the East.

Tetanus, Diphtheria, and Whooping Cough

The incidence and number of deaths from diphtheria were declining long before the vaccine was introduced, as they were from tetanus, largely because of increased attention to wound hygiene.[17] Among all the soldiers of the Second World War, only twelve cases of tetanus were recorded—a third of which occurred among soldiers who were vaccinated.[18] The great decline in deaths from whooping cough (some 80 percent) occurred *before* the vaccine was introduced.[19]

Measles

A similar pattern occurred with measles. The death rate from measles plummeted to greater than a 95 percent decline (to .03 deaths per 100,000) twenty years before the vaccine was introduced.[20]

And today, despite the fact that the United Kingdom has had the triple measles/mumps/rubella vaccine in place since 1988, and enjoys an extraordinarily high coverage of vaccination among toddlers, cases of measles recently were going up—by nearly one-fourth.[21]

Until recently, the United States was suffering from a steadily increasing epidemic of measles—the worst for decades—despite the fact that the measles vaccine in its various forms has been in effect since 1957, and the combined shot since 1975. Although the government targeted 1982 as the date of the virtual elimination of the disease, the Centers for Disease Control in Atlanta reported a provisional total of 27,672 cases of measles in 1990, the latest year for which statistics were available, which represents a virtual doubling of reported cases in 1989, which were double the number of cases reported in the year before *that*.

Although the number of measles cases fell by one-quarter (to 63,000) the year the vaccine was introduced, and bottomed out at 1,500 reported cases in 1983, the numbers suddenly swelled by 423 percent at the end of the eighties and then rose sharply, with the worst hit areas of the United States being Houston and Los Angeles County.

After the great resurgence of measles during 1989–91, cases of measles are now drastically dropping. The Centers for Disease Control happily attributes this to the tremendous push given the measles and combined vaccines at the height of the recent epidemic; vaccine coverage increased from an average of 66 percent in the years before 1985 to 78 percent in 1991.

However, a few statistics confuse this optimistic assumption. First of all, the CDC estimates that, based on retrospective surveys of coverage, approximately 800,000 to 2 million babies and toddlers who hadn't gotten their shots should have been susceptible to measles. In reality, however, only 9,300 cases were reported among this age group in 1992. Although the average age of children catching measles is dropping (from a median age of 12 in 1989, at the beginning of the epidemic, to an average lately of 4.9), nearly half of all reported cases are still among children over 5—most of whom should have been protected.

The CDC admitted that the sudden drop in cases could have something to do with "an overall decrease in the occurrence of measles in the Western Hemisphere." It also may have something to do, they say, with the cyclical nature of the disease.

HIB Meningitis

Even with the latest shot, against *Haemophilus influenzae b* (Hib) meningitis, a provaccine study group extolling the virtues of the Hib vaccine conceded that a "substantial" fall also occurred in children who hadn't been vaccinated—from 99.3 to 68.5 per 100,000.[22]

MYTH NO 2: THE DISEASES YOU ARE VACCINATED AGAINST ARE DEADLY

Increasingly, the rationale for vaccination has shifted from control of deadly disease to control of nuisance diseases such as mumps or chicken pox. In fact, a large number of the illnesses we now vaccinate against are no longer life-threatening in well-nourished children with healthy immune systems.

Measles

The zeal behind the recent measles campaign was founded on the belief that measles can be a life-threatening condition, and it seems to be one that is getting more dangerous by the year. When the British Department of Health ran its last major vaccine drive in 1989, Dr. Norman Begg, an epidemiologist of the Public Health Laboratory Service, cited the then-official statistics that one in 5,000 children contracting measles will develop acute encephalitis, an inflammation of the brain, and one in 5,000 of those will develop SSPE (subacute sclerosing panencephalitis), an almost inevitably fatal progressive disease that causes hardening of the brain.[23]

Five years later, when one columnist encouraged parents to have their children revaccinated in the countrywide measles campaign, the percentage of measles victims who might go on to develop encephalitis had shrunk to one in every 500. One in ten of these would die and one in four would suffer permanent brain damage, the columnist maintained. As the campaign intensified, other newspapers had magnified the danger even further. By November it seemed that one out of every seventeen cases of measles would turn into a case of encephalitis.

But the report of the journal geared specifically for the study of the fatal illness being worried over, the SSPE Registry, concluded that the measles-induced form of this disease is "very rare," occurring in one per million cases.[24] This rare disease also doesn't appear to be so random. A study of people with SSPE concluded that environmental factors other than measles, such as serious head injuries or exposure to certain animals, played an important part in the onset of the disease.[25]

Measles can be a killer, but it doesn't strike as randomly as medicine would have us believe. In the United States in 1990, at the height of a measles epidemic when 27,000 cases were reported, eighty-nine died. But many deaths occurred among children of low-income families, where poor nutrition played a part, as did failure to treat complications. In Africa, where children are markedly deficient in vitamin A, measles does kill. However, as study after study demonstrates, even third-world children with adequate stores of vitamin A or those given vitamin A supplements are overwhelmingly likely to survive.[26]

Whooping Cough

As WHO adviser Dr. Stewart has written: "The lesson of history—not just medical history—is that infectious diseases change in pattern, severity, and frequency through time. Whooping cough was once a serious threat to life and health in all young children. Now it is no longer so, though it is often a distressing disease and dangerous in some infants."[27]

During the whooping cough outbreaks of 1978–79 in Glamorgan, Glasgow, and Surrey, in "low-risk" areas—that is, areas of adequate nutrition—there were no cases of permanent brain damage or death among any children, nor among any babies (who are considered most at risk).[28]

Polio

Even polio is not the virulent mass killer it is always made out to be. Largely because of the 1950s epidemic (following four terms of the most highly publicized victim, President Franklin D. Roosevelt), polio is popularly thought to cut down healthy young people at random. In fact, most cases of polio are harmless infections. The current statistics estimate that only 10 percent of people exposed to polio will contract it, and only 1 percent of *those* will come down with the paralytic variety—or 0.01 percent of those exposed to the disease in the first place. Medical homeopath and noted vaccine critic Dr. Richard Moskowitz has termed the propensity of an individual to develop paralysis from this ordinarily harmless virus a "special anatomical susceptibility."[29]

MYTH NO 3: VACCINES WILL PROTECT YOU AGAINST THESE DISEASES

The big argument put forth by apologists of vaccines, particularly of those vaccines known to have substantial side effects (such as the shot for whooping cough) is that, imperfect as they may be, the benefits are worth the risk. The problem with this argument is that it assumes that vaccines actually *work*.

Whooping Cough

During outbreaks of whooping cough, half or more of the victims have already been fully vaccinated. Professor Stewart reported that, in a study of whooping cough cases for 1974 and 1978, and in 1974 in the United States and Canada, a third to a half of all children who'd caught it had been fully vaccinated. When he studied close to 2,000 babies who'd got whooping cough, two-thirds of the time they'd caught it from their fully vaccinated siblings. To Dr. Stewart's mind, "no protection by vaccination is demonstrable in infants," despite the fact that this is the very population the vaccine aims to protect—the only lives usually threatened by a nasty but otherwise mostly benign disease.[30]

"The effect of the present vaccination program is to leave the only high-risk group, the infants, at risk of both the [side effects of the] vaccine and the infection," Dr Stewart concluded.[31]

In his view, the risk of a baby's contracting encephalitis with permanent brain damage as a result of whooping cough (1 in 38,000) is comparable to the risk of brain damage (1 in 25,000) after vaccination with the shot.[32]

More recently, during a nationwide American epidemic of whooping cough in 1993, a group of researchers from a children's hospital in Cincinnati, Ohio, discovered that the epidemic mainly occurred among children who had completed the full course of DPT vaccines.[33]

About 30 percent of the children had hospital stays, although the epidemic did not claim any lives. As many of the children who contracted the disease were aged between nineteen months and six years, and so would have been vaccinated relatively recently, even scientists have begun to agree that the whole-cell pertussis vaccine on offer doesn't offer long-term protection.

Doctors are fond of pointing out that when the whooping cough vaccine was discontinued in the early seventies in Britain for a time, the number of severe cases shot up. After a U.S. documentary criticizing the DPT vaccine, the number of children being immunized fell. Health officials then claimed that cases of whooping cough rose as a result of vaccine levels falling. But when former Food and Drug Administration virologist Dr. J. Anthony Morris analyzed forty-one cases of so-called whooping cough, only five had true pertussis, and all those victims had been vaccinated. The same occurred in Wisconsin. Most of the patients didn't have whooping cough, but those who did had been vaccinated.[34]

In Britain, cases rose to "almost unprecedented heights," wrote Professor Stewart, during the 1978–79 epidemic. This figure was also interpreted as having to do with the drop in vaccination following adverse publicity. But the number of cases reported increased in all age groups, even those for which a high percentage of immunization had been achieved.[35]

Even at the best of times, when the whooping cough vaccine does work, it has only been shown to be between 63 and 93 percent effective—an extraordinarily large potential difference.[36] The latest research from Sweden and Italy has shown that the vaccine is effective in just 48 percent and 36 percent of cases, respectively.[37]

A new "acellular" version of the whooping cough vaccine now available (where the whooping cough toxin is inactivated by hydrogen peroxide, to make it safer) hasn't fared much better, either. In Sweden, where it was tested on a group of infants, one fifth went on to develop whooping cough, even after they'd been given three shots. At best the vaccine was judged to work less than three-quarters of the time.[38] In the United States, scientists working on the vaccine at the Mayo Clinic have explained that they don't really understand how much pertussin toxin is necessary to protect children; even those with high levels of antibodies in their blood seem to go on to get whooping cough.[39]

Tetanus and Diphtheria

The same seems to hold true for diphtheria and tetanus. A U.S.-sponsored vaccine review has even concluded that the diphtheria vaccine "is not as effective an immunizing agent as might be anticipated."[40]

The effects of the diphtheria vaccine seem to wear off in adulthood. In London, a quarter of blood donors between the ages of twenty and twenty-nine have been found to have insufficient immunity, while half of those between fifty and fifty-nine have lost their immunity.[41]

The New Independent States of the Former Soviet Union suffered a recent outbreak of diphtheria; in the early 1990s, more than 100,000 cases of diphtheria had been recorded. Nevertheless, even though a universal policy of vaccination was quickly instituted, it didn't appear to make any impact; one study showed that among those developing diphtheria, more than 86 percent had been vaccinated within the year.[42]

As for tetanus, the U.S. panel reviewing vaccines noted that the degree of potency of the vaccine "can vary considerably from preparation to preparation." The panel also concluded that, as the vaccine has been purified and made safer in order to prevent reaction to it, so its protective ability has diminished.[43]

Although studies of immediate response to tetanus vaccination show very high protective antibody levels, this effect quickly wears off. In one study of 84 pregnant African patients, less than a third had detectable antibodies in the blood, even though nearly three-quarters had been immunized within three years of the study.[44]

Furthermore, as in many cases of vaccination, although antibody levels may be high, this may mean nothing in terms of protecting against disease. In one study, five children between five and fifteen contracted tetanus in Finland, even though four of the five had had their full quota of shots.[45]

Once an infant has its DPT shots, medicine recommends a tetanus booster every ten years. However, there's evidence that the more shots you get, the lower your immunity: "Each additional booster reduces the sensitivity of response to tetanus toxoid antigen after three or four challenges," according to a *Lancet* editorial.[46] The elderly, who are most at risk from tetanus, have a far poorer take-up rate from the vaccine than do the young.[47]

Measles

The medical establishment has attempted to place the blame for the recent epidemic of measles on clusters of the unvaccinated, particularly among poor, nonwhite populations—but the statistics again prove otherwise. According to the government's own 1989 statistics, half the college-aged victims had been previously vaccinated. And between 1985 and 1986, more than three-quarters of all measles cases occurred in children who had been properly vaccinated.[48]

All that the measles vaccine has done has been to transform into adult diseases what were once exclusively the domain of children. In the prevaccine era, 90 percent of all measles patients were five to nine years old. Once the measles vaccine was introduced, however, 55 to 64 percent of measles patients were older than ten. The average age of patients during the measles outbreak at the University of California at Los Angeles during the recent U.S. epidemic was twenty-two.[49]

Significant numbers of these cases occurred among college-aged students, particularly those born between 1957 and 1967, when the vaccine was introduced. Students at many universities now have to provide proof they've recently been vaccinated before they are allowed to register for classes. A few years ago, the government estimated that between 5 and 15 percent of all students were susceptible.

America has tried at least four strains of the measles vaccine, and all four have significant failure rates. Study after study in the medical literature points unerringly to clusters of vaccinated children who nevertheless contracted measles.

For instance, in a 1986 outbreak of measles in Corpus Christi, Texas, 99 percent of the children had been vaccinated.[50] In 1988, 80 percent of cases of measles occurred in children who had been properly vaccinated at the appropriate age.[51] The year before that, 60 percent of cases occurred in those who'd been vaccinated.[52]

Experts in the United States and elsewhere now recommend a measles booster shot at school age or later (at about age eleven) if the earlier booster hasn't been given. But even if booster shots are offered, they often don't work, either. In a group of individuals whose measles vaccination hadn't worked, only half given booster shots ended up with antibody levels raised to a level considered protective.[53]

Rubella

In terms of effectiveness, the rubella vaccine, usually included in the MMR triple vaccine, hasn't fared much better either. In one 1970s study at the University of Pennsylvania of adolescent girls given the vaccine, more than one-third lacked any evidence whatsoever of immunity.[54] Because viruses easily mutate, the vaccine may only protect you against one strain of a virus, and not any new ones. A more recent Italian study showed that 10 percent of girls had been infected by a "wild strain" of the virus, even within a few years of being given their shot.[55]

HIB Meningitis

Perhaps the worst example of vaccine double-think concerns the Hib vaccine, which was first licensed in the United States in 1985. This is supposed to combat the most common cause of meningitis in children under five.

This form of bacterial meningitis, caused by the *haemophilus influenzae* type b, mainly strikes at preschoolers, with the peak incidence between six and fifteen months of age. The current estimates are that some 60 out of every 100,000 children will contract Hib-caused meningitis; of those, between 3 and 6.5 percent will die, and 14 percent will have continuing problems, such as deafness or seizures. Certain groups—notably Alaskan and Native American children—are supposed to be ten to fifty times more likely to contract the disease. Both groups are thought to be predisposed to the disease because of genetic factors or malnutrition.

So far, medical science has yet to produce a version of the Hib vaccine that actually works. The first vaccine introduced in the United States in 1985 was a "polysaccharide," used in children over fifteen months old, largely after one Finnish trial had encouraging results. The vaccine soon began to lose credibility after doctors reported that children were getting meningitis right after they'd been vaccinated. One Minnesota study showed that the shot *increased* a child's risk fivefold of contracting the disease.[56] The drug also didn't work on children younger than eighteen months old—the very population most at risk!

In its government-sponsored report, the National Academy of Science's Institute of Medicine confirmed that the Hib vaccine can cause Hib meningitis.[57] And in another study, where fifty-five vaccinated children nevertheless went on to develop Hib-caused meningitis, not only did the vaccine not have any protective effect (since three children died and six developed neurologic complications), but the researchers concluded that the vaccine "*increased* susceptibility to these complications" (italics mine).[58]

After 1992, when a study of 10 million children by the U.S. Centers for Disease Control showed that this version of the vaccine only protected two-thirds of children, medicine reluctantly junked the "polysaccharide" version of the vaccine as hopelessly unreliable.[59]

Once the older version was discredited, several companies came up with a "conjugate" vaccine—one that would marry the Hib portion with the tried-and-tested diphtheria vaccine (PRP-D), the diphtheria/pertussis/tetanus vaccine (PRP-DPT), or even the *Neisseria meningitidis* group b outer membrane protein complex (PRP-OMPC). The idea behind all this gobbledygook of initials was that attaching the new vaccine onto a substance known to produce antibodies would nudge the body to come up with an antibody to the Hib bug as well. Lederle Laboratories released HibTITER, and Connaught ProHIBit in 1990, to be given to children at two, four, and six months of age—the same time as the polio and DPT vaccines. The OMPC version even seemed to work on the high-risk Navajo infants.[60]

In 1993, the FDA approved Tetramune, a combination of the DPT vaccine and Hib vaccine, for use on babies and children between two months and five years old. Besides supposedly kick-starting the Hib vaccine into working better, this combination was also meant to reduce from eight to four the number of shots U.S. children had to get. Tests on nearly 7,000 children have shown that the all-in-one variety produced no significant difference in antibody response than the separate shots.[61]

Despite the medical profession's belief that it had finally cracked the problem, new evidence has popped up here and there of less-than-ideal results. In one study, children with Hib meningitis had received the conjugate vaccine at least two weeks before they'd contracted the disease. Overall, the PRP-D vaccine was reckoned to be just 74 percent effective—only slightly better than the regular Hib vaccine. The vaccine also protected only a third of the high-risk Alaskan infants, even after three doses.[62]

Furthermore, of the 164 cases of Hib meningitis reported in the UK from 1992, 43 occurred among children who'd been vaccinated. Of these 31 had had the prescribed three shots.[63]

The United States has also had problems with large numbers of bad batches of one of the leading brands of the Hib vaccine, which don't "take." The faulty batches comprised about 2 percent of the Hib conjugate vaccines released in the United States since January 1990—some 366,000 doses.[64]

Even PRP-OMPC, the most successful conjugate, has its problems. There is some evidence that the more vaccine a child receives, the lower his antibody response.[65]

Polio

As for polio, scientists are beginning to concur that one of the central premises for giving the live vaccine isn't true. In true cases of polio, the virus lives in the intestine, creating what is ordinarily a harmless infection. Problems start if it travels to the bloodstream and makes its way to the nervous system, where it can cause paralysis. The killed virus, originally developed by Jonas Salk, is injected under the skin and is supposed to travel to the bloodstream and create antibodies there that will "block" the virus before it reaches the nervous system. However, the killed polio shot does not give you "gut immunity"—that is, it doesn't raise antibodies in your intestines. That means that, while you won't get paralytic polio, the wild virus could live on in your gut and you could theoretically pass it on to someone else. Furthermore, the original Salk vaccine required three or more boosters every five years.

When first administered, the Salk vaccine was deemed a terrific success—until the polio victim rate went up in the 1960s. Coming so hard on the heels of the double-digit victim rates of the fifties, this new development was greeted as proof that the Salk vaccine didn't work, particularly amid all the hysteria to find a "cure."

The live oral (OVP) vaccine, developed by Sabin, virtually replaced the Salk vaccine in the sixties, because it not only supposedly confers lifelong immunity on its recipient, but stops him from becoming a carrier of the wild virus. And because recipients can excrete the vaccine virus for a number of weeks through the mouth and feces, the theory is that you can pass on immunity to nonvaccinated individuals, thus raising the "herd immunity." *In other words, the live oral vaccine became the vaccine of choice largely so that you or your children could act as an immunizing force for other, unvaccinated individuals.*

Scientists now realize that there is little evidence that the live vaccine actually does achieve this "backdoor" immunity among the unvaccinated. This was the conclusion of a scientific study group after an outbreak of polio in Taiwan, where up to 98 percent of young children had been immunized.[66] Even the U.S. FDA has acknowledged: "We now know that secondary spread of vaccine virus to susceptible contacts plays very little part in population immunity."[67]

There's also plenty of evidence that the polio vaccine fails. Many of today's outbreaks occur more among immunized than unimmunized populations. In 1961, for instance, Massachusetts had a polio outbreak, with more paralytic cases among the vaccinated than the unvaccinated.[68] Taiwan suffered an outbreak of 1,031 cases of paralytic polio in 1982, even though some 80 percent of infants there had received at least two doses of the oral vaccine before the age of one and at least 35 percent of the victims had been vaccinated.[69] In the 1988 outbreak in Israel of fifteen cases, twelve, or 80 percent, had occurred among vaccinated individuals.[70] As most of the vaccinated victims were between eleven and thirty, Israel's Defense Force Medical Corps concluded that this population suffered from a "gap" of immunity among those who'd never been exposed to the wild virus (as people over forty would have) and whose vaccine had worn off.[71]

Although the vaccine is supposed to be working well wherever it is introduced, the few studies carried out these days on the polio vaccine in infants in developing countries show a less-than-perfect take-up rate. The vaccine failed to give adequate protection to babies in the Gaza,[72] and less than two-thirds of Mayan, Gamian, and Brazilian infants have produced antibodies to the type 3 virus after being vaccinated, according to separate studies.[73] Some of the factors linked with vaccine failure included high levels of maternal antibodies, vaccination during the rainy season, diarrhea at the time of vaccination, and even breast-feeding. In other words, a mother's own antibodies might act to neutralize the potency of the vaccine. This leads one to speculate at how effective the polio vaccine is among infants of mothers in developed countries who choose to breast-feed long-term.

There's also some evidence that the vaccine wears off quickly. In a study of eighty-six children who'd had either doses of the enhanced killed or live vaccine, and were monitored for four years, each group showed a ten- to hundred-fold decline in antibody levels to all virus types within the first two years of follow up.[74] Furthermore, even if the vaccine "takes," you may not be adequately protected against a certain strain of the virus. During a major outbreak of hepatitis A infection in Glasgow, Scotland, blood serum of twenty-four of the victims were also tested for antibodies to polio. Only one-third of the group had an acceptable level of antibodies against one strain of the virus.[75]

Tuberculosis (BCG Vaccine)

The Heaf test is used by most school districts to measure tuberculin sensitivity. Unlike most sensitivity tests, a negative result is supposed to mean that a child does not carry antibodies to the tubercle bacillus. However, the test is notoriously inaccurate; even the American Academy of Pediatrics warns its members that the test carries the possibility of false negatives and false positives. Furthermore, no one is really sure anymore what a positive test really means. It could mean that someone is immune to tuberculosis, or had prior infections, or it could mean that someone is simply allergic or sensitive to the test.

In one study of British school districts, where 92 percent were using the Heaf test, most districts agreed on what to do with a 0 grade, which showed very little reaction (recommend immunization) or a grade 3 or 4, which indicated pronounced reaction (refer to a chest clinic for special evaluation before having the shot). The disparity occurred with those scoring grade 2. Around one-third of the districts recommended no immunization, and approximately two-thirds recommended referral to a chest clinic for special examination before going ahead with the shot. Only a single district recommended immunization at this level of sensitivity to the test.[76]

Besides the lack of agreement about which groups should or should not receive the live tuberculosis vaccine, substantial doubts exist about its effectiveness. In ten randomized controlled trials from around the world since the 1930s, the ability of the BCG vaccine to protect you has ranged from 80 percent to 0.[77] On average, the shot protects only about two-thirds of children from TB.

The problem is that BCG vaccination can only limit the multiplication and spread of the tubercle bacteria; it cannot prevent infection in people exposed to the germ. In fact, there's increasing evidence that BCG vaccines offer greater protection against leprosy than tuberculosis, particularly in Third World countries, where TB is still rife. A huge African study of 83,000 people in Malawi concluded that half were protected against leprosy, but none had significant protection against tuberculosis.[78]

The London School of Hygiene and Tropical Medicine, which conducted a special analysis, found that the vaccine is just 22 percent effective in Kenya and 20 percent effective in some areas of India. Overall effectiveness ranges from 0 to 80 percent around the world, possibly due to strain variations, genetic or nutritional differences, or environmental influences.[79]

MYTH NO 4: THE SIDE EFFECTS OF VACCINES ARE RARE AND MOSTLY MILD

Just as there is no such thing as a safe drug, there is no such thing as a safe vaccine, and we are only beginning to come to grips with exactly how dangerous each one is. The most definitive and largest study of vaccines to date, conducted by the Centers for Disease Control and Prevention, the highest government body on infectious diseases, was quietly announced to a handful of scientists with no publicity or press releases at a meeting of the Advisory Commission on Childhood Vaccines in Washington.

The low-key presentation in a small seminar on September 9, 1994, in Washington, D.C., was at odds with the spectacular nature of the conclusions: namely, that a child's risk of seizure triples within days of receiving either the MMR or the DPT vaccines.

Using database technology, the CDC monitored the progress of 500,000 children across the United States, tapping into computerized records of Health Maintenance Organizations and public insurance schemes such as Kaiser Permanente in California. In this way, the CDC was able to pull together virtually every piece of research and data on adverse reactions to the two triple vaccines. They identified thirty-four major side effects to the shots, ranging from asthma, blood disorders, infectious diseases, and diabetes to neurological disorders, including meningitis, polio, and hearing loss.

But it was the incidence of seizure that leapt off the graph, according to Dr. Anthony Morris, who attended the meeting. The rate of seizure increased three times above the norm within the first day of a child receiving the DPT shot, and the rate rose 2.7 times within four to seven days of a child being given the MMR shot, increasing to 3.3 times within eight to fourteen days.

Seizure, which covers epilepsy, convulsions, and fainting, is already one of the most common conditions in childhood, affecting an estimated one in twenty children, or 5 percent.[80] This high figure could reflect the effect of vaccination. Or the new findings could mean that vaccines will further increase that seizure rate to nearly 15 percent, affecting something close to three in twenty children.

The effects of the DPT shot were immediate, causing the incidence of seizures to increase three times the normal within twenty-four hours of the shot being given, but then falling off rapidly to just 0.06 times the norm after the first day. The MMR vaccine, however, had a far slower effect, only reaching its most dangerous period eight to fourteen days after the shot was administered.

The seizures were often serious, the CDC reported, with a quarter of all cases having to be treated in the hospital.

In measured, neutral language, the presentation concluded: "Seizures are associated with several vaccines, ignoring possible confounding via simultaneous administration. . . . Interest, via desire to minimize injections and simplify vaccinations schedules, in synergistic effects among antigens when combined or simultaneously administered."[81] What this science-speak basically boils down to is that the CDC is interested in determining whether the seizures are caused by individual vaccines, or whether the antigen stew of so many vaccines given at the same time is causing, in effect, immune-system meltdown. The CDC is carrying out further research into findings before submitting a final paper.

The findings of the study conducted by Britain's Public Health

Laboratory Service were strikingly similar. The PHLS Statistic Unit found that the MMR shot increased seizure risk three times, while the DPT also increased seizure risk threefold, usually three days after the dose was given. The peak increase rate of seizures and meningitis due to the Urabe strain of the mumps portion of the MMR vaccine usually occurred between fifteen and thirty-five days afterward.[82]

The PHLS also discovered that children given the MMR were five times more likely than expected to suffer idiopathic thrombocytopenic purpura, a blood disorder often requiring blood transfusions. The risk elsewhere has been estimated at 1 in every 30,000 vaccines.[83]

Whooping Cough

As for the individual vaccines themselves, the whooping cough, or pertussis vaccine, is acknowledged as the most overtly dangerous. Of all the adverse reactions from vaccinations now reported on the Vaccine Adverse Event Reporting System, which was set up with the Vaccine Compensation Act, a law recognizing that vaccines cause side effects and arranging for a system to provide compensation for the victims, the overwhelming majority are due to the DPT vaccine. During the period from January through August 1991, there were 3,447 reports of DPT reactions—66 percent of the more than 5,000 reactions reported in total (and this 5,000 itself is estimated to be only a tenth of the total reactions among Americans).[84]

Incredible as it seems, the safety of the pertussis drug was never adequately proved before being injected into millions of babies. Essentially, the vaccine as we know it today is no different from the first lots of it created in 1912. At that time, two French bacteriologists grew the pertussis bacteria in large pots, killed it with heat, preserved this stew with formaldehyde, and went ahead and injected it into hundreds of children. Unlike most vaccines, which are detoxified and purified versions of the germ in question, the pertussis vaccine still contains the "whole cell" of the pertussis bacteria, which is why it's called a "whole cell" or crude vaccine.[85] This means it still contains endotoxins and cell-wall substances known to be highly toxic, causing fever, interference with growth, and death in laboratory animals. Other toxins stimulate insulin production. One predisposes animals to shock and collapse; another blocks the body's recovery mechanisms.[86]

One modern difference is the addition of an "adjuvant," a metal salt (often an aluminium compound) used to heighten the effect of the drug, plus a preservative (a mercury derivative). These ingredients are used despite the fact that formaldehyde is known to be a carcinogen, and aluminum and mercury are highly toxic to humans.

The United States' new acellular vaccine, called DTaP, has been approved by the U.S. Food and Drug Administration since 1992, and now may be offered for babies, rather than simply as a booster shot for older children. The new variety is also being tested in Europe. Doctors are hoping that the results will assuage parents' fears about the dangers of the shot.

However, recent research suggests that the acellular vaccine may be no safer than the vaccine it is meant to replace. A large U.S. study called the Nationwide Multicenter Acellular Pertussis Trial, which compared over 2,000 children given either the acellular vaccine or the whole-cell version, found that the rate of serious adverse reactions—death, near-death, seizures, developmental delay, and hospital stays—did not differ between the old and new vaccines.[87]

The only safety test of the original whooping cough vaccine was conducted by the British Medical Research Council, which tried out the drug on 50,000 children aged fourteen months or older. The United States never did do tests of its own, but has always relied on these British tests conducted in the 1950s. Furthermore, the forty-two babies who had convulsions within twenty-eight days of having been given the shot were discounted and the drug assumed to be safe, even though that level of reaction translates into about one in every 1,000 children.[88]

Though the trials were designed only to demonstrate effectiveness, not safety, U.S. and British health authorities have used them as evidence that the vaccine is safe to give to babies as young as six weeks of age. This means the drug was never tested for safety at this dosage for newborns. It also means that two-month-old babies are given the same dosage as children three or four times their size.

In its government-sponsored report, the National Academy of Science's Institute of Medicine (IOM), which scoured the medical literature for seventeen health problems that have been associated with the DPT vaccine, concluded that the vaccine can cause anaphylactic shock (a severe life-threatening allergic reaction) and extended periods of inconsolable crying or screaming, sometimes lasting twenty-four hours or more.[89] According to Coulter and Fisher in their seminal work *A Shot in the Dark* (Avery), "this kind of crying, a thin, eerie, wailing sound quite different from the child's normal cry, [very much resembles] the so-called *Cri encephalique* (encephalitic scream) found in some cases of encephalitis."[90]

The IOM committee also found a link, although it was a weaker one, between the DPT vaccine and acute encephalopathy and shock, causing total collapse.[91] Encephalitis is an inflammation of the brain, often referred to as meningitis, causing a bulging and red fontanelle among infants. The American National Vaccine Information Center has amassed many reports of children who either remain brain damaged or die after these episodes. In almost every instance, the parents themselves have had to report their child's reaction to the drug because their doctor has insisted that the reaction was unrelated to the shot.

"My grandson had his first DPT shot and oral polio at his two-month well-baby checkup," says a grandmother from Washington. "After the shot he started crying. The doctor gave my daughter Pediacare (a mild infant analgesic), but it did not stop the high-pitched screaming. When the baby's temperature went down to 98, the nurse told her to feed the baby. My grandson began projectile vomiting and continued the high-pitched crying. The nurse informed my daughter this was normal. The doctor told her to give my grandson more Pediacare and, hopefully, it

*would make him drowsy. At 3 a.m. they both went to sleep.
At 7 a.m. my daughter awoke and found my grandson with
a purple color on one side of his face, clenched fists, blood
coming from his nose and mouth, and no breathing. He was
dead within twenty-one hours of his DPT shot."*

Claire from Minnesota says that after her baby daughter's first
DPT shot at her two-month well-baby clinic, she showed no
unusual behavior the first two days except that she was irritable
whenever her leg was moved (where the shot had been given).
"I checked her temperature every diaper change and it was fine.
She started having seizures two days after the shot," says Claire.
"Since then she's been put on every seizure medication there is
and was put in a coma for two weeks and is still having seizures.
She is now twenty months old and home with us having 50 to
200 seizures a day. She is very severely retarded, bedridden, fed
with a G-tube, and cortically blind."

Based on a ten-year study, the Institute of Medicine says the
vaccine could trigger an acute neurological illness in children
with underlying brain or metabolic abnormalities. Researchers
are now concerned that children can become brain damaged or
even die if they develop a severe neurological illness within a
week of receiving the vaccination.[92]

The risk of this type of neurological damage has been estimated at between 1 in every 50,000 children vaccinated.[93] Although Gordon Stewart has argued that the risk to babies of
death or brain damage from whooping cough itself is comparable
to the risk of death or brain damage from the shot, the actual
risks of the vaccine could be much worse.[94] According to the
damages paid to the families of children in Britain judged to have
been hurt by the whooping cough shot, the risk of damage over
the years 1958–79 worked out to be 1 in 30,000 children, at
least three times that for all other vaccines.[95]

Although the IOM committee concluded there wasn't enough
evidence from current medical studies to show the whooping
cough vaccine could definitely cause other serious damage, it
didn't rule this out. The possible damage includes juvenile diabe-

tes, learning disabilities, attention deficit disorder, infantile spasms, and sudden infant death syndrome (SIDS).

The FDA once sponsored a study at the University of California of children receiving some 15,000 doses of DPT vaccine. In that study, nine children had convulsions and nine had episodes of collapse, a frequency for each of these conditions of one per 1,750 immunizations. However, since each child receives three to five DPT shots, the true risk of damage could be more like one per 400 children.[96] In one study of fifty-three babies who had died of sudden infant death, twenty-seven had received the DPT shot within a month of their death. Six deaths occurred within twenty-four hours, and seventeen within a week of the shot being given.[97]

In testimony before the Senate Committee in 1985, Edward Brandt, Jr., the Secretary of Health at the time, estimated that every year 35,000 children suffer brain damage from this vaccine. Other estimates by the University of California at Los Angeles are that 1,000 infants a year die from SIDS as a direct result of DPT, which represents some 10 to 15 percent of the total number of SIDS cases in the United States.[98]

In the early 1970s, Dr. Archie Kalokerinos and Glenn Dettman, who were studying aboriginal children, were puzzled when the death rate of aboriginal children skyrocketed, in some places by 50 percent. Suddenly they made the connection: The rise in the death rate coincided with intensified efforts to immunize these children, many of whom were ill or had serious vitamin deficiencies when they received their DPT shots.[99]

As a result of this and other evidence, Sweden, Germany, and Japan have omitted the whooping cough vaccine from their regular vaccine schedules.

Tetanus

As for tetanus, the Institute of Medicine's study of vaccine damage concluded that the vaccine could cause high fever, seizures, pain, nerve damage, fatal anaphylactic shock, degeneration of the nervous system, and Guillain–Barre syndrome.[100] Tetanus boosters can also cause T-lymphocyte blood count ratios to plunge temporarily to levels similar to those of AIDS victims.[101]

Another problem with this so-called "safe" vaccine is encephalitis or damage to the nervous system or inner ear. The *Physicians' Desk Reference* warns that booster doses are more likely to increase the incidence and severity of reactions, if they are given too frequently.[102] This is probably what happened to the fourteen-year-old son of Mary. He was given a tetanus injection following a dog bite. Five days later, he had his first epileptic fit at night, and has had epilepsy ever since. Mary asked her doctor if there was any connection between the two, and like so many others, her fears were brushed aside and the boy's illness put down to coincidence. After all, her doctor said, the tetanus vaccine is known to have no side effects. "It was only when my son changed doctors, a few years ago, that his new doctor sent him for a brain scan to see if there were any underlying causes such as scar tissue," she said. "There were none."

Measles/Mumps/Rubella (MMR) Vaccine

Until recently the view of doctors and the governments of many countries was that the MMR vaccine provides "lifelong protection" against all three infections with a single shot.[103]

But in the United States from July 1990 through April 1994, 5,799 adverse incidents following MMR vaccination have been reported to the American Vaccine Adverse Events Reporting System, most requiring emergency medical treatment, with about 400 leading to permanent damage or death. And if, as the National Vaccine Information Center says, these figures represent only 10 to 15 percent of the total number of side effects (because of the massive number of cases that go unreported), the true figure could be as high as 60,000.[104]

American and British vaccine experts such as the Public Health Laboratory Service's Dr. Begg claim that the incidence of measles-vaccine-induced encephalitis is very rare, occurring in one in 200,000 children. Symptoms include fever, headache, possible

convulsions, and behavioral changes. "Most symptoms are mild,"
he says, "and the children will recover."

However, many studies report far greater risks. In one, from
Germany, 1 of every 2,500 children vaccinated had a brain complication, and 1 in every 17,650 came down with encephalitis.[105]

About one in 400 children given the shot will suffer convulsions,[106] and nearly one-fifth of young adults given measles boosters will suffer major side effects, including fever, eye pain, and
the need for bed rest.[107]

New research has made a tentative connection between the
measles shot and the sharp rise of Crohn's disease and colitis
in children.[108]

Two versions of the drug, manufactured by Merieux and
SmithKline Beecham, were withdrawn in Britain and elsewhere
in the autumn of 1992 because of the risk of contracting meningitis from the Urabe strain of the mumps portion of the vaccine.
The Japanese government withdrew its own version of the
MMR vaccine in April 1993 after discovering a link with meningitis. A year later, the Japanese authorities revealed that 1 in
1,044 children vaccinated developed aseptic meningitis.[109] The
government also found evidence that the vaccine can bring on
mumps, which can also be transferred to other children.

The U.S. National Academy of Sciences IOM report concluded that the measles vaccine can cause death from measles-
vaccine-strain-infection, thrombocytopenia (a blood condition
characterized by a decrease in blood platelets), fatal shock, and
arthritis. The committee also said it couldn't "rule out" that the
vaccine itself could cause cases of SSPE.[110]

Immediately after receiving a measles shot in 1994, Sam, a
healthy, athletic twelve-year-old, began losing his sense of coor-
dination and falling down. He also began having constant seizures—sometimes fifteen an hour. After becoming virtually
wheelchair-bound, he was eventually diagnosed as having the
fatal condition SSPE. Even though his condition is a known,
admittedly rare side effect of the measles shot, his doctors refused
to make the link. Instead they argued that the vaccine merely

set off a latent disease caused by an earlier bout of measles. The problem is, insists his mother, Sam never *had* measles.

Besides running the risk of side effects from the vaccine, your child could also contract what has become known as atypical measles, an especially vicious form of the disease that resists treatment. In a 1965 study in Cincinnati during an epidemic of measles, fifty-four vaccinated children went on to develop atypical measles. Many of these children were so ill with high fever and pneumonia that they had to be hospitalized.[111]

There is even some evidence that preventing children from getting the ordinary childhood diseases prevents their immune systems from adequately developing. When children get the measles vaccine, they often contract so-called "mild measles" with an underdeveloped rash. One study found evidence of a relationship between lack of rash in measles and increased incidence of degenerative diseases such as cancer later in life.[112] Many practitioners have reported that cancer patients have a particularly small number of infectious diseases of childhood in their medical history.

Mumps

German authorities have discovered twenty-seven neurological reactions to the mumps vaccine, including meningitis, febrile convulsions, encephalitis, and epilepsy.[113] Of all cases of mumps encephalitis over fifteen years, one-sixth were definitely caused by the vaccine.[114] Research from Canada estimated the risk of vaccine-induced mumps encephalitis at one per 100,000;[115] a Yugoslavian study concluded it was one per 1,000.[116]

As for meningitis from the mumps vaccine, the British Department of Health's recent public assurance that the risk is only one in 11,000 contradicts the long-known findings published in one of the leading U.S. pediatric journals that the rate varies from one in 405 to one in 7,000 shots given.[117]

The British government ignored these warning signals about the mumps portion of the vaccine until a surveillance study by the Public Health Laboratory Service demonstrated that an unacceptably large number of children was contracting meningitis from a certain strain of the mumps vaccine.[118] In Nottingham, a cluster of cases suggested the risk could be as high as one in 4,000 doses; the PHLS eventually concluded the risk was one in every 11,000 doses.[119]

But even when the U.K. government hastily withdrew the two versions containing the Urabe mumps virus strain—a good eighteen months after Canada did so—SmithKline Beecham continued producing vaccines containing that particular strain, "so that existing immunization programs in areas where no alternative mumps vaccine is available need not be suspended."[120] In other words, in some parts of the world it was considered better to hand out a vaccine known to pose dangers than to expose children to an illness that is mostly benign.

After her son suffered side effects after receiving his MMR, Jackie Fletcher formed a group called JABS (Justice, Awareness and Basic Support) for families of children damaged chiefly by the MMR vaccine. So far she has been contacted by 120 families whose children allegedly have sustained damage from the now-withdrawn mumps vaccine. Nevertheless, a number of cases of alleged damage being pursued in court also concern the current MMR vaccine, produced by the U.S. drug company Merck.

Rubella

A National Academy of Science report has accepted that the rubella portion of the MMR vaccine can cause long- or short-term arthritis. One manufacturer of the triple vaccine estimated that the rubella part of the vaccine causes arthritis in up to 3 percent of children and in up to 20 percent of adult women who receive it. "Symptoms [of arthritis] may persist for a matter of months or, on rare occasions, for years," the company reports—everything from mild aches to extreme crippling.[121] Adolescent girls are considered to be at greater risk of joint and limb symptoms.

As long ago as 1970, the Health, Education and Welfare Department reported that as many as "26 percent of children receiving rubella vaccination in national testing programs developed arthralgia and arthritis. Many had to seek medical attention, and some were hospitalized to test for rheumatic fever and rheumatoid arthritis."[122]

Dr. Aubrey Tingle, a pediatric immunologist at Children's Hospital in Vancouver, British Columbia, has also undertaken major research into this area. According to his own studies, 30 percent of adults exposed to rubella vaccine suffer arthritis in two to four weeks—ranging from mild aches in the joints to severe crippling. Tingle also found the rubella virus in one-third of adult and child patients with rheumatoid arthritis.[123]

Polio

With the live polio virus, the main problem is that this "attenuated" or weakened version of the vaccine virus can genetically alter in the gut, changing into its virulent form and causing paralytic polio in its recipient or those that he has recently come into contact with. These days, virtually the only cases of polio that occur in the United States are caused by the vaccine, mainly among so-called contacts—grandparents, parents, or siblings who are in some way susceptible to polio—but also among the recipients themselves.

Bernard Reis, an English professor at Vassar College and former graduate of Cornell University and Harvard, described as an energetic, athletic achiever, was happily married with a baby boy, whom he dutifully took to receive the vaccines mandated by law. A month after his little boy's vaccine, Reis became tired when attempting to climb a flight of stairs and came down with what he thought was the flu. Two days later he collapsed on his bathroom floor and, after being rushed to the hospital, was completely paralyzed, placed in an iron lung, and fed intravenously. Eleven months later he returned home in a wheelchair. "The strain of all this was too much for my marriage, which fell apart," he writes.[124] Since then, his life has been "hell in slow motion." Although able to walk haltingly, he is still extremely weak from his bout with polio. He lives on Social Security of

$300 a month in New York public housing. He has not been able to receive other government assistance or compensation.

On February 19, 1983, the first day Bob and Marjorie were to move into their new home, Bob collapsed on the sofa. The following morning he complained that he couldn't move his left arm. A few days later he was completely paralyzed. A battery of tests later, doctors finally diagnosed Bob as having paralytic polio. His daughter Chloe had received her live polio vaccine less than two months before. No doctor had warned Bob, who has Netherton's syndrome (a skin condition), that his immune system was weakened by the cortisone he takes and that he was at high risk of contracting polio from anyone vaccinated for the disease. This despite the warning to physicians on packages of the vaccine, from Lederle, the drug manufacturer. A year to the day after Bob came down with polio, he died.

There were more than one hundred cases of vaccine-induced paralytic polio in the United States between 1975 and 1984,[125] and at least ten reported cases of paralytic polio caused by the live vaccine are reported every year.[126] In the United Kingdom, thirteen cases have been substantiated between 1985 and 1991.[127] The CDC, along with German doctors from the University of Cologne, estimate the current risk for vaccine-induced polio at five per million doses given, or one case for each 200,000 first doses, which are said to be the most risky.[128] As with many official statistics, this figure could be too low; if your immune system is weakened, as it is with AIDS, or if you use drugs such as steroids, the risk is multiplied 10,000 times. In Germany, most cases of paralytic polio caused by vaccines have been among children aged two years or younger—that is, the recipients themselves.

Besides polio, your child also risks poor weight gain or other paralytic diseases with the polio vaccine. Children immunized with live agents, such as the polio vaccine, have been shown to suffer "statistically significant" reductions in their weights, compared with children of the same size who weren't vaccinated.[129] Those who were small for their ages to begin with were especially affected.

Recently, a new disease has been appearing in China, which the medical press has dubbed "Chinese paralytic syndrome" (CPS). Although it was previously diagnosed as the paralytic condition Guillain-Barre syndrome (GBS), researchers from the Second Hospital of Hebei Medical College in the People's Republic of China studied all the cases in depth and concluded that the disease, which strikes children and young adults, was a variation of polio.

Before oral polio vaccine (OPV) was introduced in the Hebei province in 1971, illness from polio was high, but diagnoses of GBS were uncommon. Then after 1971, the incidence of polio gradually fell, but that of GBS increased about tenfold. Three rises in the incidence of polio utterly coincided with three epidemics of GBS.

According to Yan Shen and Guohun Xi from the hospital's Department of Neuropsychiatry, the evidence strongly suggests that the polio virus is responsible for the cases diagnosed as GBS. "The widespread use of OPV may have led to [mutation of the virus], resulting in an alteration of [the disease] and/or to a change in the main epidemic type of poliovirus," they wrote.[130]

Cases of GBS linked to the polio vaccine also occur in the West. Cathy went to her doctor's office in July 1991 to get a routine polio and typhoid vaccination for her family's upcoming trip to Morocco. She says:

> That evening I developed a temperature, with aches and pains in my arms and legs. The pains in my legs were the most severe. About two weeks later while I was out walking one of my legs "gave out." It felt as though my legs were both weak, and they were numb. Some time after that my legs started to feel as though they were burning.
>
> My condition has steadily deteriorated over the years, and I am now at the stage of being able to take only a few steps before I experience the pains and a horrible numbness in my legs, which forces me to sit down. Any kind of movement gives me the same pain, even if I travel in a car.
>
> My hands were affected, too. They now burn when I have

done too much, and there is a weakness there. Besides the limb problems, I suffer earaches and a kind of deafness, plus frequent infected neck glands which only clear up with antibiotics. I also have serious problems with balance, unsteady walking, and falling. I have memory loss and often stop in mid-sentence.

These effects have all had a devastating effect on my life. I am now totally house-bound. I have been resting solidly for nearly five months to try to get the burning pain to ease. Although it has eased somewhat, the pain and numbness are constant when I attempt to walk.

Doctors have now diagnosed the problem as Guillain-Barre syndrome. When I contacted someone from the Guillain-Barre Society, he told me that I was the worst case he's ever seen. My doctor now admits that this was brought on by the vaccine.

Finland, like Sweden and the Netherlands, has always preferred to use the killed vaccine. However, after ten cases of polio erupted in 1985, the government organized a mass vaccination campaign with the live vaccine. A few weeks after the campaign, the Department of Pediatrics at the University of Oulu in Finland reported a cluster of twenty-seven cases of childhood Guillain-Barre syndrome, which also occurred in the United States following mass immunization for the swine flu in the 1970s.[131] Eleven of the children had been immunized before the onset of symptoms. Millions of children receiving the Salk vaccine in the 1950s and 1960s have been infected with another, potentially cancer-causing virus. This virus, named SV 40, was found to be a "fellow traveler" of the polio virus. The process of killing the polio virus was not sufficient to kill SV 40. This contaminated vaccine was then handed out to many millions of children during the initial 1955 campaign, and even later.[132] When a combined DPT and polio shot was found to contain SV 40, it was discontinued.

Meanwhile, according to new research, SV 40 and similar agents have been recovered from human brain tumors and also precancerous conditions in the brain. SV 40 has been shown to cause cancer in hamsters after the equivalent of twenty human years.[133] Numerous researchers have even attempted to link infected polio vaccine with the origin of AIDS.

Because of the risk of getting polio from the live vaccine, various governments, including that of the United States, are now considering reverting to the killed form of the vaccine (IPV), particularly as the Merieux pharmaceutical company in Europe and Connaught Labs in the United States have come up with an enhanced killed vaccine (or E-IPV, in science-speak) which supposedly gives you immunity against all three types of polio after two doses. But the new vaccine seems to be trading new problems for old. The killed vaccine has been linked with GBS, motor neurone weakness, encephalitis, meningitis, and convulsions, according to a Danish study.[134]

Hepatitis B Vaccine

The World Health Organization is considering a recommendation that hepatitis B (HB) vaccination be included in the routine vaccination schedule for babies or children all over the world by 1997, regardless of whether they are at high risk of contracting the disease, which can damage the liver and which kills one in five carriers.

Currently, thirty-three countries have national policies on HB shots. In Italy, the shot is compulsory; in the United States, the HB shot is included in the schedules for infants; in the United Kingdom, the Health Secretary has considered whether twelve-year-olds—on the brink of sexual activity—should be vaccinated against what is primarily a sexually transmitted disease.

In 1979, when a hepatitis vaccine was first released on the market, the policy of the United States was to identify and vaccinate high-risk groups, including intravenous drug abusers, the sexually promiscuous, and health care workers who handle bodily fluids and blood. Despite these efforts, hepatitis cases rose by a third between 1979 and 1989. Since the exact source of the disease is unknown, the American authorities now believe we should nip it in the bud—in infancy. *In other words, they believe we should exploit the immune systems of children to prevent the spread of what is primarily a sexually transmitted disease.*

What no one is talking about is how the old vaccine got made. No vaccine production is very pretty (whooping cough uses the mucus of infected children, typhoid the excrement of victims, and rubella has been grown on aborted fetuses), but this is one of the few that used to be derived from human blood—specifically, the blood products of homosexual men who have had hepatitis.

The vaccine was replaced in the early 1990s by a genetically engineered, or "recombinant" version of the vaccine, which is grown on yeast cells. However, the earlier plasma-derived vaccine was never withdrawn, and even those drug companies that stopped producing the blood-derived product kept selling it until it was used up. So until very recently, anyone receiving the vaccine could have received a blood-based product.

The New York Blood Center addressed this issue by studying hundreds of cases in low- and high-risk populations receiving the vaccine. Their conclusion: No one is at higher risk of developing HIV infections from the hepatitis B vaccine. Those in favor of the vaccine argue that the process that kills the hepatitis virus also kills any other viruses lurking about. But remember, at the moment, many high-level scientists, including the codiscoverer of the AIDS virus, are questioning the single-virus theory of AIDS. It's entirely possible that a number of "cofactors" in the blood causing or contributing to AIDS may not be killed by this process. The Health Secretary in his announcement called this vaccine "perfectly safe." Until we understand what causes AIDS, no one can make that statement with certainty.

The AIDS question may be why doctors, nurses, and other "high-risk" health care workers have avoided this old vaccine. In 1992, a questionnaire was sent to 595 doctors. Although most of them wrote that all doctors should be vaccinated against hepatitis B, only about half had had the shot themselves.[135]

Another problem with the HB shot is that patients who have had the vaccine sometimes give a false-positive reading on an HIV test.[136]

In 1988, New Zealand was one of the first countries to adopt a universal program of HB vaccination of newborn babies. The plan was to inoculate babies of certain mothers with hepatitis B throughout the country, and all the babies of seven districts.

New Zealand's health department proudly touted the program as "the most extensive national immunization program against hepatitis B in the world." However, they quickly took a more sober view once the program got under way. After only three months, the Hamilton Department of Health in Wellington faxed to Hepatitis B coordinators in all area health boards a message from the principal medical officers, indicating that they had received reports of allergic life-threatening shock in children receiving the HB vaccine.

A year later, the medical assessor for adverse events tallied the many side effects suffered by the children, including lethargy and malaise; diarrhea; asthma; arthritis; Guillain-Barre syndrome; faintness, pallor, loss of consciousness; and drop in blood pressure. The report noted that the incidence of adverse events could have been close to one in every fifty children after their first dose.

By April 1992, one concerned New Zealand physician reported to the health department that giving the hepatitis B vaccine at the same time as the DPT and/or polio vaccine suppressed the immune system of his patients even when the other vaccines were well tolerated on their own. A number of the babies also had prolonged postnatal jaundice, lasting up to two or three weeks.

As a result of these problems, the New Zealand health department, its tail between its legs, brought the vaccination program to an abrupt halt.[137]

Other than what we can glean from the New Zealand experience, there's a good deal we don't know about the new "recombinant"- HB vaccine. Between 30 and 50 percent of people vaccinated with three doses of the vaccine lose detectable antibodies within seven years. This could mean that you may need a booster shot every five years for the rest of your life. We also know that in 1 to 2 percent of cases—in other words, one or two out of every one hundred babies—the recommended regime doesn't take. This high failure rate has been reproduced in adults: One study showed that 10 percent of volunteers vaccinated failed to produce antibodies.[138]

Some 12,000 adverse events linked with the hepatitis B vaccine have been reported to the American Vaccine Adverse Events Reporting System between 1990 and 1994. The reports numbered some serious injuries including hospitalization or death. A large fraction included adults given the hepatitis B vaccine on its own.[139]

NEW DISEASES FROM VACCINES

Besides dangers of the individual shots, the latest problem discovered with vaccination in general has to do with ways that vaccines themselves are responsible for new diseases. Getting injected with a weakened or killed version of a virus can cause you to develop a viral "mutant" or encourage its growth in the population at large.

It has been estimated that 3 percent of babies born to mothers given the hepatitis B vaccine go on to develop a mutated form of hepatitis B.[140] In one study of a large group of babies born to hepatitis B-positive mothers and given a full immunization program against hepatitis B, in sixty became hepatitis B-positive. One in eighty of these babies showed they had a viral mutant of the vaccine. This mutant has been associated with hepatitis and active liver disease.[141] In another study, patients vaccinated with HB had a mixture of these mutants and the usual form of hepatitis B virus, as well as mild hepatitis. But those patients whose blood had the mutant on its own eventually suffered the more severe liver disease.[142]

The other problem with mutant viruses is that they often don't get detected in blood donor screening, so that this new form of hepatitis could be transmitted through donated blood. And of course the mutant may infect individuals even if they have been vaccinated.[143]

Connections have been made between the increasing prevalence of penicillin-resistant pneumococcal meningitis and universal Hib vaccination.[144]

Eradicating one strain of a virus can also encourage other forms of it to proliferate. This is precisely what's happening with the Hib meningitis vaccine. As b-type *H. influenzae* strains are being wiped out by the vaccination, mutant non-b *H. influenzae* strains are thriving.

One study looked at 408 strains of Hib meningitis. Although ninety-four percent were *H. influenzae* type b, the rest were "nonserotypable" (NST) *haemophilus influenzae* strains. The authors predicted that as more Hib vaccine was used, NST strains would cause more middle-ear infections, sinusitis, chronic bronchitis, and other mostly respiratory infections.[145]

In the 1960s, when U.S. Army recruits were given an experimental killed pneumonia vaccine, the vaccine caused unpredictable shifts in the virus type. Epidemics of disease from these mutant viruses occurred among recruits, rendering the vaccine useless and sending the scientists scurrying back to the laboratory to develop a vaccine that would knock out the mutations as well.[146]

We're also now beginning to realize that injections of any variety (including vaccinations) can increase your risk of developing polio. H. V. Wyatt of the Department of Community Medicine at the University of Leeds was one of the first to study the astonishing connection between multiple injections of any variety, particularly penicillin, given to small children and the onset of polio, particularly in developing countries where children receive more shots than those in developed countries.[147]

"Provocation polio" after a "just-in-case" injection is now long recognized and accepted in countries such as the United States and Britain. When a cluster of cases of paralytic polio occurred after a mass vaccination campaign with the live polio virus, researchers at the University of Cologne warned that DPT (diphtheria/tetanus/whooping cough [pertussium/tetanus]) shots shouldn't be given at the same time as the live polio vaccine.[148]

H. V. Wyatt has made a career of studying different populations through this century, comparing injected drug treatment

and epidemics of polio, including the injections children have
been given for congenital syphilis. He believes that multiple injections may be responsible for 25 percent of cases of paralysis
during epidemics of polio, and make children 25 percent more
susceptible to the disease during nonepidemic periods. A single
injection, he found, could increase the risk of paralysis fivefold,
and turn what might have been a nonparalytic attack into a
paralytic one. Even the World Health Organization's expanded
vaccine program of immunization "might provoke poliomyelitis," he concludes.[149]

Wyatt also believes that the risk might be cumulative—that is,
multiple injections over time might increase the risk of contracting polio at some point in the future, as may getting shots
at close intervals.

Wyatt's thesis provides much food for thought about the ori-
gins of the great polio epidemics of this century, which may
have been abetted by the introduction of widespread vaccination
and penicillin. It has also been recently validated by a new study
in Romania, by the U.S. Centers for Disease Control, showing
that the polio vaccine, given by injection, is causing outbreaks
of the disease. While the polio shot itself appeared to trigger
paralysis, the children affected had been exposed to a large number of other injections of vaccines and antibiotics. The children
were at particular risk of paralysis if other injections had been
given less than thirty days before the polio shot.[150]

Vaccines, particularly those for measles and tuberculosis, have
also been linked with the current epidemic of myalgic encephalomyelitis (ME), also known as chronic fatigue syndrome, particularly among children. Doris Jones of Ilford in Britain began
researching the link between vaccines and the disorder when her
son Stephen developed ME at the age of twelve. He'd reacted
badly to the measles vaccine when given it at a year old, undergoing repeated and prolonged screaming fits. At ten, Doris Jones
says, after having been very late at talking and walking, Stephen
caught measles and, two years later, glandular fever. Two months
after that he had another bout of measles, this time atypical, and
got ME, which he has now had for thirteen years. Mrs. Jones

has unearthed studies linking ME to vaccines against tetanus, measles, cholera, flu, and typhoid, and more recently to hepatitis B.

Some evidence suggests that symptoms of ME are partly due to a dysfunction in the body caused by antibody responses to incomplete, dead or even latent viruses—in other words, many of the "attenuated" or weakened versions of viruses administered in vaccines.[151]

In one group of studies, up to a sixth of young people with ME were vaccinated the month before they came down with the disease.[152] Vaccination appears to act as a trigger if you have a dormant infection or an exhausted or impaired immune system (either because of steroid treatment or a long-term viral infection), or even if you have allergies.

A trawl through the medical literature provides devastating proof that many vaccine programs have left us far worse off than we were before. Over thirty years, the measles vaccine has caused vicious mutations of the disease, transformed it into a disease of adults and infants, and left us with inadequate immunity to pass on to our children. Plus we now have substantial numbers of children damaged by the vaccine. But this is only the merest inkling of the repercussions of our meddling. Dr. Michel Odent and his London-based Primal Health Research Center conducted a study of long-term breast-feeding. The study started out examining whether long-term breast-feeding protects against eczema and asthma. But in the course of the investigation, the researchers came up with an utterly unexpected finding: children immunized against whooping cough were six times more likely to have asthma than those who hadn't been given the shot.[153] In virtually every category—number of sick days, cases of earaches, admittance to hospital—the unvaccinated children were healthier.

Sarah has a six-year-old daughter whose asthma seems related to her shots. "Her reaction to the first DPT shot was to scream nonstop for twelve hours, a reaction we were told was 'normal,' " says Sarah. "She was hospitalized with a high fever after the MMR vaccine, after which she developed bowel problems, and then, after the DPT booster, 'full-blown' asthma." After the complete coterie of shots, she still came down with whooping cough. Sarah continues:

> *We were talked into allowing her to be given two flu vaccinations. After that, she contracted one virus after another and numerous ear infections, so that she was constantly on antibiotics. At present she is taking twice the recommended maximum dose of inhaled steroids for children. We feel that inhaled steroids are also having side effects. She has developed thinning skin, she has gained no weight at all in eighteen months, and her feet have stopped growing.*

Generations of children with inadequate immunity may grow into adults with no placental immunity to pass on to their children, who could then contract measles as babies, when they would normally be protected by their mother's antibodies. In fact, one study showed that antibody levels are lower in women young enough to have been vaccinated than in older women.[154]

If these vaccines are providing only temporary or imperfect immunity, many of our children could grow up susceptible to rubella, mumps, or measles, all of which are far more serious as adult diseases. German measles remains a childhood disease among the self-contained Amish communities in the United States. It has increasingly become a disease of adolescence and young adulthood in the rest of the United States because of the vaccination program. Cases among the Amish community have almost always been mild, and pregnant women appear to be naturally protected.[155]

ALTERNATIVES TO IMMUNIZATION

Vitamin A and Immunization

Even for children at risk of getting serious bouts of measles, other, less drastic measures than immunization are available. When vitamin A levels are low, the outer layers of our mucous membranes become scaly and the turnover of cells decreases. The measles virus infects and damages these tissues throughout the body; blood concentrations of vitamin A, even in well-nourished children, may decrease to less than the levels usually found in malnourished children. During measles, children with marginal liver stores of vitamin A may develop an acute vitamin A deficiency, resulting in eye damage and possibly an increased risk of death from respiratory diseases and diarrhea.

In 1992, New York researchers measured vitamin A levels in eighty-nine children younger than two years old, and compared them with a control group. Among the children with measles, the vitamin A levels of 22 percent were low. Those with low levels were more likely to have a fever of 40°C (104°F) or higher, to have a fever for seven days or more, and to be hospitalized.[156] Other studies demonstrate that children with even a mild vitamin A deficiency were more likely to die of measles.[157]

Giving vitamin A to children with severe (that is, life-threatening) measles can lessen the complications or chances of dying from the disease.[158] D. T. Gerald Keusch of Boston's New England Medical Center, which conducted a study among preschool children in India, went on to say that vitamin A ought to be administered to children whenever there is evidence of a vitamin A deficiency or a possibility of complications from measles. In Africa, where measles is a killer, death rates were reduced by seven times among children under two given vitamin A.[159] Vitamin A is also reputed to offer protection against polio-type viruses.[160]

Other Preventive Measures

Besides breast-feeding your child for as long as possible, feeding him a healthy, whole-food diet and avoiding sending him to nursery or day-care facilities too early may protect him from many childhood diseases.

Current childcare practices, specifically our tendency to institutionalize children too early, have given rise to epidemics of certain infectious diseases such as meningitis. Both Dr. Robert Mendelsohn and his editor Vera Chatz were the first to warn of the dangers of "warehousing" large groups of non-potty-trained babies. Mendelsohn's suspicions were soon backed up by various studies in the medical literature, showing that day-care facilities are suffering an epidemic of Hib-caused meningitis. Researchers examining eight day-care centers found that the attack rate for this type of meningitis was 1,100 cases per 100,000—up to twenty-four times that of the general incidence among children under four.[161]

A more recent study concluded that centers most at risk included those where workers used towels or handkerchiefs (rather than disposable tissues) to wipe children's noses, or allowed children who had diarrhea or who weren't yet potty trained. Ironically, the worst places were those run as commercial businesses, rather than those staffed by volunteers.[162]

If you would feel more comfortable with some sort of booster for your child's immune system, you might want to investigate the homeopathic alternatives. There is some scientific evidence demonstrating they work.[163] In one large-scale study, more than 18,000 children were successfully protected with a homeopathic remedy (*Menigococcinum IICH*) against meningitis, without a single side effect.[164]

If you do decide to have your child vaccinated, weigh up each shot carefully as to the actual threat of the disease (is it more of a nuisance rather than a serious risk to his health or life?) versus the risk of the vaccine itself. If you opt for the polio vaccine, you may wish to consider requesting that your child receive the killed rather than the live variety. In some reports, polio live vaccines have been recommended only for use in developing countries during actual epidemics, or if the killed variety hasn't worked or been feasible.

If your child has already had his shots and is due for boosters, you can request that his blood antibody levels be checked before subjecting him to the risks of shots which, in some cases, have only a 50 percent chance of working.

You might very well be better off giving your child carrot juice and a healthy diet, rather than a knee-jerk, or, for babies and toddlers, putting your money on the oldest immunization program of all: good old mother's milk.

SEVEN

Hormonal Mayhem

Besides rooting out diseases early and trying to eliminate supposed risk factors, doctors reach for the prescription pad as a "just-in-case" measure, the idea being that you can take a pill to prevent yourself from getting ill, even while you're still healthy. The favorite preventive candy of the moment is hormone replacement therapy (HRT), and the most widespread "disease" being prevented is menopause, even in women who pass fifty-five without so much as a single hot flash. Doctors have now invented a scenario in which menopause is an illness and women are naturally "missing" a vital hormone at a certain age.

This belief—that postmenopausal women are inherently deficient in something—has bred a goodly number of ridiculous pronouncements about the post-fifty female condition. One gynecologist I know recently offered the widely aired opinion that, as women originally weren't meant to live past about forty-five, our bodies begin sputtering then because they are, in effect, past their sell-by date. He obviously has never walked in seventeenth-century graveyards to see that if people survived infectious diseases, they had a good chance of living out their three score years and ten.

Menopause results from a falling off in the production of the female hormones, estrogens and progestogens, which affect all systems of the body but particularly regulate the rhythms of women: the monthly cycles, pregnancy and birth, and the cessation of reproductive capability.

As these hormones diminish (the lower level of which the body will eventually adjust to), many women (actually less than half the female population in the West) experience the familiar symptoms of menopause: hot flashes; night sweats; vaginal dryness; cervical, vaginal, and uterine atrophy; and lack of interest in sex. These hormones also affect the density of bones; after menopause, many women experience a thinning of the bones, called osteoporosis (brittle bone disease), which can eventually result in the "dowager's hump" of female old age or even potentially fatal fractures of the spine or hips. Many doctors believe that lack of estrogen is also behind the sharp rise in heart disease in women over fifty.

HRT is being treated as the medical equivalent of the female fountain of youth. When first developed in the 1960s, hormone replacement therapy was given to women with severe menopausal symptoms. HRT employs artificial or "natural" estrogens (in some cases from the urine of pregnant mares), and more recently artificial progesterone, or progestogen—essentially the same two hormones used in the birth control pill (although in the Pill, both are synthetic). The idea is to trick the body into thinking that it is still premenopausal, in order to postpone, reduce, or eliminate the symptoms of the change. It is now available in tablets, a cream, an implant, or a patch (the last of which gets changed about twice a week, in order to provide a continual "drip feed" of hormone at the site).

In the highly successful marketing campaign for HRT, drug companies have managed to pitch the drug as an all-purpose cure-all of the bugbears of old age for all women, not just the 40 percent who have menopausal symptoms. These days, HRT is graced with a roll-call of alleged benefits, not just of menopause, but of future disease: heart disease, osteoporosis, stroke, and senile dementia.

Hormone replacement therapy has become so enshrouded in a myth of beneficence that it has been referred to more than once as "the most important preventive medicine of the century." Indeed, John Studd of King's College Hospital in London, who has probably done more to promote this drug than any other researcher in the world, is so confident of its benefits that he dismisses the need for any extra monitoring. "As all of the effects of long-term HRT seem to be protective, with the questionable exception of breast cancer, it is illogical to recommend that these women need any extra monitoring," he announced in 1992.[1]

In my view, however, future generations will look back upon HRT and other prescribed hormones such as the Pill as among the biggest medical blunders of the century. Ever since its launch, doctors have played statistical games with this drug, using loosely assembled observational studies to infer a host of future benefits such as protection from brittle bones or heart disease. These proclaimed benefits have grown ever more outlandish. Besides curing Alzheimer's disease and stroke, HRT has lately been tried out in the treatment of women with inflammatory bowel disease.[2]

THE MYTHS EXPLODED

The fact is, every one of these claims has been built upon sand. Most experts agree that the studies of women taking estrogen show increased bone density. However, the latest study of HRT and osteoporosis shows that women following the usual recommendation to take the drug for ten years upon the start of menopause are not protected any more from brittle bone disease than are those women who have never taken the drug at all. An ongoing study of women in Framingham, Massachusetts, concluded that HRT preserves bone mass only while you're taking it—and only then if you take it for at least seven years. As soon as women stop the drug, even after a decade of use, bone mineral density catches up in its rapid decline, so that by age seventy-five it is virtually the same as it is in women who have never taken the drug. This means that it affords virtually no protection during those decades of life when the risk of developing osteoporosis is greatest.[3]

To get around these problems, doctors have variously recommended that HRT should be taken forever (at which point the breast cancer risks begin to mount); or begun ten years *after* menopause, long after a woman has experienced all the menopausal symptoms the drug is supposed to alleviate; or even be given after a woman breaks her hip, which would seem to be more than a little self-defeating.[4]

At best, estrogen seems to have only a temporary effect. Although it may decrease the rate at which old bone is torn down, formation of new bone eventually decreases in some three to five years anyway. One large-scale review of thirty-one studies on osteoporosis concluded that estrogen didn't have a "significant benefit" in slowing the onset of osteoporosis.[5] Another found it didn't strengthen bones in women even when they had used it for sixteen years.[6]

In fact, there is some evidence that estrogens or progestogens actually *contribute* to osteoporosis. The spinal bone density of women under study has increased once the women stopped using medroxyprogesterone as a contraceptive, compared to no change among women carrying on taking the progestogen.[7]

Dr. Kitty Little, an Oxford researcher, has spent many years studying the effects of hormones on bone marrow. In animal experiments, Dr. Little has observed that one effect of the estrogen-progestogen combinations is to distort large cells in the bone, leading to a huge increase in abnormally sticky platelets, or tiny blood clots. These can interfere with the blood supply to the trabecular bone, the spongy bone found mainly in the spinal vertebrae.[8]

In London, Biolab's medical researcher, Dr. John McLaren Howard, has studied the levels of nutrients necessary for bone development in women with osteoporosis, particularly the enzyme alkaline phosphatase. This enzyme works with magnesium to form calcium crystals in the bone, and so is an indicator of whether new bone is being laid down. *The lowest levels of alkaline phosphatase in Dr. Howard's study were found in women with osteoporosis on HRT.*[9]

As for the cardiovascular benefits of HRT, the scientific method behind these claims is so shaky that the journals they appear in are almost apologetic about publishing them. In one major study, a group of U.S. epidemiologists selected 5,000 postmenopausal women from the American South and Midwest and measured their cholesterol levels and other supposed risk factors, from which they deduced the women's supposed risk of suffering from future cardiovascular disease. After comparing the results of those on HRT with those not on the drug, the researchers concluded that HRT could reduce the risk of heart disease by 42 percent.[10]

The researchers did acknowledge that they were making a few mighty hefty assumptions. For one thing, the study wasn't randomized—that is, the participants weren't selected randomly—so there could have been what scientists term "selection bias"; only the healthiest women with a low incidence of heart disease could have been selected to take HRT. As other researchers note, women on HRT are more likely to be white, upper middle class, educated, and thin—all factors that individually lessen their heart-disease risk in the first place.[11]

In the same edition of the medical journal, an editorial attempted to distance itself from the conclusions reached by the study. "The authors' calculation of the overall benefit . . . is speculative," said the editorial, because the study wasn't designed to tell whether HRT actually caused metabolic changes or whether they just occurred independently.[12]

And of course the entire study was based upon what may be an erroneous assumption—that a raised cholesterol level automatically leads to heart disease.

In fact, a number of researchers agree that most of the studies showing a heart benefit with HRT have been flawed. Professor Jan Vandenbroucke and his Dutch colleagues at the Department of Clinical Epidemiology, Leiden University Hospital in the Netherlands reviewed all the individual studies concerning HRT and the heart and concluded that the studies had been "biased," unintentionally selecting inordinately healthy women for the test, who may have been at lower risk of developing heart disease anyway. Furthermore, women with a preexisting heart condition were included in the studies. When you remove them from the studies, the results show similar death rates in women, whether they take HRT or not.[13] The use of HRT as a universal preventive is "unwarranted," concluded Vandenbroucke elsewhere.[14] "Perhaps we should demand some colossal well-controlled trials before we let the genie of universal preventive prescription escape from the bottle," he cautioned.[15]

Vandenbroucke and his colleagues have also disputed the entire theory that giving outside hormones will in any way protect your heart, or even that women have an increased risk in this regard. "Data on mortality from coronary heart disease shows that there is no acceleration in coronary heart disease in women after the age of fifty," he writes. "Even if there were plausible biological reasons why natural estrogens would protect against coronary heart disease, it does not follow that replacing a relative deficiency has beneficial effects."[16]

Not all studies show that HRT has a protective effect. In 1985, the Framingham, Massachusetts, study—the same one that showed the catch-up osteoporosis risk after coming off HRT—suggested that the risk of heart disease with HRT use was actually *increased*.[17] In another major study, the effect of estrogens on deaths disappeared after the researchers had corrected their statistics for diseases already present when the study started.[18] In two others, favorable benefits couldn't be attributed to HRT.[19]

Most important, virtually all the trials were conducted with oral estrogen alone, whereas most women who haven't had hysterectomies now take an estrogen combined with progestogen (progestin in the United States) in order to counteract what are now known risks of endometrial cancer with estrogen-only preparations.

But adding progestogens appears to reverse some of the supposedly favorable effects of estrogen on blood cholesterol levels, by blunting the rise in high-density lipoprotein cholesterol,[20] although one study showed the reverse.[21]

"If the addition of progestin reverses even 5 to 10 percent of the relative benefit of the estrogen-replacement therapy with regard to ischemic heart disease," write Drs. Lee Goldman and Anna Tosteson, of Brigham and Women's Hospital in Boston, who have studied the subject, "its net effect as compared with unopposed estrogen therapy would probably be detrimental even if the entire increase in the risk of endometrial cancer is eliminated."[22]

The latest study, dubbed PEPI (Postmenopausal Estrogen Progestin Intervention), claimed to find a benefit on the heart of combination HRT. However, the trial also discovered that progestogen increases levels of the fat triglyceride, which is a known risk factor for heart disease, particularly in women. This triglyceride effect could make HRT an even more dangerous option for diabetics.[23]

Furthermore, when actually tested in a population, HRT either does nothing or actually increases the risk of heart disease, particularly in women with a low risk of heart disease. In Italy, where there is a low level of heart disease anyway, researchers found that HRT was increasing the risks of heart disease by .88 times after five years.[24] And one of the first randomized, placebo-controlled trials into HRT and heart disease found that there were more cases of heart disease in those taking hormone supplementation than those given a placebo.[25]

Undeterred by the lingering doubts of a tiny minority, researchers are now experimenting with HRT to treat existing heart problems. So far, the studies have mainly looked at the effect of estrogen on animal arteries or human arteries obtained during cardiac transplants. But in one study on humans, German researchers from Hannover Medical School discovered that absorption of the drug was highly variable, and that artery diameters remained unchanged in women with low absorption of estrogen. They are still unclear whether the ability of estrogen to relax arteries actually means anything significant in terms of treating heart disease.[26]

And now a recent study has undermined the entire assumption that estrogen offers natural protection against heart complaints. The study, conducted by the University of California at San Diego's Department of Family and Preventive Medicine, tracked fifty-year-old women over a nineteen-year period, before and after menopause. The study made the astonishing discovery that the women's natural levels of estrogen gave them no special protection against heart disease. Women with heart disease didn't have lower levels of estrogen than those with healthy hearts; *in fact, estrogen levels did not alter to any great degree after menopause.* (Cholesterol levels and blood pressure weren't major factors in heart disease, either.)[27] Another study showed that HRT has no beneficial effect on reducing the level of blood angiotensin converting enzyme, which is supposed to help in heart disease.[28]

Yet another study, conducted in the Netherlands of over 11,000 women over nine years, found that women who went on to develop heart disease didn't have levels of estrogens that were any different from others in the study population.[29]

This discovery kicks away one of the main platforms of hormone therapy—that it protects women from heart attacks. It also means that post-menopausal women aren't "missing" estrogen that needs to be "replaced."

Another frequent claim made about HRT, without a shred of convincing evidence, is that it reduces the risk of stroke. Not even the studies demonstrating protection from heart disease could find a change in the risk of stroke. Far from being protective, HRT may bring on strokes (as does its closely related cousin, the Pill).[30]

At forty-five, Maria was put on HRT by her doctor. From the day she took her first pill, she started to bleed. Her doctor told her that the drug simply "needed to get into her system" and told her to double up on the dosage. After she did, she began passing out and her left leg turned purple.

"When I began having pains in my stomach and chest, a doctor called out on emergency told me to stop the pills immediately. Nevertheless, I continued to pass blood clots." At this point, Maria's doctor told her that she was losing so much blood because the drug was "now leaving her body." Once it did, he assured her, everything would return to normal.

A month later the pain had traveled up Maria's body to her arm joints. She could neither bend nor breathe, and her chest felt like it was caving in. She was then given prednisolone, a steroid, and penicillin, and began vomiting so much that nothing would stay down. After a week she had to call her doctor to pay her a home visit because she couldn't move, but lay on the floor on a mattress in her living room.

"My left side felt paralyzed, my head flopped, I couldn't see, and my speech was slurred. The doctor said I'd had a reaction to penicillin, but thought the steroid would counter any ill effects. He left me lying on the floor," said Maria. Many tests later, the medical consensus was that Maria had suffered a stroke brought on by the HRT.

Hormones may well be able to stave off temporarily some of the confusion and woolly-headedness induced by falling hormone levels, and some women do feel very well on estrogen. Many pro-HRT organizations claim that "new research" suggests that HRT can prevent Alzheimer's disease. However, a recent fifteen-year study found that HRT has no effect on keeping your brain sharp. Any reduction in cognitive function has been shown to be the same, regardless of whether or not women use estrogen.[31]

A LITANY OF SIDE EFFECTS

Without all these claimed benefits, all HRT offers is a grocery list of potentially fatal side effects. Doctors haven't yet worked out the best way to administer this drug, and there is little control over the amount of estrogen that gets released into the bloodstream. The most popular way to take HRT is by mouth. However, via this route, women experience a number of gastrointestinal symptoms—nausea, vomiting, abdominal cramps, bloating—and may even develop jaundice.

This may be one reason why medicine came up with the skin (transdermal) patch, which bypasses the liver, resulting in higher levels of estrogen being absorbed by the body. However, a fifth of patients experience blistering, hyperemia (increased blood flow in the area), and discoloration of the skin using this method. Consequently, an increasing number of doctors now use estrogen implants, which require a small outpatient operation to insert the pellets under the skin.

Estrogen implants (and even patches) appear to create a "tolerance" for estrogen that some doctors warn is similar to addiction; a woman will have higher-than-normal levels of estrogen in her bloodstream, but nevertheless complains of the return of menopausal symptoms at increasingly frequent intervals. Although these implants are supposed to last for six months, many users complain of a return of symptoms three to nine weeks later. This phenomenon—called "tachyphylaxis" (which means, literally, "too much prevention")—occurred in three out of every hundred women in a study by the Dulwich Hospital Menopause Clinic in London.[32]

After examining a number of such studies, Dr. Thomas Bewley, former president of the Royal College of Psychiatrists, and Dr. Susan Bewley, a gynecologist at University College Hospital, London, concluded that this dependence "occurs in 15 percent of cases," largely for psychological reasons. As they explained: "Estrogens are psychoactive. They lift mood, can be given by injection, and their use has powerful psychological effects."[33]

HRT proponent John Studd has written that women who have psychiatric problems require larger-than-normal estrogen levels anyway. "These women may need higher levels [of estrogen] to obtain symptomatic relief, since many were originally treated for premenstrual syndrome (PMS) or depression [during menopause]" he wrote.[34] Elsewhere he has said that it is "by no means rare" for patients to require an increasing dose of hormones. "It may just mean they are addicted to feeling better," he says.[35]

It may simply be that the estrogen-sensitive cells in the body, continually blasted with high doses of the hormone, lose the ability to respond.[36] Or it could be that early use of estrogens, whether in HRT, to control PMT, or as included in the Pill, may set up an increased need for replacement therapy. It may be that HRT creates artificially high levels of estrogen in the body, triggering a hormonal "crash" when these levels fall even slightly, and thereby exacerbating ordinary menopausal symptoms.

Ordinarily, the body's pituitary glands and ovaries work in exquisite tandem, constantly adjusting estrogen levels to fit the body's need of the moment, like a car set on automatic, says Dr. Ellen Grant, author of *Sexual Chemistry* and a long-time critic of HRT and the Pill.[37] HRT, which delivers a constant level of estrogen, she says, is like having a car struck in a single gear.

Another problem with estrogen implants is endometrial stimulation—a potential cancer-causing reaction. These days, it is acknowledged that using estrogen-only preparations on a woman who still has a uterus can increase by up to twentyfold her chances of getting endometrial cancer after several years. This is because estrogen causes rapid proliferation of endometrial cells (as it does in pregnancy). To counteract this, most women are given progestogen for ten to twelve days per month, which imitates the second half of the menstrual cycle, producing withdrawal bleeding.

Endometrial stimulation in women given the implants occurs for an average of two years after they finish taking supplemental estrogen.[38] What this means is that, in order to lower your risk of getting endometrial cancer, you have to commit yourself to taking oral progestogen for two years or more after you finish taking estrogen.

Proponents of HRT constantly attempt to make light of the proven breast and endometrial cancer risks of HRT. In John Studd's view, the breast cancer risk is increased if a woman takes HRT, but since several studies have shown that fewer women die from HRT-caused disease than ordinarily, he doesn't see this as such a big deal. "There is not enough information to suggest that breast cancer risk is a valid reason to withhold estrogen therapy," he has written, and many medical practitioners would tend to agree with him.[39]

However, almost every study to date about HRT suggests a

significant cancer risk; the only thing disputed is exactly how substantial this risk is.

- Thirty-seven studies of breast cancer risk, analyzed together, showed that long-term estrogen use increases a woman's risk of getting breast cancer by 60 percent.[40]

- An analysis of sixteen studies of HRT concluded that, after fifteen years, the risk of getting breast cancer increased by 30 percent in women using estrogen-only HRT, and more than doubled in those using the combination (estrogen and progestogen) drug. This risk increased with every year of use. Based on 1987 usage, this would translate as 4,708 new cases of breast cancer and 1,468 deaths among American women every year.[41]

- A six-year Swedish study of 23,000 women using HRT found an 80 percent increase in the risk for women using estrogen-only HRT. However, the highest risk was incurred by those using the continuous combination estrogen-progestogen drug. Far from being protective, drugs with progestogens more than quadrupled the risk.[42] While no other study has been able to duplicate the level of risk identified by the Swedish researchers, other reports have shown that the addition of progestogens in HRT adds to the risk of breast cancer.[43]

- The landmark Nurses' Health Study, produced by the Harvard Medical School and backed by the American Cancer Society, which examined 725,550 woman-years of follow-up and nearly 2,000 cases of breast cancer, found that women using estrogen-only HRT had a 30 percent increase in breast cancer. This risk increased to 41 percent for those using the estrogen-progestogen mix. The most startling figures of all, however, concerned longer-term use. Those using HRT for more than five years had a 46 percent increased risk of breast cancer (and a 45 percent risk of dying from it if taking estrogen-only HRT). For women over sixty the risk leapt to 71 percent. The study concluded that "the significant increase in the risks of breast cancer and of death . . . suggests that the risks and benefits of hormone therapy among older women should be carefully assessed"—which, in the guarded tone of scientific papers, would appear to amount to a virtual damnation.[44]

As for endometrial cancer, estrogen alone increases the risk from three to twenty times; adding progestogen may increase your risk of getting endometrial cancer from 30 to 80 percent over those who don't take HRT.[45]

And new evidence from Washington State shows that combination HRT drugs that add progesterone fail to protect against endometrial cancers at certain doses. In the trial among over a thousand postmenopausal women, although the risk of endometrial cancer was quadrupled among those who took opposed estrogen, the overall risk remained at 1.4 times among those who took combined HRT. The study also found progesterone needed to be taken for up to twenty-one days a month before it had any appreciable effect. Whenever it was taken for ten or fewer days a month, the cancer risk remained at 3.1 times, compared with someone not taking HRT.

The benefits also seemed to reduce over time. After five years, even those taking progesterone for up to twenty-one days a months had a 2.5 times risk of developing endometrial cancer.[46]

Professor Klim McPherson, a noted British epidemiologist from the London School of Tropical Diseases who has participated in both Pill and HRT studies, found in the British study in which he participated that breast cancer risks increased by 60 percent. However, after reviewing all the studies and taking the most conservative line, he concluded that the best estimate is that HRT increases the breast cancer risk by at least 30 percent.[47]

Janette had a close friend who found a lump in her breast after being on HRT.

After the lumpectomy, she was told it was cancerous and, two weeks later, she had a mastectomy. However, the cancer had spread to the axillary lymph nodes (which were removed).

A course of radiotherapy followed, plus radiation of the ovaries and tamoxifen tablets. She continued to have pain on the right side, where she'd had the mastectomy, due to problems with the nerves and also the radiation. The cancer spread to her liver. Now she is undergoing chemotherapy.

At forty-five, now with two daughters, eighteen and twenty-one, Janette's friend is preparing to die.

HRT, like the Pill, has always been touted as a "protection" against ovarian cancer. But the latest discovery by the American Cancer Society is that women who stay on HRT for more than ten years increase their risk of developing fatal ovarian cancer *by 70 percent*. In the ACS study, which tracked more than 200,000 menopausal women, the risk increased the longer the women were on HRT, although most were using twice the dosage currently used today.[48]

Most pro-HRT literature concentrates on the supposed euphoria experienced by women on the drug. What it doesn't discuss is that 70 percent of women experience a host of side effects with estrogen or progestogen, and that half of all women stop taking the drug after six months.

Katie was one such woman:

I became incredibly ill while using HRT. My symptoms included indigestion, bloating, lethargy, extreme tension, and violent headaches. My heart thumped all day, particularly when I tried to move about. My chest wall tightened, with pains down my arms, almost like a heart attack. Besides symptoms of panic, I was so ill I couldn't concentrate or even watch anything on TV, particularly emotional scenes. I came off the drug nine months ago; I am not out of the woods yet, to put it mildly. My doctor wouldn't accept that I could still be adversely affected three weeks after stopping HRT, and wanted me to see a psychiatrist! On top of everything, of course, my hot flashes have returned with a vengeance—no doubt due to having been suppressed by the HRT.

Besides monthly, periodlike withdrawal bleeding, which many women find objectionable, progestogen causes a plethora of other side effects. These include PMS-like symptoms—breast tenderness, bloating, abdominal cramps, depression, anxiety, and irritability[49]—in short, many of the symptoms HRT is supposed to treat.

In an attempt to minimize these side effects, particularly withdrawal bleeding, some doctors give women continuous progestogen. However, this commonly leads to breakthrough bleeding and, of course, nullifies the supposedly long-term protective effects against endometrial cancer. In one study of patients who'd used the continuous combined estrogen and progestogen therapy, 15 percent had episodes of breakthrough bleeding, 5 percent had benign endometrial tumors, and another 5 percent had endometrial cancer.[50]

Doctors like to maintain that the estrogens of HRT don't pose the same risk of thrombosis as those estrogens used in the Pill. The prevailing wisdom is that the same estrogen (albeit a different dosage) placed in the contraceptive pill and acknowledged to cause cardiovascular incidents does not cause this problem when placed in fairly similar form in hormone replacement therapy. As the *British Medical Journal* put it: "Many doctors have been surprised to discover that a hormonal treatment they had learned to avoid in women at risk of cardiovascular disease is now being specifically advised in this situation."[51]

In fact, the continuous estrogen-progestogen combination has demonstrated an ability to cause worrying changes in the blood. In one study of women on the combination drug, changes were observed in the ability of their blood to clot and also their body's ability to break up blood clots. Two women developed thrombosis. The researchers believed this could signal an increased risk of stroke.[52]

This has been confirmed by a recent major British study in Oxford, which found that women on HRT increase their chances of thrombosis nearly four times. The risk can increase if doses of HRT are raised, and reached nearly seven times if the women were taking as much as 1.25 milligrams or more a day.

The Oxford researchers found the risk was greatest during the first year of use.[53]

Those at greatest risk of venous thromboembolism are so-called "premenopausal" women—women over forty who are still ovulating and so still producing estrogen. The addition of HRT produces a massive overdose of estrogen, which can lead to thromboembolism. This is worrying, in light of the increased tendency among doctors these days to offer HRT to women at their fortieth birthday, whether or not they are still ovulating.[54]

Progestogens can also alter your glucose and insulin levels,[55] cause higher than normal levels of calcium in the blood, hepatitis, liver cancer, urinary tract infections,[56] jaundice, excess fluid (with or without heart failure), and virilization—such as an increase in facial hair, and deepening of the voice—which can be irreversible. HRT also exacerbates endometriosis.[57]

Hormone supplementation is also linked with increasing the severity of migraines, because it causes an overreaction in the arteries and veins.[58] Patients have reduced their incidence of headaches tenfold when they stopped both smoking and taking hormones.[59]

This is in addition to all the other side effects of estrogen: at least a twofold increase in the risk of gallbladder disease,[60] elevated blood pressure, enlarged and tender breasts, changes in the shape of the eyes, and depression.

Harriet was first prescribed HRT for severe menopausal symptoms and to prevent osteoporosis. She was told by the hospital doctor who took her X ray, and also by her own doctor, that there was no alternative and that her bones would crumble if she didn't take it.

> *After three weeks I felt wonderful, but during the fifth week not only did all my previous symptoms return with a vengeance, but I also experienced urinary incontinence [and difficulties with my vision], speech, memory and motor [co-ordination]. At times my vision appeared as though I was looking through the wrong end of binoculars (everything appeared much smaller). My speech at times was an incoherent jumble; I could not remember*

my name or address or recognize people or objects, and there were long gaps in the day which I could not explain. Some days I could not walk unaided, and often my husband had to drag me out of bed and make me move because my body felt encased in lead. I also became severely dyslexic. I stopped taking the tablets immediately after the first symptoms occurred, but my condition continued to deteriorate. My doctor just did not believe me because I could only visit his office on "good" days. I was told that all I needed was "counseling." I declined and turned to alternative therapies. Within eighteen months my central nervous system was almost back to normal—walking more than a hundred yards was still a problem. However, the HRT had left me with a serious intolerance to petrochemicals. Many toiletries, household cleaners, new fabrics, [and] new buildings caused asthmalike attacks, bouts of severe aggression or depression, or muscle collapse, all accompanied by tissue swelling. A strict diet and nutritional supplements (including a course of intravenous vitamins and minerals) has helped to re-store my immune system, and now I do not have severe attacks.

But HRT and the Pill aren't the only hormones being investi-gated. A young Australian woman with a seventeen-month-old baby asked the Key Centre for Women's Health in Victoria, Australia, to help her to breast-feed her nephew temporarily since she had weaned her own child two months before. Doctors gave her a synthetic oxytocin nose spray made by Sandoz, in an at-tempt to stimulate milk production; oxytocin, a peripheral hor-mone produced by the pituitary gland, is known to help with the ejection of milk.

Although the oxytocin did increase her milk supply, the baby was unsatisfied, and after two days the woman quit trying. She did report, however, that two hours after she'd been sprayed with the hormone, she experienced intense sexual desire and, after intercourse with her partner, heightened orgasms. Appar-ently, the key to this aphrodisiac effect was the progestogen-only birth control pill she was taking. Twice afterward she tried the nose spray, once on the Pill and once after she'd stopped taking it. It worked only when she was also on the Pill.

Quickly forgetting the baby, who may never, in the end, have gotten fed, the Australian researchers realized they were onto a good thing and rushed into print an article about "hormones and sexual arousal" and oxytocin as a potential aphrodisiac.

One only has to imagine how this single finding could quickly get distorted into a new medicine, which may soon generate headlines about "new hope for frigid women," and after that "new hope for marital difficulties," and before long, "keep your marriage alive," "keep your woman begging for more," and even "the essential hormone after menopause." It may not be long before this drug gets thrown in with the usual cocktail of estrogens and progestogens for every woman over fifty or tucked in with the birth control pill, eventually getting us that much closer to total surrender of the hormonal control of our bodies to modern chemistry.

ALTERNATIVES TO HORMONE REPLACEMENT THERAPY (HRT)

If you decide that all these risks aren't worth taking just to rid yourself of hot flashes, there are many alternatives. Many nutritional doctors, including those with great experience in treating women during menopause, argue that the kind of menopause you experience, like your degree of morning sickness or PMS, simply reflects your nutritional state. They believe that a difficult menopause *is* a "deficiency disease," but not of estrogen. The root of the problem is deficiency in one of a number of vital micronutrients, food intolerance, or the inefficient function of certain organs. According to Dr. Ellen Grant, "Hot flashes are not a sign of estrogen deficiency . . . [but] a result of an allergic reaction." Flashes are very similar to headaches, migraines, and rises in blood pressure.[61] John Mansfield, a British allergy specialist and author of *Arthritis: The Allergy Connection* (Thorsons) and other books, concurs that many menopausal symptoms are related to food sensitivity. "Once we put women on an elimination diet, the severe symptoms stop. In some cases, we find the women have a candida albicans overgrowth."

Patrick Kingsley, another nutritional specialist who has had success with illnesses as diverse as cancer and multiple sclerosis, finds that a whole-foods diet and supplement program helps relieve many menopausal symptoms.

Besides avoiding calcium megadoses (which interfere with the absorption of zinc and iron), Dr. Grant suggests that menopausal women take the following supplements: magnesium (500 milligrams), zinc (at least 30 milligrams), boron (3 milligrams), which helps the body make its own estrogen, at least 10 milligrams manganese, and 1 gram vitamin C per day. You also need vitamin K if accelerated bone formation is desirable, vitamin D, folic acid, at least 50 to 100 milligrams of B_6 (or 50 milligrams pyridoxal-5-phosphate, the first metabolite of B_6), essential fatty acids, and "first-class protein."

In his experience with American patients, nutritionist Dr. Leo Galland finds that 400 units per day of vitamin E and six capsules of 500-milligram evening primrose oil per day will help ovaries maximize their output of estrogen during the early stages of menopause.

Evening primrose oil and vitamin E will help maintain libido, but the most effective method of maintaining interest in sex and keeping the vaginal canal lubricated is to have regular sex. Dr. Kingsley says the idea that women get old and haggard after menopause is "absolute rubbish." "Although there is slightly more estrogen diminution after menopause, the body is still producing it from the adrenal glands," he says. "Leading a pleasurable and exciting life also helps maintain sexual energy."

Nutritional pioneer Dr. Stephen Davies, author of *Nutritional Medicine* (Pan), believes that, since the adrenal gland, the major organ involved in adaptive changes in the body, has the highest concentration of vitamin C and pantothenic acid of any organ, it's wise to ensure an abundance of these two essential nutrients. It's also good practice for your practitioner to make sure that your thyroid is functioning normally.

If supplements and changes to your diet don't sort you out,

you can try several alternative approaches. Dr. Galland says that controlled scientific studies have shown that 1,000 to 2,000 milligrams a day of hesperidin-derived bioflavonoids, taken on an empty stomach, work in treating hot flashes. The amino acid beta alanine has also been found extremely useful in relieving hot flashes.

Patrick Kingsley has had success with the homeopathic preparation Lachesis (30c potency), used four times a day for a few days, reducing gradually to once a day just before bedtime. It will immediately abort a hot flash, he says, if taken at the first sign. An alternative homeopathic remedy is silver nitrate (30c).

Increasingly, naturopaths are showing interest in food and plant sources of female hormones. Rhubarb and hops both contain estrogen-like hormones, known as phytoestrols, which have been shown to relieve menopausal symptoms—without the dangers or the side effects of HRT. Soybeans and soy products—such as tofu and miso—are also good sources of estrogen.

Phytoestrogens are compounds that have a similar molecular structure to estrogen, and their effects are comparable, although weaker than those of estrogen itself. Other sources of phytoestrols include anise, celery, fennel, ginseng, alfalfa, red clover, and licorice.

Japanese women—with their high-soy diet—have a much lower frequency of hot flashes and other menopausal symptoms than women in the West. One study found that Japanese women on a traditional low-fat diet had plant estrogen levels in their urine up to 1,000 times higher than those of American women.[62]

However, food sources of phytochemicals are a far cry from natural progesterone, which is being sold as a cream and touted as the solution for being female and over forty with little evidence that it is safe to take. Although it is called "natural" because it is derived from yams, natural progesterone is made in the test tube. Our bodies produce a basic steroid skeleton, or molecular blueprint, from which all hormones are derived. This skeleton goes through a number of natural processes, governed by enzymes from different organs, to transform into individual hormones such as progesterone. Chemists making so-called "natural" hormones imitate this process by extracting a number of chemical processes in the test tube, tacking on extra parts of molecules here and there, to end up with a substance with more or less the same molecular structure as that which our bodies produce. But all such progesterones must go through this chemical processing, and all share similar side effects. There are no proprietary progesterone drugs licensed by the FDA in America, although there are in many European countries. For Gestone, one licensed progesterone in the United Kingdom, side effects include loss of vision, double vision, migraine, changes in the cervix or breast, insomnia, and changes in menstrual flow or cycle, to name a few.[63] Some epidemiologists believe that high levels of progesterone may be a risk factor for breast cancer.[64]

Progesterone in creams is sold as a "cosmetic" in the United States. As such, manufacturers are not obliged to go through the safety testing required by the Food and Drug Administration for drugs. Because there are none of the usual FDA regulations that apply to drugs, any manufacturer can put in any amount of the hormone he wishes. One laboratory, which analyzed nineteen body creams containing progesterone sold in the United States, found that the creams contained anything from less than 2 milligrams to 700 milligrams per ounce. Furthermore, not everyone absorbs progesterone in the same way, and those spots where you've rubbed in the cream can have far higher doses than your blood levels.[65]

For longer-term problems such as osteoporosis, the solution is far more complicated than simply wolfing down glasses of milk or calcium pills, as most doctors now recommend. American nutritional researcher Dr. Melvyn Werbach, author of *Nutritional Influences on Illness* (Third Line Press) and other excellent summaries of the scientific evidence of nutritional information, has examined most of the main studies purporting to show that calcium slows osteoporosis. He believes that many calcium studies showing a daily need of a gram or more have been criticized as being subject to inaccuracies. And calcium intake is disturbed by the high phosphorus content of the typical Western diet.[66]

At London's Biolab, Dr. McLaren Howard has found in his

studies of osteoporotic patients that not one woman with osteoporosis, compared with healthy controls and even menstruating
women, has suffered from low levels of calcium.[67]

American researcher Dr. Guy Abraham has also demonstrated
that most cases of osteoporosis are not caused by calcium deficiency and cannot be prevented by calcium megadosing. Instead
he found that magnesium deficiency plays a key role because this
mineral is necessary to activate bone enzyme alkaline phosphatase.

In his own study, Dr. Abraham gave magnesium to nineteen
women taking HRT.[68] After eight months, the bone mineral
density in the women taking the supplements had increased by
11 percent, compared with no increase in the women taking
HRT alone. Although fifteen of the nineteen women had bone
mineral density below that considered likely to cause fractures,
after a year, only half still had bones that were too thin. Bone
mineral levels were still improving after two years.

In Dr. McLaren Howard's study, besides the enzyme alkaline
phosphatase, women with osteoporosis were found to be low in
magnesium, zinc, manganese, and vitamin C.

Regular, weight-bearing exercise has consistently been shown
to stave off bone loss, even in women past menopause, despite
the usual medical claims that if you don't exercise before forty,
you can't do anything to improve your bones. Regular exercise
has been shown to halve your risk of hip fracture,[69] and twice-
weekly high-intensity exercise has been shown to increase bone
density and to improve muscle mass, strength, and balance in
postmenopausal women—all important points if you want to
avoid fracture. Cigarette smoking accelerates the destruction of
estrogen and so hastens the onset of both menopause and osteoporosis. If you stop smoking, you reduce your risk of hip fracture
by 25 percent.[70]

Another reason we in the West may be plagued with osteoporosis is our tendency to eat excessive amounts of protein. As
calcium is needed to metabolize protein, a high-protein diet
means calcium is constantly leeched from the bones. Osteoporosis

is virtually unknown in places such as Africa, where the inhabitants eat far fewer proteins.[71]

Besides a well-varied whole-food diet rich in fruits and vegetables, it is wise to restrict meat and excessive protein, caffeine, and salt. If you wish to take supplements, have yourself assessed by a qualified nutritionist to find out which supplements you need. Not getting the balance right could be an expensive and possible dangerous waste of time. Also be sure to get your digestive function checked since low stomach acid can be responsible for low absorption of calcium. You may wish to take a supplement of vitamin D_3, which increases the uptake of calcium in the diet, and small supplements of boron, which help to metabolize vitamin D_3.[72]

— IV —

TREATMENT

EIGHT

Miracle Cures

ANTIBIOTICS

I owe my life to antibiotics. In 1942, when my mother was twenty-four, her dentist unwisely extracted a tooth while she had the flu. Within days her neck ballooned with a streptococcus infection, and she was rushed to the hospital. My father, then her fiancé, wept helplessly at her bedside while priests filed past him after administering the last rites.

And then the wonder drug arrived. As a last resort, my mother was given penicillin, still in experimental use then. Within a day or two the swelling that had almost obscured her face simply melted away. My ordinarily doubting father rushed off to church and humbly knelt before the altar, convinced that he had witnessed a miracle.

In those days, antibiotics were being tested to combat deadly bacterial infections. As a result of the work of Alexander Fleming and others, penicillin began to be used gingerly during the Second World War, against such life-threatening illnesses as septicemia, meningitis, and pneumonia. There is perhaps no other family of drugs that has so revolutionized—indeed defined—modern medicine.

Nevertheless, fifty years later this century's wonder drug has become one of the most abused substances in modern medicine. What was once reserved for life-threatening illnesses such as lobar pneumonia is now routinely handed out at the doctor's office for athlete's foot or colds—anytime a benign infection is suspected, or even suspected of developing one day. Up until now, an unnecessary antibiotic was only thought to cause a tummy upset or a reaction in the approximately 5 percent of those truly allergic to them. But a growing body of opinion believes that repeated courses of antibiotics can so disturb a person's internal ecology that it begins a process of disease that could end in chronic fatigue syndrome, diabetes, or even cancer.

With the notable exception of antibiotics (so long as they are used very judiciously), the fact is that drugs do not make you better. At your next dinner party, try playing the following game. Challenge everyone around the table to produce a single drug that can cure people of an illness, other than antibiotics. If you come up with anything, stop whatever you're doing and call me.

After many years of wracking my brain, trawling through the information on thousands of drugs on the market, I cannot think of a single category of drug besides antibiotics that will do anything more than what drug companies call "maintenance"—that is, making the patient more comfortable with his illness, or trying to prevent the disease from getting worse, often at the risk of developing a number of other conditions potentially far worse than the one being treated.

Medical science has devised a number of amazing preparations that are capable of cleverly interrupting certain processes—depression, wakefulness, stomach acid production, ovulation, hormone production, inflammation, pain, even the electrical signals controlling your heart. They've managed to come up with certain crude replacements for the body's delicate machinery, as insulin does for people with diabetes, or steroids for people with Addison's disease. Medicine is good at interrupting psychotic behavior or the menstrual cycle—in effect, at blocking tab A from slotting into slot B.

What twentieth-century medicine isn't very good at, though,

is curing. There isn't one single drug out there besides antibiotics that is capable of clearing up even the most benign condition. In fact, since the development of the big breakthroughs in medicine—antibiotics and cortisone—in the 1940s, medicine hasn't come up with one drug that represents a major type of cure in medical science (unless you count acyclovir, which appears to prevent cold sores, if not the underlying infection that causes them to periodically erupt). In the main, virtually all the drugs developed supposedly to treat the big chronic diseases such as asthma, arthritis, eczema, and the like at best alleviate some symptoms but in many instances leave millions of people far worse off than they were before.

This is because medicine, in the main, doesn't understand why we get ill. Doctors understand *how* most diseases progress in minute detail, but rarely *why* they start. Consequently, the drugs developed to treat these diseases are crude and clumsy, suppressing one or more symptoms of a disease or, in some cases, as with asthma, blocking what may be a healthy immunological defense.[1] And because medicine doesn't know how to cure anything besides some infections, many new types of preparations get pounced on as soon as they are released, as a sort of flavor of the month, and tried out on an ever-widening circle of illnesses to see if they will be the one to do the trick. Cyclosporine is the current fad in medicine, being used to treat every autoimmune disease from arthritis to lupus erythematosus to psoriasis. Originally developed to stop the body from rejecting transplant organs, it acts by lowering the immune system T-cells and brings with it a host of dangerous side effects such as skin cancer and other types of malignancies. It's also associated with liver and kidney damage.

Because its natural domain is waging war in an emergency setting, medicine uses this selfsame weaponry against even everyday or chronic ailments. But this approach doesn't work as well on your everyday problem like hemorrhoids or PMS—and too often resembles using a sledgehammer to swat a flea.

It is nothing less than astonishing how little we know about many of the drug treatments we take for granted. Doctors freely admit they've never known exactly how aspirin works. Because they're stumbling around in the dark, they also often don't know when drug therapy is virtually useless and when to leave well enough alone.

Because of the highly sophisticated tools available to epidemiologists (the scientists who study disease in populations), doctors appear to have lost the ability to make the simple connection between giving people a drug that can, say, cause cancer, and the incidence of cancer going up. Their conspiracy of faith in medicine may be why doctors like to pretend that drugs don't have side effects. My mailbag is full of stories from exasperated patients describing how their doctors have insisted that the obvious, demonstrable side effects of a drug are "coincidental." But the statistics disprove any coincidence. Some 659,000 Americans aged sixty and older were hospitalized in 1990 after reacting to a drug, to name just one statistic.[2]

DRUG TESTING ON THE PUBLIC

The simple fact is that the true nature—and dangers—of any drug are only fully understood after it has been released on the market. Drugs companies are obliged by the Food and Drug Administration to conduct animal and human studies before releasing drugs. To prove its safety, quality, and efficacy, a drug has to pass through several stages before a license to market is granted. The first stage usually involves animal testing—a highly unreliable test in any event—which is supposed to give a crude indication of the therapeutic effects and dosage; the second is an early study on healthy human volunteers to assess more accurately the required dosage; the third, the most exhaustive and expensive, involves clinical trials.

Sometimes a trial tests a new drug against a placebo, but there are no set guidelines as to which kind of trial needs to take place. A test group can range from as few as 18 people to 1,500 strong. This is a remarkably low number compared to the tens of thousands being unwittingly tested with a drug, once it has received a license. Some tests are aborted early and the drug is assumed to be effective and safe if the test response seems particularly favorable, as it did with the anti-AIDS drug AZT, which was later discounted as preventive medicine in the Concorde tests after it had been handed out to thousands who were HIV-positive but still healthy as "prevention."[3]

In the United Kingdom, the antiarthritis drug Opren was tested at the usual dose on only 116 people, mostly for less than three weeks. On the basis of this information, plus some trials in the United States, a license was granted in the United Kingdom (whereas the Food and Drug Administration decided to wait for the results of further tests). As it turned out, to date over 4,000 Britons, many elderly, have contacted the Opren Action Group alleging some injury, mainly persistent increased sensitivity to light; eighty-three deaths have been associated with the drug. The drug was withdrawn in 1982.

There is immense pressure on the drug company to produce a successful trial. By the time a drug is ready to be tested on humans, it may have been researched and developed for a decade or more, costing the company as much as $250 million. This none-too-subtle pressure is one factor in what is becoming a wealth of poorly performed drug testing. The Food and Drug Administration has discovered "serious deficiencies" in 11 percent of all clinical trials in the United States. A recent review in the prestigious *Science* magazine found that the conclusions reached by researchers are often flawed by the most basic errors in design and analysis. Besides failing to randomize subjects properly, the researchers often scour their data and divide it into smaller and smaller subgroups in order to come up with the desired result. They're also often guilty of removing data from their analysis or substituting misleading numbers, again in order to come up with the "right" conclusion.[4] "Much poor research arises because researchers feel compelled for career reasons to carry out research that they are ill equipped to perform, and nobody stops them," wrote Douglas G. Altman, head of the Medical Statistics Laboratory of the Imperial Cancer Research Fund.[5]

DATA TORTURE

An even larger potential problem is fraud, or "data torture," its newest euphemism. No one knows the exact extent of fraud in medical research, but approximately 40 percent of the deans of the major U.S. graduate schools say they know of confirmed cases of scientific misconduct occurring in their own institutions within the last five years. More than one-quarter of the scientists surveyed by the American Association for the Advancement of Sciences admitted that they had personally encountered at least two instances of research that they suspected was falsified, fabricated, or plagiarized in the previous decade.[6] Because many journals don't employ a statistical "referee" to review a paper before it is published, it is relatively easy to get a fraudulent study into print.

For twenty years, U.S. congressional committees have been occupied with investigating the recurrent problem of fraud in research. A shudder recently went through the medical community about fraud, sparked by the U.S. lumpectomy trials, where Dr. Roger Poisson of St. Luc Hospital in Montreal fiddled with data and included women who blatantly should have been disqualified. When found out, it transpired that Dr. Poisson was misguidedly acting from the best of motives; he felt that the largest number of his patients "deserved the best treatment." To ensure this, he fabricated a wealth of data, including information on the size of their tumors. However, his actions betray an inability, typical among many in medicine, to act as an impartial scientific judge without fear or favor: he already believed a certain course to be the best one, and manipulated his data to support his beliefs.[7]

Fraud and misconduct are so rife that even a number of rising stars in the scientific community have been implicated. Dr. John Darsee, noted for his research in cardiology at Harvard Medical School, was found to have published the results of a number of studies that had never in fact taken place. Dr. Stephen E. Breuning, a professor at the University of Pittsburgh, became nationally recognized for his work with the mentally retarded and for his published studies supposedly showing that mentally retarded children improved markedly when taken off certain tranquilizers. For years, Dr. Breuning crisscrossed the United States, expounding on his theories, until it was eventually discovered that much of his data had never existed, or his subjects ever been tested. Eventually Dr. Breuning pleaded guilty to two felonies and served time in a halfway house prison. Nevertheless, even after his public exposure a number of scientific journals attempted to prevent his coauthors from publicly retracting the results of articles in which he'd been involved.[8]

Now, in the computer era, fraud may be even more difficult to detect. The fraud squad of the FDA used to be able to inspect the actual raw data in paper notebooks and lab reports. But these days, digital imaging allows scientists to "clean up" their data by means of electronic cameras, which record even the most elementary cell slides. In this digital format, the image can be changed to match whatever outcome the researcher is hoping to achieve.[9]

Even if done properly, drug tests are usually short term, demonstrating only either short-term safety or benefits. It is only after the drugs are released and studied in people like you and me (if, indeed, that happens) that drug companies get a picture of how safe or dangerous a drug really is. As Sir William Asscher, former chairman of the Committee on Safety of Medicines, put it, "by the time a drug is licensed, we really know very little in the case of a new chemical entity about its possible risks."[10] And America has a highly inadequate adverse events reporting systems, reliant upon the goodwill of doctors to admit to side effects of drugs they themselves give to their patients.

Even if drugs were studied more thoroughly before being tried out on patients, most drug approaches to treating illness take the nature of a giant experiment. For all the big chronic problems—asthma, psoriasis, arthritis, eczema—drug treatment is given largely on a suck-it-and-see (or inhale-it-and-see) basis, ending up with the patient taking a medicine cabinet of drugs whose side effects range from blindness, cancer, and mental disorders to death. This sort of approach usually indicates that your doctor is hoping that, by throwing a load of drugs at a problem, it may eventually go away.

TOO MUCH OF A GOOD THING

The problem with antibiotics is a problem often seen in medicine, the philosophy of excess: If one is good, two must be twice as good, and what works in an emergency must be doubly good for your everyday ailment. Study after study in the medical literature of the last decade points to massive and incorrect overuse of antibiotics. A 1981 audit of antibiotic use in the United States, published in the *Review of Infectious Diseases,* claimed that in half of all cases where antibiotics were prescribed, the medical condition didn't warrant them, or the prescribing doctor prescribed the wrong drug, the wrong dosage, or the incorrect duration for taking the drug. In Britain, these prescribing habits were paralleled in two studies published in *The Wrong Kind of Medicine?* (Hodder & Stoughton) by Charles Medawar, director of the consumer organization Social Audit, which showed that antibiotic use in three British hospitals was inappropriate in about two-thirds of cases.[11]

The fact is, in the overwhelming majority of cases, antibiotics are prescribed for conditions they cannot treat. In 97 percent of cases, antibiotics are given for viral ear, nose, and throat problems or for what is assumed to be cystitis but may only be thrush—conditions which, in most cases, do not respond to antibiotics.[12] In the doctor's office, reckons allergy specialist Dr. John Mansfield, in "three out of four instances" antibiotics are used as "placebos": to "cure" such things as colds. In 1983, more than half of the more than 32 million Americans who saw doctors for treatment of the common cold were unnecessarily given a prescription for an antibiotic. But, as any medical student knows, viral infections (the cause of colds and flu) do not respond to antibiotics.

Besides respiratory infections, the next most common use of antibiotics (about a quarter) is for childhood middle-ear infections. Although these infections (referred to as otitis media) are usually self-resolving, the rationale has always been to use the antibiotics as a just-in-case measure—in case meningitis or mastoiditis develops. In the United States, antibiotic prescriptions to children under ten more than doubled between 1977 and 1986, and now account for around half of all antibiotic pediatric prescriptions.

This meteoric rise in prescriptions for ear infections has paralleled a similar rise in the number of cases of ear infections for children under three (more than two-thirds of all American children will suffer one or more bouts of middle-ear infection). In other words, despite the wholesale attack on these infections with antibiotics, the incidence of them is rising. Except when real pain is present, there is no evidence that antibiotics do any good at all. In fact, a number of studies show that antibiotics actually make things worse. Children not given the drug tend to have fewer recurrences, compared to those given antibiotics.[13] Other research shows that in three-quarters of cases, repeated antibiotic therapy may eliminate bacteria, but not middle-ear fluid, suggesting that bacteria isn't the source of the problem.[14]

In a shocking number of cases, the doctor himself doesn't know that penicillin won't cure a cold or flu. But in many cases your doctor hands you a prescription just to get rid of you. Anyone doubting this should take a peek at the cover of the February 1, 1991, for-doctors-only *MIMS* magazine, whose cover line blares out: "Otitis Media: Can You Stop Prescribing for the Mother?"

In the inside pages, one David Grieg, a British doctor, writes:

> . . . *we often need a placebo. Yes, I really do mean need. Any mother who has sat up half the night with a crying child needs something to placate her. Any child whose excruciating earache has caused all this fuss needs a let out. Especially if it magically disappears as they reach the doctor's [office].*[15]

Even if a doctor believes an antibiotic is truly necessary, he usually prescribes it before he knows for sure. In most instances, the doctor might take a lab sample of the suspected infection, but he'll also hand the patient a course of antibiotics to start immediately. The patient could be halfway through the course before he discovers he's taken the wrong drug, or taken it for no reason.

This makes sense in life-threatening cases where a patient might be dead in the thirty-six or seventy-two hours required to get results back from the lab, but not with more benign problems, particularly when clinical diagnoses so often are wrong. In only half of all so-called cases of true cystitis, for instance, are *Escherichia coli* bacteria, the cause of true cystitis, actually present, says Professor Ian Phillips, a microbiologist at London's St. Thomas Hospital.[16]

Hospitals also tend to overuse antibiotics as a just-in-case measure for surgical patients "in case" they develop infections during surgery. "For instance, it's known that antibiotics are helpful during surgery of the large bowel to prevent infection," says Phillips. "This gets extrapolated into completely clean surgery like hysterectomies or appendectomies where there is no clear indication," he says. Hospitals even routinely administer antibiotics to premature newborns, "just in case" they fall prey to bacteria.

Up till now, doctors haven't worried about overprescribing because they figured the drugs do little harm to patients other than perhaps a little tummy upset. Only 5 percent of the population was thought to be seriously allergic to penicillin.

But a glance at the *British National Formulary* reveals many potentially crippling side effects of antibiotics: Prolonged use of neomycin to treat liver disease can cause the liver to malfunction; tetracycline can permanently stain a child's teeth yellow; chloramphenicol can interfere with the bone marrow's production of red blood cells and cause irreversible, potentially fatal bone-marrow depression.

Even more worrisome, repeated courses of antibiotics appear to seriously disturb our immune systems in ways that medicine doesn't yet understand. Health writer Geoffrey Cannon, author of *Superbug* (Virgin Publishing), refers to the current use of antibiotics as the "Domestos theory of human health—if there are bacteria present in the gut then they must be blasted out." Allergy specialist Dr. John Mansfield, who regularly treats immune system disorders such as candida albicans, believes that "undoubtedly the most common cause is the broad-spectrum antibiotic. Three or four courses can often push a patient over the precipice into chronic illness."

Because antibiotics wipe out good bacteria and bad, once the good bacteria in the gut are eliminated candida or one or another opportunistic yeasts or molds in the gut can overpopulate, so the theory goes. The toxins they send out can inhibit T-lymphocytes, the main search-and-destroy cells in the immune system. This in turn can weaken the body, Dr. Mansfield says, leaving it open for more serious problems: gastrointestinal or hormonal disorders, severe allergies, psoriasis, or even multiple sclerosis. Many such cases can be treated with dietary and medical management. But even if a patient is lucky enough to find a sympathetic and knowledgeable doctor, there is no guarantee that his immune system won't be permanently damaged. There are even some speculative arguments that continually stripping off the friendly bacteria and mucosa in the gut could lead to Crohn's disease and irritable bowel syndrome.

We also don't yet know the long-term effects on this generation of children, who receive many courses of antibiotics before they even reach their teens. Sally Bunday, of the Hyperactive Children's Support Group, claims her group sees a definite correlation between antibiotic use and hyperactivity among children—a relationship supported by the findings of American allergist Dr. William Crook.[17]

In Sally's case, her son was given four years' courses of antibiotics by their doctor to cure persistent catarrh. "And he was five before we had a decent night's sleep and the problem was diagnosed," she says.

Other connections have been made between overuse of antibiotics and childhood developmental problems. A nine-month survey by the Developmental Delay Registry of 800 families in the United States, most of whom have children with developmental problems, found that children who had taken more than twenty courses of antibiotics between the ages of one and twelve years were fifty percent more likely to suffer some developmental problems, from autism to speech difficulties. Conversely, children who'd been given three or fewer courses were half as likely to have developmental problems. Nearly three-quarters of the affected children had been developing normally up until the age of one. The affected children were far more likely to have had ear infections or to have had grommets placed, which gives added credence to the antibiotics link because so many pediatricians use the drug to treat the condition.[18]

Sally experienced this with her child, Luke:

> *Our son was using about a dozen words by seventeen months.*
> *Then he fell ill with a respiratory infection and was prescribed*
> *the antibiotic amoxycillin. Suddenly Luke lost his vocabulary.*
> *In fact, he did not speak again for almost eight years.*

Sally attended a medical conference two years later, at which doctors reported observing children between the ages of one and two regressing, losing their speech, and developing signs of withdrawal and behavioral problems after being administered antibiotics. Antibiotics have also been linked with hearing loss in children. In developing countries, up to two-thirds of hearing loss among children is reckoned to be caused by the indiscriminate use of antibiotics such as streptomycin and gentamicin.[19]

More worrisome, antibiotic overuse may possibly even lead to illnesses such as diabetes. Dr. Lisa Landymore-Lim of Australia, while studying for her chemistry doctorate, decided to examine all patients with diabetes whose disease was diagnosed before age twenty-three. She discovered that the more antibiotics a child was exposed to, either in the uterus or at the beginning of his life, the more likely he was to develop diabetes at an early age.[20] In one of many similar cases, a six-year-old who'd ended up developing diabetes had been given amoxycillin five times before his first birthday, twice during his second year, and three more times during his third and fourth years. Besides nine other course of antibiotics, he received cephalosporin, antihistamines, a powerful antivomiting drug, and one for gastrointestinal spasms, and Bactrim, a very potent antibiotic. This sort of revolving-door prescribing for children is becoming virtually commonplace today.

Repeated courses of antibiotics only encourage the development of supergerms in your body that will resist treatment from the antibiotics, so that when you really need the drug, it won't work. This kind of "transfer resistance" can also affect the population at large, as it has with gonorrhea and staphylococcus infections. A moderate course of penicillin used to cure both these diseases easily. Now it takes two giant doses of penicillin, often in combination with another antibiotic, to do the job. In some parts of Africa and in the Philippines, penicillin won't work at all.

Resistance rates of the staph germ have been isolated in hospitals in Athens, where antibiotics are enthusiastically prescribed, and have been found to have increased in a single year by about 50 percent to all drugs but penicillin, where resistance was already at 80 percent.[21]

ASTHMA DRUGS

Despite greater diagnostic skills, better identification of the causes of the disease, and ever more sophisticated drug cocktails with which to treat it, doctors and asthma associations are stymied by the fact that the epidemic incidence of asthma and asthma-related deaths continues to go up. The latest U.S. figures compiled by the government, which analyzed data for 1982–92, show that the annual death rate for asthma in young people between the ages of five and thirty-four has increased a whopping 40 percent, to over 5,000 deaths per year.[22]

These days, it's difficult to determine whether the disease or the "cure" is responsible for killing off patients. Beta-agonists administered by a metered-dose inhaler, specifically albuterol and fenoterol, have been associated with an increased risk of death or near death.[23] The marked rise in asthma deaths during the 1960s in many countries coincided with the introduction of high-strength isoprenaline inhalers.[24] When the inhalers were withdrawn, mortality fell to previous levels. But the problems haven't been due just to beta2-agonists. In many countries a rise in asthma deaths occurred in the 1980s, particularly in New Zealand, which two studies showed was linked to the popularity of fenoterol, a type of beta2-agonist, but also oral steroids and theophylline, another type of asthma drug.[25]

Regular inhalation of beta2-agonists has also been shown to cause "hyperresponsiveness"—that is, excessive constriction of the bronchi,[26] and potentially fatal abnormal heartbeats, or the spread of the allergen to more remote airways, thus increasing inflammation or even causing the bronchial muscles to constrict to a fatal degree.[27]

Over time, these drugs may also make the disease worse. In one study, patients receiving fenoterol four times a day had worse outcomes after six months than those given inhaled drugs only as needed.[28] Regular use of certain beta2-agonists also causes a greater decline in lung function than does "on-demand" use.[29] And some patients have had symptoms improve once doses of inhaled beta2-agonists were reduced.

Inhalers such as Ventolin have many established side effects, including sudden lowering of blood pressure, swelling around the heart, and collapse. Allen and Hanburys, Ltd., the manufacturer of Ventolin, also warns doctors that the drug often has a "paradoxical effect"—that is, it causes bronchospasms, the very situation it is meant to prevent.[30]

Deaths from asthma are often due to very high doses of drugs from inhalers. In a recent Canadian study, asthmatics who inhaled thirteen or more canisters of fenoterol in a year increased their risk of dying *ninety times*. As for salbutamol, those who used twenty-five or more annual doses in smaller-sized canisters were forty times more likely to die.[31] Although both doses far exceed the recommended limit, asthmatics can grow very dependent on inhalers, reaching for them at the first sign of shortness of breath.

In fact, the risk of death begins to increase dramatically when only 1.4 canisters a month of inhaled beta-agonists are used, particularly among users of fenoterol.[32] The new long-lasting, high-potency beta2-agonists such as salmeterol (Serevent), which control asthma symptoms for twelve hours at a puff, could also exacerbate the problem.

STEROIDS

Steroids are fast catching up with antibiotics as the most abused class of drugs in your doctor's black bag. There's no doubt that the discovery of steroids half a century ago was a major advance in medicine—a lifesaver for those like the late President John F. Kennedy, who suffered from Addison's disease, a disease of the adrenal glands causing insufficient hormone production. Steroids mimic the action of the adrenal glands, the body's most powerful regulators of general metabolism. John Stirling, director of the vitamin company Biocare, credits a very short course (three injections) of steroids with jump-starting his failing adrenal system after anaphylactic shock, thereby saving his life.

The problem is, like antibiotics, steroids appear to be a miracle "cure." Patients with crippling arthritis or asthma seem to be instantly better on steroids. The wheeze, the swelling, the pain go away. So doctors turn to steroids as the first, rather than last, line of attack for their anti-inflammatory and antiallergic effects.

As with antibiotics, what was once reserved for the extreme emergency is now being used on the most trivial of conditions. Steroids are now handed out as readily as antibiotics, even to babies, at the first sign of inflammation of any sort. In Europe, the latest drug set to replace more benign, over-the-counter remedies for babies with croup is a steroid (budesonide); hydrocortisone is included in the latest over-the-counter medication for hemorrhoids. Steroids make up many over-the-counter skin drugs, and are considered the drug of choice for asthma, eczema, arthritis, back problems, bowel problems such as ulcerative colitis—indeed, for any and all inflammations or allergic reactions—and new uses are still being invented. The sole exception is Addison's disease, where steroids act as a replacement therapy to cortisone, much as insulin is given to diabetics.

Far from being a wonder drug "cure all," steroids cannot cure one single condition. All they do is suppress your body's ability to express a normal response. In a few instances, this type of suppression will give the body a chance to heal itself. But more often, the effect is immediate, devastating, and permanently damaging. And we are only now realizing just how quickly damage can occur. Doctors have always assumed that patients can only suffer side effects after long-term use. However, we are lately discovering that *there is no such thing as a safe dose*. Permanent debilitating damage can occur weeks after you've begun treatment, even on low doses. A randomized, double-blind, placebo-controlled study conducted in the Netherlands showed that prednisone has a major effect on the bone mineral density of the lumbar spine. Those patients taking only 10 milligrams of prednisone (prednisolone in the United Kingdom) daily suffered a decrease in bone density of 8 percent after only five months of using steroids. Once the patients were off the drugs, their bone density increased somewhat, but not to pretreatment levels. This bone loss was considered comparable to that suffered by women who had had their ovaries removed.

The level of bone loss was similar to that reported at much higher doses of the drugs, which suggests that when it comes to dosage, more is not necessarily any more dangerous than less. The Dutch researchers concluded that "the use of prednisone should be limited as much as possible to short periods of time."[33]

Even low doses of inhaled steroids (400 micrograms per day) reduce bone formation.[34] Rub-on steroids have caused Cushing's syndrome in children as soon as a month after treatment has begun[35] and inhaled steroids slow growth in children after six weeks.[36]

Although steroids are used for virtually all types of inflammatory and autoimmune illnesses, they have not been subjected to long-term scientific study to find out how or whether they work for specific conditions. Septic shock and adult respiratory distress syndrome are two conditions for which steroids were widely used as treatment—until scientific trials demonstrated that they were not only of no benefit, but may actually have been doing harm.[37]

Unlike with antibiotics, steroids are *all* broad-spectrum—that is, they don't affect simply the area of the body you wish to treat, but scatter their effects through every cell: the central nervous system, cells in the bone, smooth muscle, blood, liver, and a number of other organs of the body.[38] Doctors have been trying to rearrange the chemistry of cortisone to make it more specific to certain parts of the body, but so far this goal has proved elusive.[39]

Doctors seem to have a particular blind spot about these drugs, oblivious to the terrible carnage that even the manufacturers admit steroids are capable of. For thirty years we've known that steroids can routinely cause overactivity of the adrenal hormones, which produces Cushing's disease, characterized by a fat abdomen and face, a "buffalo hump" in the back of the neck, high blood pressure, and muscle weakness. They can also cause muscle wasting, hyperglycemia, water retention, skin atrophy, bruising, stretch marks, insomnia, serious mood changes, symptoms of schizophrenia or manic depression ("steroid psychosis"), osteoporosis, cataracts, glaucoma, menstrual problems, impotence, loss of libido, allergic shock, recurrent thrush of the mouth, and diabetes.

The Incidence of Side Effects

The British association GASP (Group Against Steroid Prescriptions) recently polled its 15,000 members to document just how common these side effects are. In their study, they discovered that at least 70 percent or more of the group suffered weight gain, bruising, pain (to the back and legs—even though steroids are routinely prescribed for back pain), muscle weakness, and mood swings. Two-thirds polled complained of moon face, headaches, fluid retention, slowness in healing, thinning skin, and depression. A full half reported they'd developed osteoporosis, and the same percentage memory loss, sensitivity to light, and loss of sex drive. A third complained of buffalo hump, stretch marks and high blood pressure. Almost a quarter had cataracts, and a quarter had period problems. Others complained of psychosis, damage to the immune system, angina, and hair loss.

Most significantly, more than half the members had never been warned of these potential side effects. In another survey of 104 patients, less than two-thirds recalled receiving any advice from their doctor on potential side effects.[40]

The most worrying aspect of steroids concerns the possibility that your pituitary gland will stop producing ACTH, a hormone that regulates the adrenal glands, needed by the body during stress and to fight infections. Once you're on steroids, it can be impossible to stop.

Patients on steroids for prolonged periods can turn into steroid "junkies" unable to withdraw from taking the drugs; when the body is flooded with extra cortisone, the adrenal glands decrease their own output—sometimes to zero.

Deaths from lack of adrenal gland function have occurred when patients have switched from oral to inhaled steroids without overlapping the drugs. Doctors now know that you must gradually withdraw steroids, so the adrenals have a chance to start making cortisone on their own again. But this process is extremely slow: For patients on long-term use, it could take up to two years for the body to produce enough adrenal hormone to respond to extra stress from an illness or an accident. Surgeons often give steroids to such patients before operations, but this means that weaning has to begin all over again.

Doctors also sometimes maintain that if you inhale or rub on steroids, you are less likely to suffer side effects. But new evidence shows that inhaled steroids are not as harmless as previously supposed. The consensus up until now has been that beclomethasone dipropionate (BDP) of 400 to 800 micrograms daily is appropriate for the three- to five-year-old age group. However, a group of pediatric consultants from various hospitals in Britain showed that this dose was every bit as powerful as 200 times more of the oral variety (80 to 160 milligrams) in suppressing the adrenal and pituitary glands.[41] This dosage has also produced significant growth retardation in children.

Steroids in Children

The use of steroids in children is difficult to justify. For thirty years we've known that prolonged use for asthma and eczema retards growth in children[42] and delays puberty. Many studies of children with juvenile chronic arthritis given steroids show they suffer growth retardation.[43] Children given topical and inhaled steroids are prone to the same side effects, such as stunted growth and adrenal suppression.[44]

Steroids may also affect a child's cognitive performance. In one study, where children on combination steroid drugs were given tests of visual retention association, the performance of children on the drugs (some six to eight hours after receiving steroid medication) was significantly worse than that of a group of nonasthmatics. Although these differences disappeared a day or so after the medication was given, they may nevertheless be constant for those children permanently on the drugs.[45]

Evidence also suggests that topical and inhaled steroids can cause cataracts and glaucoma, ordinarily only associated with oral steroids.[46]

Bone mineral density has also been found to be lower with children the longer they stay on steroids.[47] And even inhaled drugs for such diseases as asthma are found to have adverse effects on bone metabolism and adrenal function at higher dosages (more than 1,000 micrograms per day).[48] Steroids can even cause death of the mass of bone (osteonecrosis), necessitating joint replacement.[49]

Even with the so-called dramatic effects on such crippling conditions as rheumatoid arthritis, new research demonstrates that these anti-inflammatory effects appear to wear off in time, leaving sufferers worse off than before. Patients at the Royal University Hospital in Saskatchewan, Canada, taking prednisone (1 to 23 milligrams) for an average of 6.9 years, had similar rheumatoid arthritis symptoms (joint swelling, reduced mobility) after five years to those who'd never taken the drug. After ten years, the condition of the group on prednisone was *worse* than the nondrug group, with increased fractures and cataracts.[50]

Medicine has even turned this state of affairs into a syndrome, called "steroid-resistant asthma," which includes patients who don't respond to normal doses of cortisone and in whom the drug, in some cases, makes the asthma worse.

Many otherwise benign infections become life-threatening in children on steroids. In the summer of 1992, nine-year-old Lexie McConnell was diagnosed as having toxoplasmosis. Although there was no imminent danger of the disease affecting her sight, and the illness might have resolved itself, it was affecting an area near Lexie's retina and, in the view of her doctor, ought to be treated. Her father Art explains:

> Within twenty-four hours of commencing steroid treatment, Lexie was deeply ill with side effects; immediately her face ballooned. We were told that she should lead a normal life, so we sent her to school, and swimming, although she was often too ill to stay. By November, she had put on an enormous amount of weight and had terrible pains, holes in her tongue and black stools, which we later found out indicated internal bleeding.
>
> Finally, when she was in excruciating pain, we took her to the hospital. After many hours, she was eventually found to have chicken pox. The doctors also mentioned that she could have had a disseminated herpes simplex infection.

It was only then that Art and his wife learned that the drugs had basically left Lexie without an immune system and that she could die from anything, even a cold sore.

"By Saturday, she went into intensive care and lost consciousness," says her dad. "An hour later, she died."

Drugs for Eczema

With eczema—another illness doctors don't understand—physicians reach for one or another powerful drug to stamp out the inflammation, but not the problem. The drugs of choice are steroids, the immune-suppressant cyclosporine, or even oral psoralen photochemotherapy (oral PUVA), a treatment option for psoriasis that is linked with genital cancer.[51]

As with inhaled steroids, rub-on steroids have long been touted as the "safe alternative" to systemic steroids, but there's little evidence to back this up. Increasingly, topical steroids are showing themselves to be every bit as dangerous as their orally delivered cousins. Rub-on corticosteroids can produce an array of serious skin problems,[52] damage bones and organs,[53] and cause permanent adrenal suppression.[54] They've also been implicated in Cushing's syndrome in children, as soon as a month after treatment, and, like the oral variety, may impair the responses of the pituitary and adrenal glands, thus requiring yet more (oral) steroids during illness or trauma.[55]

Like asthmatics, children with eczema are prone to the side effects of long-term use of steroids, such as stunted growth and adrenal disease.[56] One child covered with eczema from head to foot from eighteen months of age was treated once a day from age six with a layer of betamethasone ointment over his entire body; by age thirteen, he was about nine-and-a-half inches smaller than average. Although he experienced some catch-up growth once the steroids were discontinued, he never recovered what was estimated to be his likely size.[57]

Even hydrocortisone cream, supposedly so mild it is often prescribed for babies, is known to have a myriad of side effects, including thinning of the skin, especially on the face, stretch marks, delayed healing or ulceration of wounds, suppression of the adrenal glands, and sugar in the urine.

In fact, increasing evidence is emerging to suggest that topical and inhaled steroids can cause eye damage—cataracts and glaucoma—of the kind ordinarily associated only with the use of oral steroids.[58] Cases of psychotic episodes with inhaled steroids, again assumed to be caused only by the swallowed variety, are also coming to light.[59]

ARTHRITIS DRUGS

With arthritis, medical treatment has an air of desperation. Doctors not only don't know how to sort out the problem but often make a hash of things, throwing a load of potentially lethal drugs at the condition and then prescribing new drugs to deal with the side effects caused by the "treatment." Conventional medicine tends to take the view that there is no known cause or cure for arthritis, and so all that it can do with certainty is to alleviate your pain.

The most common frontline drug for both rheumatoid and osteoarthritis used to be aspirin at high doses. This has now been virtually replaced by the "nonsteroidal anti-inflammatory drugs," or NSAIDs, as they're known in the trade. In the United States there are at least fourteen such drugs on the market; several years ago one of them (ibuprofen) got taken off the list of prescribed drugs and was made available over the counter. Increasingly doctors now turn to NSAIDs as a first port of call; in 1984, nearly one in seven Americans was treated with one of these drugs, a figure that is now grossly out of date, as they are prescribed for everything from headaches to period pains. Arthritis offers drug companies a $10 billion industry in NSAIDs alone.

These drugs mainly work by inhibiting the synthesis of prostaglandins, and thus suppressing inflammation. (They also do a number of other things, such as interfere with enzyme production, the ramifications of which we don't yet understand.) The problem is that the drugs don't just inhibit the prostaglandin that concerns your joint pain; they roadblock all formation, particularly at such high doses. Since this substance plays a major role in normal gastrointestinal function, NSAIDs, not surprisingly, interfere with it. This can result in gastric erosion, peptic-ulcer formation and perforation, major upper gastrointestinal hemorrhage, and inflammation and changes in the permeability of the intestine and lower bowel.[60]

Once you begin taking NSAIDs, you multiply by seven times your chances of being hospitalized due to gastrointestinal adverse effects.[61] These statistics could be very conservative; the Food and Drug Administration's own best estimate is that 200,000 cases of gastric bleeding occur each year, with 10,000 to 20,000 deaths. In the United Kingdom, some 4,000 people die each year from taking NSAIDs—twice the number of deaths from asthma.

The elderly, or those with a history of peptic ulcers, are at particular risk. The FDA now places a warning on each NSAID prescription: "Serious gastrointestinal toxicity such as bleeding, ulceration, and perforation can occur at any time, with or without warning symptoms, in patients treated chronically with NSAID therapy."

With or without warning symptoms. Because NSAIDs reduce pain, particularly at high doses, they also often mask any indication that something is wrong. For many patients, the first sign that they have an ulcer is a life-threatening complication.

Besides ulcers, even the "safest" of NSAIDs, ibuprofen, can cause colitis; the drugs indomethacin, Naproxen, and a sustained-release preparation of ketoprofen may cause perforations of the colon.[62] Because these drugs decrease the mucosal prostaglandins, they may cause a leaky gut, resulting in an increased susceptibility to toxins passing through—a recipe for conditions like colitis.[63]

NSAIDs can also cause blurred or diminished vision, Parkinson's disease, and hair and fingernail loss; they can also damage the liver and kidneys. Doctors from several medical centers, including New York's Beth Israel and Harvard Medical School in Boston, reported seven cases of "significant hepatitis" and one death from diclofenac (Voltaren), although they didn't know whether this drug was alone in causing these problems or whether any of the others could as well.[64]

Arthritis patients taking NSAIDs have had false-positive results in tests for hepatitis, indicating possible damage to the liver.[65]

NSAIDs can also increase the risk of high blood pressure (hypertension), especially if taken in large doses. In one study, of nearly 10,000 patients in Boston, who'd recently started on medication to lower their blood pressure, 41 percent were found to have been taking NSAIDs during the previous year. These results showed that NSAIDs more than doubled a patient's odds of developing hypertension.[66]

Colitis and Crohn's disease remain mysteries to most doctors. One likely cause still unrecognized by most gastroenterologists is the link between nonsteroidal anti-inflammatories and the development of these diseases, even though NSAIDs are well known to injure the mucosa of the colon and to cause ulcers. Of the sixty new cases of colitis and colon problems seen between March 1991 and June 1994 at the General Hospital in Jersey, the British Channel island, twenty-three (or 38 percent) had developed while the patient was taking an NSAID. None of those twenty-three patients had a preexisting inflammatory bowel disease.

Although a large number of NSAIDs were implicated, diclofenac and mefenamic acid were the most common culprits. The drugs had usually been taken orally, but even the rectal and intramuscular variety caused colitis within a few days of therapy.

In some instances, the colitis was mild and would rapidly improve once the drug was withdrawn and yet another drug such as sulfasalazine or mesalazine (mesalamine in the United States) was administered. But some patients developed full-blown ulcerative colitis, requiring systemic and topical steroids, and one needed to have his colon surgically removed after developing toxic megacolon in the wake of intramuscular doses of diclofenac.[67]

For all their side effects, NSAIDs have no advantage over simple analgesics such as aspirin or Tylenol (acetaminophen). In one study, large (2,400-milligram) and small (1,200-milligram) daily doses of ibuprofen worked just about as well as high daily doses (4,000 milligrams) of acetaminophen in controlling pain and inflammation.[68]

Besides using NSAIDs for inflammation and pain, doctors try to treat arthritis with what are called the antirheumatic drugs or slow-acting, antirheumatic drugs (SAARDs). The hope (for that is all it is) is that SAARDs will act to stop whatever autoimmune destruction is going on. In every case, treating is a decidedly hit-and-miss affair, with doctors stumbling upon something that seems to work in the course of treating something else. Many of these drugs are powerful immunosuppressants and cell-blockers, such as sulfasalazine, gold, antimalarial drugs, derivatives of penicillin, chemotherapy, and drugs used during transplant operations and developed to treat more serious and life-threatening conditions. Specialists do not understand how SAARDs work—if and when they do—but accept they can be highly toxic and even life-threatening.[69] Lack of research into their long-term effects means the patient has to play a game of Russian roulette to discover whether he will develop symptoms from the "cure" that are worse than the condition he's being treated for.

Even after suffering any reaction, the patient may be no better off. The benefits have seldom been put to proper, long-term scientific scrutiny. One of the few double-blind studies that tested the second-line treatments against a placebo among 3,439 arthritis patients concluded that the benefits of the drugs were uncertain.[70]

Gold is the traditional, and favored, SAARD, even described by some rheumatologists as "the gold standard"—a surprising title for a highly toxic treatment that can lead to fatal bone-marrow suppression.[71] As it has been administered since the 1920s, it is staggering that there has never been a long-term trial to test for reactions.

It became the treatment of choice only because researchers misunderstood the causes of arthritis. German bacteriologist Robert Koch had shown that gold and other heavy metals could fight tuberculosis and other infectious diseases. As it was believed arthritis was an infection, the theory was that gold could treat it as well. Even though we've known differently for a long time, no one in medicine has stopped to question the use of this treatment.

If you're having this drug injected, as is typical, your doctor should be monitoring you carefully for early side effects such as skin rashes and mouth sores. More serious side effects include kidney problems and bone-marrow suppression. Because of these concerns, gold tablets were developed. Early studies show they cause fewer side effects than injections,[72] but also don't work as well.[73] About a third of patients suffer side effects severe enough to stop the treatment.[74] In fact, gold is considered so toxic that many specialists are turning to methotrexate—originally developed as a cancer drug—as the safer option![75]

In the wrong hands, however, methotrexate is a potential killer, causing liver and kidney damage, lung disease, and bone-marrow suppression.[76] Although improvements have been noted in between 30 and 70 percent of patients,[77] the typical side effects of stomach complaints, nausea, and anorexia can worsen dramatically if the dose is increased or the drug mixed with another. Damage to the liver and lungs has been reported,[78] as has death among arthritis patients on high doses, especially if the patient takes the dose daily instead of weekly.[79]

Even sulfasalazine, from the family of cytotoxic drugs that block the growth of cells, has gotten in on the act, although it can suppress bone marrow and cause infertility, cancer, or birth defects.[80]

DRUGS FOR HYPERTENSION

Hypertension is another area where a mountainous concoction of drugs rarely does any good against a condition that can usually be cured with judicious diet and exercise. Doctors have plowed through a variety of drug treatments—diuretics, beta- and calcium channel-blockers, reserpine, clonidine, methyldopa—without apparent success. In the United States, only a fifth of patients on drugs managed to reach what are considered modest blood-pressure goals (less than 140 mm Hg systolic and less than 90 mm Hg diastolic) set by the U.S. Nutritional and Health Examination Survey.[81] In England, a study of 2,000 patients with high blood pressure from thirteen general practices in England showed that only a little more than half of those taking drugs for hypertension had achieved what is considered even a moderately healthy level.[82] As for Europe, in a survey of 12,000 patients across five countries, only a third managed to achieve the blood-pressure target set by their doctors.[83]

If there isn't much evidence that blood-pressure drugs do much good, there's plenty to show they do great harm. One particularly worrisome side effect is hypotension—or a sudden drop in blood pressure when one stands up—which can cause dizziness and falls.

Hypertensive drugs are also the major cause of hip fractures among senior citizens.[84] Although all varieties of blood pressure drugs have been implicated in various disorders—depression, sexual dysfunction, tiredness, and appetite disturbances—diuretics (supposedly the "safe" blood-pressure drugs) have been shown to cause an eleven-fold increase in diabetes,[85] beta-blockers may be one cause of cancer deaths in elderly men,[86] ACE inhibitors can cause potentially fatal kidney damage[87] or death if given too soon after a heart attack,[88] and calcium channel-blockers have been linked to severe skin conditions such as Stevens-Johnson syndrome.[89] Doctors even use these drugs to treat women with hypertension during pregnancy, in spite of the fact that beta-blockers are thought to have a harmful effect on fetal circulation,[90] and ACE inhibitors to damage or kill the developing fetus if given during the second or third trimesters of pregnancy.[91]

Beta-blockers may even affect certain kinds of memory. A team at the University of California at Irvine divided a healthy group of volunteers into two subgroups, giving one propranolol and the other a placebo an hour before they were shown slides that told two stories. Tests taken just before the stories were shown demonstrated that all the drug takers were fully beta-blocked.

The first story factually told in pictures the scene of a child visiting his father's workplace with his mother. The second, however, was designed to arouse strong emotions; on the way to the workplace, the child was hit by a car and badly injured. A week after seeing these images, when all the subjects were given a surprise memory test, both groups showed similar results when recounting the first story. However, the propranolol group had significantly worse recall of the second, emotionally charged story.[92]

Although the study examined the effect of a single dose of beta-blocker on healthy subjects, rather than on heart or migraine patients, animal studies have demonstrated that memory of emotionally charged events requires activating the beta-adrenergic systems, which of course are blocked by beta-blocking drugs.

COMBINATION HEART DRUGS

Most doctors think if one drug does some good, then two will double the benefits. The beta-blocker/calcium channel-blocker combination has become very popular for patients with coronary artery disease. The thinking behind this is that a low dose of the two drugs will decrease the number and severity of attacks of angina (pain around the heart during exertion) more effectively than a high dose of one of the drugs alone, and with fewer side effects. Since many factors influence the balance between the supply of oxygen to the heart and its demands, and a single drug can only counter a few of these factors, doctors have simply assumed that a second heart drug with different chemical actions might work in a complementary fashion. Because drugs for angina often cause rebound circulatory effects, which work against their effectiveness, the other assumption has been that these unwanted effects can be counteracted by a second drug. However, these two assumptions have never stood up to scientific scrutiny. According to one review of the results of a number of controlled clinical trials, combining a calcium channel-blocker with a low-dose beta-blocker rarely has any additional benefits for angina patients, and can increase adverse reactions by up to 60 percent.[93]

The other problem is that most doctors don't really understand how each of these drugs relieves angina on its own. Beta-blockers work by blocking the receptors in the heart from receiving impulses from chemicals released during effort, or stress. Because this action inhibits the rise in heart rate and blood pressure during exertion, it has always been assumed that the drugs relieve angina and other symptoms of coronary artery disease by decreasing heart-oxygen demand. Because electrical impulses from the heart (which control the contraction and relaxation that occur with every beat) are channeled through calcium ions, calcium channel-blockers—which work to slow down these electrical instructions—theoretically slow down your heartbeat. They also help to dilate arteries, increasing the flow of blood and supposedly easing the work the heart has to do to pump blood through the body. Consequently, many doctors have operated under the assumption that calcium-blockers relieve areas in the body with blocked blood vessels by increasing the supply of oxygen to the heart. This notion—that beta-blockers and calcium-blockers somehow work in tandem by increasing heart oxygen supply and lowering demand—is behind the strong support among the medical community for their combined use. However, both drugs actually alleviate angina through strikingly similar effects—including reducing the heart's oxygen consumption, limiting the rise in heart rate, redistributing the blood flow from the heart, and relaxing the blood vessels.

In fact, recent observations show that the two drugs don't necessarily interact well together. Although calcium-blockers can stop the arterial constriction in the heart caused by beta-blockers, this may only occur in areas of the body with normal blood flow, and may only further reduce blood flow in those areas of the heart already under threat. By the same token, while beta-blockers may prevent the rapid heart rate induced by calcium-blockers, this may do nothing to prevent the lowered blood pressure calcium-blockers frequently cause. Calcium-blockers may even worsen angina if blood pressure falls markedly.

In many other ways, the two operate antagonistically. Beta-blockers can increase the lowering effect on blood pressure of the calcium-blockers, and so increase the risk of poor blood supply to the heart. The combination can also exacerbate angina if the two drugs combine to cause rapid heartbeat. Beta-blockers can also cancel out the ability of calcium-blockers to relax the blood vessels. Abnormally low blood pressure, causing dizziness and sudden falls, worsening heart failure, and conduction defects (that is, problems with electrical instructions from the brain) may occur more often during combination therapy than with single drug therapy.[94]

Presently, American doctors have been warned to stop prescribing the calcium channel-blocker nifedipine. The National Heart, Lung and Blood Institute has warned doctors that shortacting nifedipine "should be used with great caution, if at all." The warning is based on the study of sixteen scientific trials of short-acting nifedipine involving more than 8,000 patients.

The risk of dying increased with the dosage; the mortality risk is 1.06 times greater than the average with dosages of between 30 and 50 milligrams a day, increasing to nearly three times greater when the daily dose is 80 milligrams. Another study the Institute considered showed that patients on calcium channel-blockers were 60 percent more likely to suffer a heart attack than those taking either diuretics or beta-blockers. Nifedipine was found to be the most dangerous of the calcium channel-blockers.[95]

DRUGS FOR EPILEPSY

With such a spectacular array of drug therapy at their fingertips, doctors aren't particularly good at doing nothing—at adopting a wait-and-see attitude, to see if a condition clears up by itself. Although medicine these days claims to be more cautious about automatically handing out anticonvulsant drugs to children with mild blackouts and seizures, the conventional wisdom among most doctors is still that, unless suppressed by drug treatment, epileptic seizures will recur, and that drug treatment can affect the course of the disease, reducing the risk of early epilepsy turning into an intractable disorder.

The problem is that epilepsy is hopelessly overdiagnosed. Experts at Birmingham Children's Hospital in Birmingham, Great Britain, concluded that about half the cases of so-called juvenile epilepsy are wrongly diagnosed.[96] This is significant, as more than half of the 340,000 cases of chronic epilepsy in Britain are believed to have begun in childhood. Dr. Michael Prendergast, child psychiatrist at Birmingham Children's Hospital, examined 311 children referred to the hospital for suspected or diagnosed epilepsy and discovered that 138 of them (44 percent) didn't actually have it. His results are nearly identical to those of a Scottish study completed in 1896 by the Royal Hospital for Sick Children in Glasgow. In that study, Dr. John Stephenson, the hospital's pediatric neurologist, found that 47 percent of the children referred there did not in fact have epilepsy.

Jacqui, now thirty-six, was diagnosed as having epilepsy when she was eleven after suffering several blackouts. She was immediately placed on anticonvulsants, although the first convulsion didn't appear until *after* she'd been on the drugs. She has spent years battling the myriad of drug side effects, including blackouts and convulsions. From 1988, when she began reducing the dosage of the drugs she was taking, her seizures have correspondingly dropped in number, from 200 to several dozen a year.

David Chadwick, professor of neurology at the Walton Centre for Neurology and Neurosurgery in Liverpool, Great Britain, argues that epilepsy is an umbrella term referring to a group of disorders and not a single, homogeneous disease. In some cases of epilepsy, such as "benign rolandic epilepsy" in children, where seizures (affecting only the face, throat, and arm) occur only during sleep, there is strong evidence that the seizures stop by themselves by midadolescence. Furthermore, the preliminary data suggesting that people are better off getting drugs as early treatment is far from "definitive."[97]

Among the very few longer-term studies examining which factors predicted at least a five-year seizure-free remission, one found that developing epilepsy before age sixteen and having no evidence of brain damage, tonic-clonic (grand mal) seizures, or spike wave abnormalities on an electroencephalogram (EEC) were all factors that tended to favor remission, whether or not drugs were given.[98] (It should be noted that David Chadwick says the situation is very different with other forms of epilepsy, such as juvenile myoclonic epilepsy, where patients who've had grand mal seizures have a high probability of relapse if the drugs are withdrawn. In this group, epilepsy drugs can be lifesaving.)

It's very difficult to know whether drugs given early make any difference, because untreated epileptics are difficult to find. But those studies that have been performed suggest that drugs make virtually no difference. In one, after twenty years half the group not on drugs had gone into "remission." This is an equivalent percentage of those who go into remission after years of taking drugs.[99] Similarly, in a group of patients in Africa and others in Ecuador whose treatment was delayed, six-month remission rates were the same as they were in populations given early drug treatment.[100]

New evidence shows that children who suffer their first-ever seizure are no worse off for having any treatment delayed to see if a second seizure occurs. Delaying treatment does not reduce the chances of controlling the seizures later, nor does it affect possible remission when the child grows. The only advantage of starting immediate treatment is that it can delay the next seizure, but doctors and parents who insist on it after the very first attack will never know if it was going to be the only one.[101]

Much evidence about early treatment suggests that patients taking drugs may actually be worse off. In one study, patients with seizures after a head injury who took the epilepsy drug phenytoin had more seizures than those taking a placebo.[102] In a recent Italian study comparing patients on a drug against those on a sugar pill, although the treatment group supposedly runs only half the risk of having a further seizure, thus far there has been no difference between the two groups in terms of remission time.[103]

Doctors really don't have enough information to encourage early treatment with certainty, particularly as all epileptic drug treatment carries a host of potentially lethal effects. In one recent study, side effects were so serious that nearly a quarter of patients on phenobarbital (phenobarbitone in Britain), and 11 percent of those on carbamazepine, had to be taken off the drugs.[104] In one of the first-ever medical trials to assess the safety of antiepilepsy drugs on children, 9 percent of children given phenobarbitone to treat their epilepsy had to come off it because of the serious side effects they suffered. The researchers, from King's College Hospital in London, found a similar problem with phenytoin, and at least 4 percent of children reacted to either valproic acid or carbamazepine.[105]

Indeed, all epileptic drugs are potentially lethal; the manufacturer of valproic acid (Depakene or Depakote) warns that patients on the drug have died from liver failure.

This is what may have happened to twelve-year-old Helenor

Bye, who was given valproic acid—at the time thought to be a safe drug. Her mother writes:

> Within months she started wasting away before my eyes. She was getting thinner and started hallucinating. Eventually her hair started to fall out. The doctor was convinced she was emotionally disturbed, and that she was enjoying the attention.
>
> Her condition continued to deteriorate until she was just half of her normal body weight. Still, the doctor thought she was just a spoiled child, twisting round her fingers two doting parents.
>
> After eight months, she became delirious and was rushed to the hospital. She died a few days later, weighing just three stone. She had to die to prove to them she was ill.

ANTIDEPRESSANTS

Drug treatment is also highly subject to flavor-of-the-month fads. Once doctors get enthused over a new compound that has seemingly done wonders in one area, they like to try it on every illness. The latest wonder drug is the "selective serotonin uptake inhibitor," or 5-HT drug—the active compound in Prozac.

One cause (or outcome) of depression and suicidal behavior is believed to be low levels of the brain chemical serotonin, as happens in those with lowered cholesterol levels. Prozac (or fluoxetine, its generic name) works by increasing the availability of serotonin in the brain; this is accomplished by slowing the passage of this neurohormone into nervous system cells. Prozac has been sold as an amazing improvement over the older "tricyclic antidepressants" because it is not a sedative, it does not impair thinking or physical activity, and it has fewer side effects for more patients.

Hailed in the media in the late 1980s as the breakthrough for depression we've all been waiting for, Prozac quickly became America's bestselling antidepressive and, after the sell-out publication of Listening to Prozac, America's bestselling happy pill.

Enthusiasts are already planning to widen the uses of these types of drugs for overweight patients, those with cancer experiencing nausea from anticancer drugs, people with obsessive compulsions, and even PMS. In addition, because there is some evidence that this kind of drug reduces dependence (unlike Valium and other benzodiazepines) by stimulating the reward mechanism in the brain, doctors are discussing the possibility of using it to help control smoking and dependence on other drugs.

The glossy press about Prozac passes lightly over the more than one hundred lawsuits the manufacturer, Eli Lilly, faced from patients claiming that Prozac led them to suicidal and homicidal thoughts and actions. In one case, a Prozac user killed five and wounded twelve others at his place of work. In another, a woman attacked her mother by biting her, ripping out more than twenty bite-sized pieces of flesh. Eli Lilly has now reached a settlement with the families of the victims killed and injured by Joseph Wesbecken, who went on a shooting rampage while on the drug.[106]

Although the FDA cleared Prozac from this association with violence, a recent study suggested that of all types of antidepressants, the highest number of suicides have been recorded for those patients on serotonin inhibitors.[107]

According to Eli Lilly's own published warnings on the drug, some 10 to 15 percent of patients in initial clinical trials reported anxiety and insomnia; 9 percent, particularly underweight patients, report significant weight loss or anorexia. In one study, 13 percent of patients on the drug lost more than 5 percent of their body weight.[108] In other words, about one in ten patients experiences the same symptoms from the drug that the doctor is trying to treat.

Prozac has also been known to affect nearly every system of the body, including the nervous, digestive, respiratory, cardiovascular, musculoskeletal, and urogenital systems, and the skin and appendages. These side effects include, most commonly, visual disturbances, palpitations, mania/hypomania, tremors, symptoms of flu, cardiac arrhythmia, back pain, rashes, sweating, nausea, diarrhea, abdominal pain, and loss of sex drive. Less common effects include antisocial behavior, double vision, memory loss, cataracts or glaucoma, asthma, arthritis, osteoporosis, stomach bleeding, kidney inflammation, and impotence. Prozac also, albeit infrequently, can cause abnormal dreams, agitation, convulsions, delusions, and euphoria.[109]

Although it's known as the happy drug by some zealots, Prozac may need a new sobriquet soon with the discovery that it may also cause sexual dysfunction in up to a third of users. In an overlooked research paper published in the *Journal of Clinical Psychiatry* in 1992, F. M. Jacobsen found this sort of level of sexual problems among people taking fluoxetine. A paper published in the same journal a year later found that the rate of sexual dysfunction while on the drug was as high as 75 percent.[110]

Migraine

Besides depression, serotonin inhibitors are being investigated for everything from cholesterol-lowering to PMS. Sumatriptan is a new migraine drug, called a 5-HT agonist, that supposedly works by reducing the swollen blood vessels around the brain.

It is chemically related to 5-hydroxytryptamine (serotonin), and was developed after scientists revised their thinking about what causes migraine. Dr. Frank Clifford-Rose of Charing Cross Hospital in London, who helped coordinate many of the studies of sumatriptan, says that migraine, rather than being initiated by the blood vessels in the brain itself, is now believed to be a biological disease of the nervous system, and that serotonin plays a key role. It has long been known that 5-HT can cause headaches, and experiments have shown that 5-HT is released during migraine attacks.

Glaxo was the first pharmaceutical company to come up with a drug that was chemically related to 5-HT but was supposed selectively to block the brain's receptors for this hormone. This would cause the blood vessels in the brain to constrict without affecting what could be as many as fifteen other 5-HT receptors, which help with blood clotting, activity in the lungs, and the gastrointestinal system.

In 1991 Glaxo enthusiastically launched sumatriptan as "a revolutionary acute therapy in migraine" after a number of studies showed highly promising results. Among 1,600 patients, within two hours, 81 to 86 percent reported that their headaches had disappeared or lessened to the point of being mild.[111]

In the wake of a great deal of noisy fanfare, medicine has begun to retrench now that reports are flooding in demonstrating that patients taking this drug may be trading one health problem for another. At least 5 percent of users of sumatriptan experience chest pain. Because the drug works on blood vessels, it has always been assumed that the chest pain had to do with the heart. But new evidence shows that the pain may start in the esophagus (the canal from your mouth to your stomach).[112] The results of one study of patients taking sumatriptan showed no electrocardiogram changes, whereas contractions of the esophagus were shown to increase significantly with the drug. A fifth of the patients included in this study developed chest pain, lasting between two and forty-five minutes, although there seemed to be no relation in time between the onset of the pain and the abnormal recordings of the movements of the esophagus.

These study results should be regarded with caution, particularly since the changes were seen only when three times the normal amount of the drug was given. However, changes in the blood have also been shown in patients taking the standard therapeutic dose of sumatriptan; blood pressure in the lungs and aorta rises by 40 percent and 20 percent, respectively, which could mean that chest tightness arises from the veins in the lungs or those running along the breadth of the body rather than in the esophagus.[113] In rare cases, people on sumatriptan have experienced arterial spasms in the heart.[114] There is also a small risk of poor blood flow to the heart:[115] angiographies of patients on sumatriptan showed that the drug does indeed constrict arteries.[116] One woman with no previous history of vascular disease suffered a fatal heart attack after injecting herself with sumatriptan,[117] and at least two patients developed serious irregular heartbeat.[118] In some patients the chest pressure or pain radiates out to the left arm and head, in the manner of angina.[119]

The other problem with sumatriptan is the possibility of rebound migraines, which cause patients to have increased dependence on the drug. The Gothenburg Migraine Clinic in Sweden found that over half of patients given sumatriptan by injection had recurrences of migraine within five to ten hours after nearly every treated attack. In another study, all but one of the patients had a headache the next day.[120]

In Germany, after an average of nine months a group of patients had reached the point where they had to use the drug nearly every day to prevent their headaches from recurring. One fellow who'd suffered from migraines only once a month began getting them every morning after he'd begun taking sumatriptan.[121]

Glaxo denies that there is any evidence of dependence on the drug, and points out that the drug is only approved for short-term intermittent treatment of acute migraine attacks, and not for daily prevention.

In the Gothenburg Clinic, 70 percent of patients experienced one or more side effects, including neck pain, chest symptoms, tiredness, tingling, and a reaction at the injection site. The oral variety can also cause nausea and vomiting.

Besides this multitude of side effects, a question mark hangs over sumatriptan's genuine effectiveness in times of need. Although as many as 90 percent of patients have responded over three treatment courses, studies have shown that only about 50 to 60 percent will respond to it during any one attack.[122]

DRUGS FOR HYPERACTIVITY

Ritalin (methylphenidate) is America's other miracle drug, taken by as many as a million children in the United States to control hyperactivity and attention deficit disorder (ADD). Up to 12 percent of all American boys aged between six and fourteen are being prescribed Ritalin to treat a range of behavioral disorders. In 1990, worldwide production of the drug was less than three tons; just four years later that figure had virtually tripled. About 90 percent of total prescriptions were for American children.

Recent media attention has focused on it as a drug that can "unlock" a child's potential, compared with the supposed limitations of the dietary approach to hyperactivity. This is despite the fact that in many instances a child is given the drugs before it has been demonstrated that he could benefit from it. A team of researchers from the United Nations International Narcotics Control Board looked at the records of nearly 400 pediatricians who'd prescribed Ritalin, and found that half the children who'd been diagnosed with attention deficit disorder had not been given any psychological or educational testing before receiving the drug. The UN concluded that frustrated parents or educators and doctors were too ready to affix a label of ADD to a host of behavioral difficulties.[123]

The view espoused by Ritalin promoters is that the drug, an amphetamine, works by correcting biochemical imbalances in the brain. Not only is there no evidence of this view, but no evidence that Ritalin makes any lasting change. As CibaGeneva Pharmaceuticals (the manufacturer) admits, there are no long-term studies on Ritalin's safety or effectiveness.[124] Furthermore, The American Textbook of Psychiatry shows a 75 percent improvement with Ritalin compared with a 40 percent response with a placebo, suggesting that half the response to Ritalin could be purely suggestive.[125]

What we do know is that it suppresses growth, makes a child more prone to seizures, and causes visual disturbances, nervousness, insomnia, anorexia, and toxic psychosis. It's worth remembering that this drug is a class II category controlled substance, such as barbiturates, morphine, and others with a high potential for addiction or abuse. Uppers supposedly have a paradoxical effect on children, quieting them down, but often the effect is mixed. Children get subdued during the day, but stimulated at night, unable to sleep. The entry for Ritalin in the U.S. Physicians' Desk Reference carries a warning of drug dependence and psychotic episodes: "Careful supervision is required during drug withdrawal, since severe depression as well as the effects of chronic overactivity can be unmasked." Numerous cases of suicide after drug withdrawal have been reported. One study showed that children treated with stimulants alone (rather than with counseling as well as drugs) had higher arrest records and were more likely to be institutionalized.[126]

Peter Breggin, author of *Toxic Psychiatry* (Fontana), notes that long-term use of Ritalin causes irritability and hyperactivity—the very problems the drug is supposed to treat.[127] Brain atrophy was evident in more than half of twenty-four adults treated with psychostimulants.[128] In another study in Johannesburg, of fourteen children only two responded to the drug. One child showed some deterioration, and another marked deterioration.

CHEMOTHERAPY

If antibiotics and steroids are the Sherman tanks of medical chemical warfare, chemotherapy for cancer is its nuclear warhead. No other illness is subject to the sophisticated combinations of chemicals that have been developed for cancer treatment.

Chemotherapy was first proposed as a treatment for cancer directly after the Second World War, when research on mustard gas demonstrated that it has the ability to kill living cells, particularly those that rapidly divide, such as those in the intestinal tract, bone marrow, and lymph system. Doctors soon came up with the idea that they could use mustard gas to poison cancer, which constitutes the most rapidly dividing cells of all. In fact, many of the drugs we use today are close cousins of mustard gas—one reason we find them so toxic.[129]

In the early 1970s, medicine discovered that certain rare cancers would respond to chemotherapy and result in a person living longer. These include combinations of drugs for Hodgkin's disease, certain non-Hodgkin's lymphomas, some germ cell tumors, testicular cancer, and certain cancers in children, such as Wilm's tumor, acute lymphocytic leukemia, and choriocarcinoma, in which fetal cells transform into cancer and threaten the mother's life.

However, twenty-five years later it is safe to say that virtually no progress has been made since then–U.S. president Richard

Nixon declared the "War on Cancer" in 1971. No cancer incurable then is curable today. Chemotherapy's modest successes are almost identical to what they were then.[130] Since then, all the billions of dollars of research we've thrown at cancer haven't influenced survival one little bit. *For most of today's common solid cancers, the ones that cause 90 percent of the cancer deaths every year— breast, most lung, colon and rectal, skin cancer, liver and pancreatic and bladder—chemotherapy has never been proved to do any good at all.*[131]

After surgery, giving out chemotherapy as a "just in case" measure to kill any "secret" pockets of cells has appeared to improve the survival prospects of certain groups of patients with breast, colon, or lung cancer. Recurrence rates are supposed to be reduced by a third, and survival improved.[132]

However, this evidence is only empirical (that is, only based on observation, not scientific studies). It is very likely that it was other factors that helped the survival of these patients. In one of the few reviews of all studies comparing chemotherapy against another form of treatment, chemotherapy proved no better than tamoxifen alone in women over fifty with breast cancer.[133]

Chemotherapy has been shown to increase the survival of patients with ovarian and small-cell lung disease, intermediate and high-grade non-Hodgkin's lymphoma, and localized cancer of the small intestines—although, again, this is not proven beyond a shadow of a doubt.[134] Sometimes these advantages are major, as with ovarian cancer, where it has been shown that it may extend the lives of patients for years. More often the effect is modest, as with lung cancer patients, increasing survival by only a few months.[135]

The other problem is that cancer doctors define "cure" and "response" in different terms than you or I might. In the main, oncologists look only at "response"—that is, shrinking the tumor—as a measure of success, without considering whether this increases survival or improves quality of life. Dr. Ralph Moss, former employee of the prestigious Sloan-Kettering Institute, has made it his life's work to examine the scientific evidence of orthodox and alternative cancer treatment. He describes a textbook on medicine in which a top National Cancer Institute

(NCI) scientist said that for most forms of cancer, many patients initially respond. But in only three forms of cancer—ovarian, small-cell lung cancer, and acute nonlymphocytic leukemia—did any appreciable percentage survive without disease, and even then this percentage represented, at best, less than a sixth of the total group of patients. In all the other types of cancer, disease-free survival was rare.[136]

Major chemotherapy manufacturer Bristol Myers discloses that only 11 percent of patients taking carboplatin, and 15 percent of patients taking cisplatin, had a complete response to these drugs; remission lasted, on average, about a year, and both types of patients survived, on average, only two years. And this is for the two major drugs given primarily for ovarian cancer, which is one of the cancers that most responds to chemotherapy![137]

In the majority of studies, the most important question of all—*Does chemo help you to live any longer than you would have done if you hadn't had the treatment?*—is never even asked! In the rush to be seen to be doing something about cancer, the FDA has now officially sanctioned that new drugs for cancer can be fast-tracked on the market so long as they show they shrink tumors. There is no need to show that they lengthen the survival of cancer patients.[138]

You'd never know any of this if you talked to the average oncologist. Most would talk of the great strides made in chemotherapy, the new drugs, the new protocols (that is, combinations of drugs). But the measure of how much this constitutes the treatment of desperation is the language used—"rescue" therapies and "salvage" operations—and also the types of treatments being resorted to. The latest are termed "rescue," as in rescuing you from the brink of death. Doctors harvest bone marrow from the patient before launching into treatment, then administer high-dose chemotherapy in the hope that replanting the bone marrow will somehow "rescue" the patient before he dies from the drugs! Other researchers are experimenting with growing immune-system cells in the test tube in a last-ditch attempt to restore blood formation in patients who have undergone murderously high doses of chemotherapy.

Recently, one doctor returned from an autopsy with the proud announcement that his patient, who'd had widespread, disseminated cancer, had died "cancer-free." What he did not mention was that it was the lung disease, induced by chemotherapy, that killed him.

In oncology, more is always considered better. After the success with Hodgkin's disease with a quartet of cancer-killing drugs and steroids, medicine has applied this protocol to many other types of cancer, even though there is no evidence that it does any good at all. For many forms of cancer, multiple use of drugs appears to be no more effective than single drugs, which carry many fewer side effects. In one of the only studies of its type, reported at a meeting in Dallas of the American Study of Clinical Oncologists, a double-dose of chemotherapy given to breast cancer patients was found to be no more effective than the standard dose.[139]

But even when medicine admits that drugs haven't a prayer of curing, chemotherapy is given as palliative cure (that is, to improve the time the patient has left). This argument, of course, ignores the terrible effects of chemotherapy, which can hardly be said to improve the quality of life.

One of the most-used chemotherapy drugs is cyclophosphamide, which comes from mustard gas. It can cause nausea, vomiting, hair loss, and anorexia, and can damage the blood, heart, and lungs. Another drug, cisplatin (Platinol), made of the heavy metal platinum, can damage nerves and kidneys and cause hearing loss and seizures. It can also cause deafness, irreversible loss of motor function, bone marrow suppression, anemia, and blindness.

Mechlorethamine, an analogue of mustard gas (the "M" of MOPP treatment, the standard protocol for Hodgkin's disease), is so toxic that those administering the drug are advised to wear rubber gloves and avoid inhaling it! A most-dreaded complication is mucositis (or inflammation of the mucous membranes, particularly of the gut and mouth), possibly leading to life-threatening infection.[140] Various types of chemotherapy can cause heart problems, destroy bile ducts, cause bone tissue death, restrict growth, cause infertility, lower white and red blood cell counts, and lead to intestinal and lactose malabsorption.

If a patient is lucky enough to be one of the few for whom chemotherapy actually does treat the illness successfully, chances are high that it will cause a worse cancer to develop many years later. In one study, one third of women treated for Hodgkin's disease as children, for instance, ended up developing breast cancer by the time they were forty. This risk is at least three times greater than among the general population.[141] Adults who had chemo as children also have a risk of bone cancer. Thus far, some 13,000 children who'd survived cancer for three years have been identified as bone cancer victims.[142] By using chemotherapy to treat cancer, many survivors could be trading one type of cancer for a more deadly one later on.

Before your doctor writes you a prescription for any drug, it's a good idea to check if another drug isn't causing your problem in the first place. According to the Health Research Group, the lobbying organization founded by consumer advocate Ralph Nader, fifteen categories of drugs can bring on depression: barbiturates, tranquilizers, beta-blockers, heart drugs (particularly those containing reserpine), including drugs used to treat cardiac arrhythmias, ulcer drugs, high blood pressure drugs, corticosteroids, antiparkinsonian drugs, amphetamines, painkillers, arthritis drugs, anticonvulsants, antibiotics, and drugs used to treat slipped discs or alcoholism. If your feelings of depression have come on about the time you started on a new drug, look first to that drug as the cause.

Unfortunately, in too many cases the treatment for drug-induced depression is an antidepressive, which can react with the original drug and cause further physical or mental problems. The only treatment for this kind of depression is to stop or gradually cut down on the original drug or, if absolutely necessary, to switch to a similar-acting drug that will not cause depression.

DRUGS TO TREAT THE SIDE EFFECTS OF DRUGS

With so many drugs causing so much illness, an entire medical industry has grown up just to counteract the ill effects of medical "treatment." There are now drugs to combat the nausea caused by chemotherapy, and drugs to counter the terrible side effects of transplant drugs. Zantac, or ranitidine, is one of a family of drugs called histamine-2 receptor antagonists. They work by blocking the H2 nerve receptors in the stomach, which histamine ordinarily stimulates to produce gastric acid. By inhibiting this action, the H2-blockers reduce both the amount of gastric acid in the stomach and its pepsin content. They also block the effects of the hormone called gastrin, produced in the stomach to stimulate the production of stomach juices. The drug is relatively long-acting, suppressing gastric acid secretion for twelve hours at a stretch. In most cases, claim Glaxo Laboratories, "healing occurs in four weeks" or, in those who don't initially respond, four weeks after that.

NSAID-caused ulcers have been a lifesaver for drugs such as Zantac. Recently it was discovered that most ulcers are caused by the *helicobacter pylori* bug and can be cured with a one-time, largely antibiotic drug treatment. Because of ulcers, Zantac was the bestselling drug in the world. The *H. pylori* breakthrough may strike a major financial blow to ulcer-drug manufacturers such as Glaxo, who rely on a steady stream of users taking Zantac indefinitely as "maintenance." Consequently, the ulcer-drug makers have been searching around for new long-term uses for what are some of the biggest money spinners of all time.

Lately, Glaxo has been specifically advertising Zantac for NSAID users to take as preventive medicine for ulcers. (As for healing NSAID-induced ulcers that are already there, there is less convincing evidence. In one study, under a third of NSAID patients healed after four weeks; about half after eight weeks.)[143]

The problem with using H2-blockers as a just-in-case measure is that patients have to stay on them (as well as NSAIDs) long term and risk suffering one or more of a long list of potential side effects: headaches (often severe), insomnia, vertigo, depression, hallucinations, blurred vision, irregular heartbeats, pancreatitis (inflammation of the pancreas), diarrhea, nausea/vomiting, abdominal discomfort, hepatitis and other liver disorders—even death. Other problems include blood count changes (usually reversible); rare cases of agranulocytosis (a severe blood disorder) have been reported, as have occasional cases of impotence, hair loss, and anaphylactic shock. Taking H2 antagonists may mask any warning symptoms that you've got cancer of the stomach and so delay your diagnosis. I wonder how long it will be before there is another drug developed to counteract the effects of the drug taken to counter the effects of the first drug.

A DRUG CHECKLIST

As with medical tests, before you take *any* drug it is vital that you learn as much as you can about it—indeed, more than even your doctor knows. Every drug marketed in the U.S. has a listing in the *Physicians' Desk Reference,* which is essentially a profile of the drug at a glance, listing when it should or shouldn't be taken and also its side effects and any specific warnings imposed by the FDA. This volume and other, more consumer-friendly versions published by the same company are available at any large bookstore.[144]

Once you've read up on the drug being proposed for you (or asked your doctor to photocopy the entry in his *PDR*), put the following questions to your doctor:

- **Is drug therapy really necessary for this problem?** Many conditions, such as premenstrual tension or depression after a bereavement, can be treated by diet or the loving attention of friends and relatives. A new study finds that people suffering from major depression can be aided just as well by help in facing up to and solving their problems as by taking antidepressants.

   Unless you can be persuaded that your condition will definitely worsen, why introduce a substance that could also introduce a whole new set of problems?

* **What will happen if I don't take the drug?**

* **What is this drug supposed to do for me? How will it do that? How are you going to monitor the use of the drug? Do your instructions differ from those in the PDR?**

* **What sorts of drugs or substances (including nonprescription drugs, food, or alcohol) should I avoid when taking this drug?**

* **With what other drugs does this drug dangerously react?** Although one drug used alone might carry a small risk, when combined with another drug that risk can be multiplied several times over, as can the strength of the toxicity.

* **What are the known side effects of this drug, as reported by the manufacturer?** (Don't settle for vague assurances from your doctor; request that he read out from the *PDR*.)

* **What are the latest reports in the medical literature about this drug's side effects?** Magazines such as *The Lancet* publish new studies all the time demonstrating that the risks of a certain drug are far higher than the manufacturer originally thought. If your doctor doesn't know, go to a science reference library. Another possibility is to do a Medline search, a computerized version of the *Cumulated Index Medicus,* a summary of most scientific studies performed on most treatments. If your library doesn't have Medline, they probably have the *Index Medicus* itself, an unwieldy set of volumes that fills most of a shelf.

    Otherwise visit a large medical bookshop. Many useful

books about medications can also be found in general book-shops. Your best source for full information about a drug's side effects is to own your own copy of the *Physicians' Desk Reference*.

- **May I discontinue any other drugs I am currently taking?** The Health Research Group suggests that if you are taking other drugs, you have a "Brown Bag Session" with your doctor—that is, you place all medication you're taking (including nonprescription drugs) in a brown bag and take it to your doctor's office on the next visit so that you and your doctor can determine if any complicate the effects of the others. (It also makes sense to write out a list of all the drugs, including the frequency with which, and times of day when, you take them—so that you don't mix up what you are taking.)

- **Under what conditions and how should I stop taking this drug if I notice certain side effects? What sorts of tests are available to monitor my reactions to the drug?**

- **If I don't wish to take this drug, what other possible therapies are there for me to consider?** Here you might have to prod your doctor gently into enumerating the possibilities he's heard of, not just to offer his opinion. Many doctors will tell you they simply don't believe in nondrug therapies—when in fact, very few doctors know anything about them.

If all else fails, contact the FDA. Anyone around the world has right of access to information about drugs licensed by the FDA, courtesy of the American Freedom of Information Act. Write a letter to the address below, asking for a Summary Basis of Approval (SBA) on the drug in question (make sure to find out the generic and, if possible, the brand name). An SBA will include detailed summary of the data, including results of any clinical trials, which influenced the FDA's decision to approve the drug.

Also ask for Adverse Drug Reactions (ADRs)—unverified reports of any side effects reported—including new MedWatch reports (the new database of drug reactions recently set up by the FDA). Finally, ask for any reviews or assessments of the ADRs, which will put these isolated reports of reactions in context. (Bear in mind that American drugs can be licensed in different doses than British ones, and for different conditions.)

You will be charged $3 per request, after the first one hundred pages of photocopying and first two hours of research, which are free, you are charged 10 cents per page of photocopying and a fee of $13–46 per hour, depending upon the grade level of the person required to do the research. (In your letter you can ask for an estimate of how much your search will cost.)

The address to write to is:

Food and Drug Administration
Freedom of Information Office
5600 Fishers Lane
Rockville, MD 20857

They must respond within ten days, if only to say that your request is being investigated.

WONDER DRUGS

The problem with wonder drugs is that they breed in the public mind a sense that medicine can and always should work miracles, even with benign problems. What gets forgotten is the price we always pay by tampering so totally with mother nature.

Many benign problems will clear up by themselves. When my daughter was small and still nursing, I suffered from a couple of bouts of severe mastitis. I phoned my hospital and convinced my doctor, who usually treats the problem with antibiotics, that I wanted to wait twenty-four hours to see what happened. During that time (and on subsequent occasions) I bathed the affected breasts with heat. My daughter, as if sensing my problem, nursed more than usual on the affected breast. A day later I was back to normal.

Other than for emergencies, where orthodox medicine comes into its own with the most brilliant of modern technologies, there are invariably better and far less invasive ways to treat—and often cure—most medical conditions. And most of these unorthodox methods have as much, if not more, scientific evidence of success than what we consider the "tried and tested" conventional route. For arthritis, asthma, eczema, hypertension, hyperactivity, and migraine there is solid evidence that such cases have mostly to do with food allergies or nutritional deficiencies. Locating both can alleviate, if not cure, the condition.[145] Even mental illness such as depression has been shown to respond to nutritional medicine.[146] With epilepsy, much progress has been made at such orthodox medical centers as Johns Hopkins Medical Center in Baltimore, using a high-fat diet to control seizures. In one review of fifty-eight cases, seizure control improved in two-thirds of patients.[147] Some researchers speculate that the high fat intake helps to repair the myelin sheath around the nerves.

Although an all-out cure for cancer remains elusive, many alternative methods have some scientific evidence of success—certainly more than either chemotherapy or radiation.[148] In fact, simple surgery alone without follow-up just-in-case chemo or radiation can be the treatment of choice for certain early cancers.[149]

NINE

Dental Medicine: Safe Until Proven Dangerous

What would you say if you heard that doctors had selected one of the most toxic substances known to man, hadn't bothered to do any safety testing before placing it permanently in your body, and continued to maintain steadfastly that there was no danger whatsoever that any of it was doing you any harm?

AMALGAM FILLINGS

The American Dental Association continues to insist, as it did in 1984, that "when mercury is combined with the metals used in dental amalgam, its toxic properties are made harmless." However, this position has been based upon reverse logic: that amalgam fillings are safe because the evidence does not prove irrefutably otherwise.

Although we refer to our fillings as "silver" or mercury, amalgam is actually made up of about 52 percent mercury, with the remainder copper, tin, silver, and zinc. At the end of the nineteenth century, amalgam, which literally means "mixed with mercury," was discovered as a cheap compound to replace gold, which was too expensive, and lead, which was considered too dangerous, as a dental filling. It was introduced in the United States in the late 1820s. The National Association of Dental Surgeons (ADS), the dental association of the time, held a debate as to whether dentists should use mercury amalgam fillings. The Association came out against mercury, and said it should be eliminated. But because amalgam was so much cheaper than other materials of the times, it became the filling of choice, particularly among dentists whose patients were poor, and in fact was promoted as a political issue—the filling everybody could afford. Most dentists chose to ignore the warnings about and known toxicity of mercury, arguing that those who favored gold did so solely for pecuniary reasons and were denying medical help to patients on lower incomes. By 1840, the ADS had disbanded, undermined because of what heated up to a raging battle over the amalgam issue.[1]

Nearly sixty years later, a new dental association, the American Dental Association (ADA), was established, which endorsed mercury amalgam as safe—a position the current ADA has maintained ever since. Dr. Murray J. Vimy, clinical associate professor of the Department of Medicine at the University of Calgary in Canada, who has spent fifteen years studying the effects of amalgam, makes the point that amalgam slipped through the cracks of safety regulation because it has been around so long. Drugs or substances such as this, which prefigured regulatory agencies like the Food and Drug Administration, are said to be "grandfathered" into practice if they were used before safety testing began. "If the information we have about the effect of amalgam fillings were presented before the Food and Drug Administration today, they would not pass it for use because it hasn't even passed the required animal tests, let alone the human ones," says Dr. Vimy—referring to the animal trials required by the FDA today.[2]

In 1993, the Public Health Service issued a report evaluating the safety of dental amalgam. The report allowed that small amounts of mercury vapor are released from your fillings and can be absorbed into the body, and that these could cause small responses in that rare group of allergic individuals. Nevertheless, it concluded that "there is scant evidence that the health of the vast majority of people with amalgam is compromised, nor that removing amalgam fillings has a beneficial effect on health."[3]

The FDA's position continues to be that there is no valid data to demonstrate clinical harm to patients, nor that removing a patient's amalgam fillings will prevent any adverse health effects or reverse the course of existing diseases.[4]

It's a position that is proving at variance with the doctrine of several other countries. In Germany the Federal Health Agency (Bundesgesundheitsamt, or BGA) decided in early 1992 that amalgam fillings should be used only for molars. The BGA also announced that amalgam containing gamma-2, a compound of tin and mercury, should be banned because of its inherent insta-bility and the risk of mercury being released while a tooth is being filled. The German government has been cagey, denying there is scientific evidence that amalgam can cause long-term disease other than for people who are allergic or have electro-chemical reactions. Nevertheless, they also say that amalgam shouldn't be used for pregnant women, patients with kidney fail-ure, or toddlers.[5] The Germany Federal Registry of Dentists has sent a letter to the Minister of Health, requesting that he rule that no dentist in Germany be allowed to use dental amalgam.[6] The Swedes have taken the first step in an outright ban of amal-gam fillings, to be in place by 1997. Austria has plans afoot to ban amalgam by the year 2000. And some German companies such as Degussa, one of the world's largest manufacturers of den-tal amalgam, are stopping the production of amalgam—even though it represents, at the time of writing, half their turnover—and moving into the manufacture of composite fillings (the plastic alternative to amalgam). In a recent British television report on amalgam, Dr. Matthias Kuhner, a senior manager at Degussa, admitted that one consideration for their move was potential lawsuits.[7]

The Canadian and American Dental Associations claim that dental amalgam exposure is minuscule compared with dietary exposure—that people get most of their mercury, in effect, from tuna fish. However, when the World Health Organization assembled some of the world's authorities on mercury poisoning, they concluded, after reviewing the scientific literature, that the public's highest daily exposure to mercury comes from dental amalgam fillings. They determined that human daily retained intake is from 3 to 17 micrograms a day from dental fillings, compared with about 2.6 micrograms a day from fish and seafood, and other food, air, and water.[8] The committee also concluded that, regarding mercury vapor, a "specific no-observed-effect level (NOEL) cannot be established"—which means that no level of exposure to mercury vapor, however slight, has been found to be completely harmless. Dr. Lars Freiberg, chief adviser to the World Health Organization on mercury safety, and perhaps the world's leading authority on mercury poisoning, has said: "There is no safe level of mercury."[9]

A Timed-Released Poison

Without a doubt, mercury is extraordinarily toxic to humans. The well-respected Toxicity Center at the University of Tennessee, which rates poisons for their lethal toxicity to humans, scores mercury at 1600—plutonium, the most deadly, scores 1900. This rating places mercury among the most toxic substances known to man.

Dentists themselves show overwhelming evidence of mercury poisoning; autopsy reports of a group of dentists showed higher concentrations of the metal in their pituitary glands and double the number of brain tumors than among the ordinary population.[10] Female dentists and personnel are at least three times more likely to suffer sterility, stillbirth, and miscarriage,[11] and all dental employees have a higher concentration of mercury in the central nervous system, kidneys, and endocrine system.[12] More worrying, amalgam appears to cause subtle brain damage in dentists exposed regularly to amalgam fillings. Several years ago in Singapore, the neurological functions of a group of dentists were assessed and found to be less efficient than those of a similar group who hadn't been exposed regularly to amalgam, although the dentists did just as well as the control group on intelligence tests. The higher their exposure to mercury, the worse their performance on the neurological tests.[13] Dr. Diana Echeverria, a neurotoxicologist at the University of Washington, also tested American dentists to see whether they showed any evidence of mercury poisoning. Her study found subtle losses of manual dexterity and concentration—both evidence of central nervous system disorders.[14]

Further proof of the highly toxic nature of mercury comes in the form of the meticulous recommendations by the American Council on Dental Materials and Devices concerning its storage and use. This organization recommends that dentists use tightly sealed containers, avoid any contact with the mercury, and perform annual mercury level tests on all dental personnel.

The party line of both the British and American Dental Associations is that the mercury in amalgam fillings becomes inert, or "locked in," when mixed with the other metals and placed in the mouth.[15] But numerous researchers have proved that mercury vapors are continuously released from the fillings, particularly when you chew or eat hot or acidic foods. The University of Calgary in Canada, which has been at the forefront of amalgam research, found that chewing increases the "intra-oral" (within the air of the mouth) mercury content sixfold if you have amalgam fillings, making it fifty-four times higher than the intra-oral mercury content of patients without amalgam fillings. The greater the number of fillings, the more mercury vapor was released.[16] At a conference at Kings College, Cambridge, Professor R. Soremark of the Department of Prosthetic Dentistry of the Karolingska Institute of Sweden announced: "The absorption rate is close to 90 percent, 74 percent of which is retained by the lungs. In ten minutes, 30 percent of the mercury absorbed in the lungs is transferred to the blood."[17] Mercury can "corrode" in the mouth, which is to say, rust, as metallic ions and vapor form on the amalgam surface—once it comes into contact with heat, saliva, and such elements as fluoride or large gold fillings. Although most of these products get excreted, about 10 percent accumulate in the various organs and tissues of the body. Furthermore, the five metals contained in amalgam can combine to produce some sixteen different corrosion products, all floating around in the body to unknown effect. Professor J. V. Masi of Western New England College in Springfield, Massachusetts, who has studied this issue in detail, has written that all metals used as restorative dental materials are capable of corroding.[18]

A Body of Evidence

Although much of the evidence about mercury has an element of speculation about it, there is growing proof that this released mercury settles in tissues in the body. Until recently, although we knew that mercury was released by chewing, we didn't know where it ended up. In December 1989, Dr. Murray J. Vimy of the Department of Medicine, along with numerous other medical researchers from the Departments of Radiology, Medicine and Medical Physiology at the University of Calgary in Canada, published a study in which radioactive amalgam fillings were placed into the teeth of adult sheep. (Using radioactive amalgam effectively "labeled" the mercury so it could be easily traced. It also eliminated the need for a control, as mercury present in food, air, or water wouldn't be so labeled. Sheep were chosen because their physiological responses were thought to be most like those of humans.)

Within twenty-nine days, substantial quantities of mercury appeared in the lungs, gastrointestinal tract, and jaw tissue of the sheep. Once the mercury was absorbed, said the study, "high concentrations of dental amalgam rapidly localized in the liver and kidneys."[19] Over the course of the twenty-nine days, the mercury vapor measurements taken from the mouths of the sheep closely approximated those taken from people in previous studies. The brain, the heart, and several endocrine glands also contained substantial quantities of mercury. The study concluded:

> Our laboratory findings in this investigation are at variance with the anecdotal opinion of the medical profession, which claims that amalgam tooth fillings are safe. Experimental evidence in

support of amalgam safety is at best tenuous. . . . From our results we conclude that dental amalgams can be a major source of chronic [mercury] exposure.[20]

Dr. Vimy and his colleagues have spent more than a decade examining the effects of amalgam fillings on sheep, monkeys and, more recently, humans. Although 12,000 papers have been published to date on the dangers of amalgam, it is only because of the interest of respected medical departments like that at the University of Calgary, and their devastating findings, that the issue began to heat up, particularly in North America.

The evidence that Dr. Vimy and others have published demonstrates that mercury from amalgam fillings migrates to tissues in the body, causing harm—a type of "timed-released poisoning," as Vimy has called it.

The extent of the harm is still under study. "The evidence shows there is some risk, we're not sure of the extent of the risk, but it certainly is prudent to study and consider it," Vimy says.[21]

In Dr. Vimy's initial experiments on sheep, the radioactive mercury landed in the stomachs, liver, left and right kidneys, in the oral cavity, the lungs and the gastrointestinal (GI) tract, the brain, the heart, and the endocrine glands. "The denser the tissue, the larger the volume of mercury which collected there," Vimy said.[22]

Sheep were originally chosen for the University of Calgary's study because they are especially ruminant—that is, they chew all day. Dr. Vimy's team felt that, if the mercury didn't go into the tissues and organs of sheep, it wouldn't go into the tissues or organs of any other living creature. "Sheep," they summed up, "were a worst-case scenario."[23]

Although sheep have a physiological response similar to that of humans, Dr. Vimy and his colleagues were ridiculed for using sheep because they have a higher frequency of chewing than humans and more than one stomach, and so more bacteria for digestion. (The medical press tended to disparage the findings with such headlines as: "Sheep Baaad Amalgam Recipients"). So Dr. Vimy's group decided to repeat its experiment, this time using monkeys. They chose monkeys because their rate of chewing is more similar to that of humans, as are their teeth, diet, feeding frequency, chewing pattern, and organ physiology. They found the same pattern of mercury deposits in these monkeys—in the oral, lung, and GI tract—as they had seen in the sheep.[24]

Vimy's animal studies were vindicated by the work of Professor H. Vasken Aposhian, head of the Molecular and Cellular Biology Department of the University of Arizona in Tucson. Aposhian and his team counted the number of amalgam fillings of volunteers, from which they were given an amalgam score. The study participants were then given a salt of 2,3-dimercapto-propane-1-sulfonic acid (DMPS), a chelating agent that binds to mercury and removes it from the body through the urine. An analysis of the results showed that the more amalgam in the teeth, the higher the amalgam in the body as excreted with the DMPS. Aposhian's team was also able to show that two-thirds of the mercury excreted in the urine of those study participants with dental amalgams came from their fillings.[25]

In 1990 Dr. Vimy and his researchers conducted another sheep experiment to find out the effect of mercury's migration around the body, primarily on organs such as the kidneys. After placing regular (rather than radioactive) fillings into the mouths of several sheep, Vimy's group measured the flow rate of inulin, a starch, through the sheep's kidneys. This is a standard index of kidney function, since inulin is neither secreted nor absorbed. "Thirty days after the placement of amalgam fillings, kidney function and its filtration capacity was reduced by 50 percent," Dr. Vimy said. A control group of sheep given white plastic fillings showed no change in kidney function.

The research team found a rapid rise (by 300 percent) of sodium in the urea, even though the sodium diets of the animals were restricted. This indicated that substantial amounts of sodium were being lost. They also found a rapid decline in albumin excretion—by 68 percent.[26] This showed that the reabsorption of urea was impaired and that kidney blood flow was reduced. Noted Vimy: "That's like walking around with one kidney."[27]

POSSIBLE DISEASES FROM MERCURY AMALGAMS

There is no conclusive proof that amalgam fillings produce certain diseases, particularly since whether mercury will be toxic to any given person has a lot to do with genetic predisposition, length of time in the body, other environmental factors, and so forth. However, a number of new studies and clinical observations show a possible relationship between amalgam and a number of diseases.

Mercury and the Immune System

Mercury from amalgam fillings appears to lower T-lymphocyte cells, one of the most important components of our immune system.

The immune system contains T-lymphocyte cells and B-cells. Very generally speaking, of the numerous kinds of T-cells the most important are the T-4 lymphocytes, called the "helper" cells, whose job it is to identify foreign bodies and cancer cells for the B-cells to engulf and destroy. Without these helper cells, the B-cells cannot do their job. Hence, in the case of AIDS, although B-cells are available to attack the offending viruses, there aren't enough T-cells around to label them the enemy.

The T-8 lymphocytes ("suppressor cells"), on the other hand, keep the B-cells from attacking normal body tissues. Any lowering of the total T-cell population or disturbance in the delicate T-4:T-8 ratio can lead to autoimmune diseases such as multiple sclerosis, lupus erythematosus (a chronic inflammatory disease), inflammatory bowel disease, and the like.

In what he terms a "preliminary report," David Eggleston, a California dentist who has studied the effects of mercury exposure, measured the T-lymphocytes of three patients before and after removing their amalgam fillings. In all three cases their percentage of T-lymphocytes went up substantially (from 47 percent to 73 percent in one case, an increase of 55.3 percent). Eggleston then reinserted amalgam in the dental cavities of two of the patients and measured the percentage of T-cells. In both cases, the percentage of T-lymphocytes decreased again (in the above-mentioned patient, to 55 percent—a 24.7 percent decrease). Finally, when Eggleston removed the new amalgam and put in a nonamalgam filling, the T-cells were up again in all patients—72 percent in the case mentioned above, an increase of 30 percent.[28]

At a 1990 conference, Eggleston announced thirty such trials with an average improvement in T-cells of 30 percent. Colorado dentist Hal Huggins, author of *It's All in Your Head* (Avery), who has himself studied the toxic effect of amalgam fillings on patients, claims that number is conservative. "At the University of Colorado, I've measured T-cell rises of 100 percent to 300 percent after fillings were removed," he says.[29] These findings could mean that amalgam may have a role in causing or exacerbating allergies, autoimmune diseases, and even leukemia. In fact, white blood cell level abnormalities such as those found in leukemia have been shown to normalize when the patient's fillings are removed properly.[30]

ME and Multiple Sclerosis

There may also be a relationship between mercury poisoning from amalgam fillings and ME (myalgic encephalomyelitis), and also multiple sclerosis (MS) and other sclerosing diseases, such as ALS, the wasting disease that afflicts cosmologist Dr. Stephen Hawking. In one study, conducted in Sweden, the mercury levels in MS patients were on average 7.5 times higher than in the control group. In many cases, treatment with antioxidation therapy (that is, vitamins A, D and E, selenium, and/or removal of amalgam fillings) helped patients to improve—sometimes completely.[31]

Hal Huggins and the United Kingdom's Dr. Patrick Kingsley, noted for his work with MS and cancer patients, have both treated hundreds of MS victims, almost always find evidence of mercury toxicity. Furthermore, many patients sensitive to amalgam report classic symptoms of MS: numbness and tingling in the extremities, facial twitching, tremors or shaking of hands and feet. In 1984, a Swedish patient with numerous neurological problems was diagnosed with ALS, thought to be invariably fatal. The dentist, who recognized many symptoms similar to those of mercury poisoning, suggested that the patient have her copious amalgam fillings replaced, particularly as she could date her neurological problems from the placement of the fillings. Six weeks after the fillings were replaced, the patient was able to walk up stairs without experiencing back pain. Four months later she returned to the same University Hospital at Umea, Sweden, which had diagnosed her illness, for a week-long follow-up investigation. The following notation was placed in her medical records: "The neurological status is completely without comment. Hence the patient does not show any motor neuron disease of type ALS. She has been informed that she is in neurological respect fully healthy." The hospital concluded that the problem had been to do with mercury in the spinal cord. Nine years later, this woman is still in good health.[32]

Frequently, mercury poisoning also causes unexplained chronic fatigue. Hal Huggins says that over 90 percent of his 2,000 patients have ME-like symptoms of fatigue that improve when their fillings are removed. Biologically, says Huggins, this is easily explained. Mercury interferes with the oxygen-carrying capability of red blood cells; in most of his patients, who are given an "oxyhemoglobin" test, the oxygen-transport ability of the red blood cells is about half what it should be. This explains why they are chronically tired even though they have normal hemoglobin levels.

Amalgam in Pregnancy

Mercury fillings in pregnant women may also affect the growing fetus. In another University of Calgary study, Vimy and his colleagues placed radioactive-tagged amalgam fillings in the twelve molar teeth of five pregnant sheep on their 112th day of pregnancy. As early as three days after the fillings were placed, mercury was evident in the blood of the fetuses and amniotic fluid; sixteen days later it was evident in fetal pituitary glands, liver, kidney, as well as part of the placenta. By thirty-three days later (around the time of birth), most of the babies had higher levels of mercury than the mothers did. And during breast-feeding the mothers had eight times as much mercury in their milk as in their blood.[33] In Sweden, mercury use is banned in pregnant women, in marked contrast to the practices of other countries like Britain, which encourages women to have dental work done during their pregnancy.

More recently, a study on humans showed that mercury from a mother's fillings can cross the placenta and pollute the brain of her unborn child. Professor Gustav Drasch (a forensic toxicologist) and his colleagues at the Institut fur Rechtsmedicine in Munich examined the brains, liver, and kidneys of dead babies and of fetuses aborted for medical reasons. They found that the level of mercury in the babies significantly matched the number of amalgam fillings in their mothers. The babies were even found to accumulate mercury in their kidneys from the amalgams to the same degree that adults do from their own fillings. As most of these children obviously were not breast-fed, or if so were fed for only a short period, the researchers concluded that the mercury must have crossed the placenta.[34]

Fertility

There's also evidence that amalgam fillings may affect fertility. A group of German women with hormonal irregularities were studied to see whether they had excessive levels of any environmental agents such as mercury, pesticides, or industrial chemicals in their bodies. By far the most common problem was mercury contamination, levels of which again significantly matched the number of the woman's fillings and the amount of mercury released while chewing.[35]

Hair Loss

Mercury fillings may even affect hair loss. In one study, nearly half of women with unexplained hair loss had evidence of elevated mercury in their bodies; in two-thirds the condition disappeared once they'd had their fillings removed.[36]

Allergies Caused by Mercury

Although there is no hard scientific evidence that mercury in some way contributes to allergies, there are copious case studies among dentists whose patients suffering from food or environmental ailments improved in some way once their fillings were removed.

Tara, a Swedish patient, had suffered with allergic problems—including eczema—from birth. At five she had developed severe asthma and had to take daily medication. During the whole of her adolescence she was often hospitalized. She also suffered from severe headaches and double vision. At three, Tara had had her first amalgam filling; she was ultimately to have seven fillings in total over eleven surfaces. Researchers, on examining her history, realized that her asthma had come on following the placement of two deep fillings. They also realized that her mother had received a large amalgam filling during her pregnancy.

Tara and her mother consented to have all their amalgam fillings removed. Six weeks after the procedure was completed, Tara's eczema began to disappear and she no longer required asthma medication. Seven months later, both conditions completely cleared up, and stayed clear over the eight years her progress was followed.[37]

The closest we have to a scientific study is a consolidated report of six separate studies of patients who had their amalgam fillings replaced. Eighty-nine percent of the nearly 1,600 participants reported cure or improvement of thirty-one types of conditions. In the studies compiled from data from four countries, 83 percent reported improvement in general gastrointestinal problems and 76 percent in urinary tract problems; 87 percent cured or improved their migraines, and 75 percent of those with multiple sclerosis reported that they were better or cured.

If this data were extrapolated to all Americans with amalgam fillings, 17.4 million would have conditions like allergies improve or disappear simply by having their mercury dental fillings exchanged for nonmercury ones.[38]

Even though there are many success stories, Hal Huggins cautions that, unlike his MS patients, 85 percent of whom improve, only 60 percent of his "environmentally ill" patients get better, suggesting that mercury is only one of many contributory factors.[39]

Upset in the Gut

What has been studied scientifically is mercury's ability to upset gut bacteria and create a resistance to antibiotics. The University of Calgary team combined forces with Dr. Anne O. Summers and her colleagues at the Department of Microbiology at the University of Georgia in Athens, who are expert in matters concerning the gut. Calgary sent their raw statistics on the six monkeys to Summers and her colleagues to analyze in terms of the effect of mercury on intestinal flora.

The University of Georgia researchers found increased mercury-resistant bacteria in the gums and intestines of the monkeys, once they'd had amalgam fillings placed. In earlier work, Dr. Summers had shown that when there is a high mercury resistance in gut bacteria, there is also a high level of resistance to antibiotics. In her study, the mercury–resistant bacterial strains such as streptococci were also resistant to ampicillin, tetracycline, streptomycin, kanamycin, and chloramphenicol.[40]

To simplify greatly, the presence of mercury creates a change in the chemical makeup of the 1.15 kilograms (2½ pounds) of "friendly" bacteria living in the intestine, making it resistant to antibiotics. This means that the bacteria, which are essential for the smooth operation of the immune system, are, in effect, "otherwise engaged" and no longer able to keep fungi such as candida albicans (which causes thrush) in check. The altered bacteria also enhance the reabsorption of mercury vapor as it migrates from the teeth. This sets up a basic dysfunction in the gut, upsetting protein metabolism and gut flora, and leading to a situation whereby food particles go undigested. Dr. Vimy believes that amalgam fillings could be responsible for candida and the proliferation of allergies suddenly developing in people in their middle years, as well as for the general problem of resistance to antibiotics present in the population at large.

Alzheimer's Disease and Mercury

Although Vimy showed only that mercury from fillings travels to the brains of sheep, we now have evidence that it settles in the brains of humans, too. American dentist and researcher David Eggleston spent months in the local county morgue examining the accumulation of mercury in the brain tissue of eighty-three accident victims with amalgam fillings, and discovered that the number of amalgam fillings correlated with the level of mercury in the brain.[41] Patrick Störtebecker of the Störtebecker Foundation for Research in Stockholm has described studies demonstrating that mercury poisoning reaches the brain directly from the nasal cavity.[42]

When considering the possibility that Alzheimer's disease could be an environmental illness, the finger of blame has always been pointed at aluminum. But increasing evidence shows that it is mercury, rather than aluminum, that is found in greatest concentration in the brains of Alzheimer's disease victims. W. R. Markesbery and his medical research team in the departments of Chemistry, Pathology, and Neurology at the University of Kentucky and also the Sanders-Brown Center on Aging in Lexington, Kentucky, have been investigating Alzheimer's disease and its association with mercury for several years. In their most recent study they examined the brains of ten autopsied Alzheimer's patients for concentrations of trace elements. The trace element found in the highest concentration was consistently mercury; the study also noted diminished zinc and selenium levels in the subjects examined.[43] In the view of the researchers, a high level of mercury in the brain of Alzheimer's patients is the most important of the imbalances they observed. But they also consider the lower zinc levels significant, since zinc and selenium are known to protect against heavy-metal toxicity.

Minute doses of mercury in the brain produce identical changes to those seen in Alzheimer's.[44] Tubulin is a protein needed for the healthy formation of neurofibrils, or connective nerve tissue. Alzheimer's patients have impaired tubulin, which causes what is known as a "neurofibril tangle," where messages in the brain don't connect properly. Professor of Medical Biochemistry Boyd Haley and the other colleagues at the University of Kentucky fed rats aluminum but observed no change in tubulin levels, whereas mercury-fed rats displayed a diminished tubulin level similar to that of typical Alzheimer's patients.

Vimy and his team at the University of Calgary Medical School also used rats to show that mercury markedly inhibits tubulin levels. In fact, concentrations of mercury in the brains of these rats were similar to those recorded in monkeys twenty-eight days after placement of dental amalgam fillings.[45]

Jim, now eighty, had a mouth full of fifteen large amalgam fillings, some covering virtually the entire tooth. Periodically his dentist of thirty-five years had replaced old silver fillings with new ones. Five years ago, his wife, Martha, noticed that Jim's motor skills began deteriorating. By last summer his walking had become quite poor; when he fell over at a party she was astonished to realize that he didn't remember how to get up and refused to cooperate with friends attempting to assist him. Later that summer, Martha also noticed that a "fog" seemed to have descended over Jim. He couldn't walk or climb stairs without assistance. During a vacation in Austria he seemed to have forgotten how to swim—formerly a favorite activity. "Mentally, he just wasn't with it at all," she says.

In September, Martha took Jim to a geriatrician who diagnosed Alzheimer's disease and predicted that Jim would need to be placed in a nursing home in three months' time. The shock of this diagnosis jolted Jim into listening to his wife, who'd been trying to get him tested for amalgam poisoning for years. Positive test results showing high amalgam levels persuaded Jim to have the fillings out.

Jim had the fillings removed in two sessions at the dentist. On his way there, Jim needed to hang on to Martha to climb the several flights of stairs to the dental office; after the final session, he walked down the stairs unaided. Soon after the fillings were removed, his doctor agreed with Martha that Jim had "woken up." Five months later, once he'd undergone a detoxifying program to get the amalgam out of his system, Jim now goes out again by himself. He is once again able to prepare his and Martha's tax returns and to write letters. Although his walking can be poor, it is getting better, and, most important, Jim now recognizes when he isn't walking properly and corrects himself.

Some among the antiamalgam lobby consider that aluminum may well be a red herring in the quest to find the cause of Alzheimer's. Nevertheless, it is difficult to dismiss mounting evidence of some role for aluminum in the development of the disease.[46] It could be, as some suggest, that a brain depleted of zinc and overwhelmed by mercury is susceptible to the depositing of aluminum, but that aluminum itself doesn't cause the problem. Or it could be that both aluminum and mercury contribute. Although aluminium is ever present—in our water, commercially prepared orange juice, food, cosmetics, drugs, deodorants, cooking utensils, and flip-top cans—the amounts of aluminum we are exposed to from these sources is nothing like the concentrated dose of mercury we receive when it is placed in our mouths and inhaled with every chew.

MERCURY LAWSUITS

Even if the dental associations in United States and Britain have not alerted the public about the dangers of amalgam, companies that manufacture amalgam (and which could be most open to liability claims) recently had to take the warning signs seriously. A new law in California (Proposition 65) aims to protect Californians from being unwittingly exposed to chemicals known to cause cancer or birth defects. Any work environment containing such potentially harmful materials must carry a warning.

The Environmental Law Foundation decided to test this by taking Jeneric, one of the biggest manufacturers of dental amalgam, to court on this issue. The court ruled in favor of the ELF, and Jeneric became the first such company to issue health warnings on its product, in the form of an alert to dentists, dental staff, and patients in California about the potential dangers of birth defects from exposure to mercury.

Jeneric has added warnings to all amalgam containers shipped to California and agreed to supply dental offices with a warning sign to be displayed prominently in their waiting areas: "This office uses amalgam filling materials which contain and expose you to mercury, a chemical known to the State of California to cause birth defects and other reproductive harm. Please consult your dentist for more information." It also agreed to stop selling mercury fillings to dentists who fail to put up the warning notice.

After the Jeneric ruling, ten other dental amalgam manufacturers banded together and challenged it. A federal court judge decision overturned the earlier one, on the grounds that the regulatory authority for amalgam was not Proposition 65, but the FDA, which of course has ruled that mercury fillings are safe. "For every one step forward," says Vimy, "we take ten steps back."[47]

In the summer of 1996, the lower court ruling was overturned upon appeal by the ELF. The appeal court ruled that the lower court had erred in granting the reversal; since Proposition 65 is a law passed by California voters, FDA regulation does not preclude the Proposition's mandate of a warning to patients. This means that at the time of writing California dentists must disclose to their patients that fillings contain mercury.

REMOVING YOUR FILLINGS

Not everyone should get their fillings removed. If you do suspect that your fillings are making you ill, it might be wise to get proof of it, by undergoing a series of tests demonstrating mercury sensitivity. At Chelsea and Westminster Hospital in London, Drs. Don Henderson and Michele Monteil of the Department of Immunology have developed a simple blood test to determine if your fillings are making you ill.

The test, called a Metal Specific Memory T Cell Test (MSMT), determines your immune system's "memory" of dental and other metals. When your body is exposed to a foreign invader (say, a virus), your body mounts a defense and kills the infection. The next time you get exposed to the same virus, your body can attack it more quickly and powerfully, because of its immunological memory—the antibodies it has developed. These immune-system responses can actually be measured.

As for metal, although all people will demonstrate immunological memory of a variety of metals, including mercury, only those who have a serious reaction—for instance, those who get a rash from nickel—will show a strong memory response. A test like this to measure industry exposure to heavy metals has been available for years. Drs. Henderson and Monteil have demonstrated that the strength of immune-system response to mercury and other dental metals can also be graded.[48] You should also be assessed for potential mercury toxicity on the basis of a comprehensive clinical medical and dental history. In addition, each individual filling should be tested for electrical potential with a *millivoltmeter,* since each filling is a potential battery. Some clinical ecologists will perform this function.

According to Jack Huggins, the most important aspect of removing fillings is removing them in the right sequence, that is, taking out the most negatively charged ones first.

Many of the patients rushing to have their amalgam fillings replaced are getting more ill because no protocol is being observed to protect them from the onslaught of mercury vapors released. This happened to John, a British scientist, who almost died after having his fillings carelessly removed.

Potential health problems with alternatives to amalgam certainly exist, but are fortunately much rarer in most people. Nevertheless, it's doubtful that any holistic dentist would describe any dental material as being completely without potential risk.

We do know that composites can make teeth sensitive when first placed. But some patients experience continued sensitivity when their filling is "leaking"—that is, a gap exists between the tooth and its filling. With composite fillings, which are all based on resin-based materials, moisture like saliva, blood, or gum fluids can adversely affect its ability to bond properly.

When liquid composites are placed in the mouth, these plastic substances must be "cured" or polymerized, which hardens and sets the plastic through the use of a curing light. When the material is cured, the filling can shrink between 2 and 5 percent. If the bond is inadequate, the composite will shrink and have a marginal gap between filling and tooth, which will never improve. According to Dr. Stephen Dunne, Senior Lecturer and Consultant of the Department of Conservative Dentistry at Kings Dental Institute in London, 60 percent of curing lights in general practice are operating below manufacturer's specifications.

Composites have always been expected to last only half as long as amalgam fillings. However, Carl Leinfelder of the University of South Carolina, who performs materials-testing on humans, says that the "ideal" restorative materials least resistant to wear (even over fillings made of gold, classically considered the hardest substance) are certain makes of resin-based polymers placed in by a careful layering process.

Dentists using this method tend to etch the cavity, sealing it with a resin-bond layer. Next, they place in a soft, self-hardening substance of glass ionomer; over that goes more resin bond, then a macrofill material of high polymerization, which needs to be cured with the dentist's light. Another layer of bond follows and then a microfill substance after that, of high strength and low wear.

If you are contemplating having resin-based fillings, choose a dentist who uses a rubber dam and meticulous isolating procedures prior to placing the filling, as well as a reliable curing light. Most of all, he should have plenty of experience and lots of contented patients.

With your children's teeth, the best course of all is prevention. Breast-feed if you can, avoid giving them sugary drinks and too many sweets, provide them with a whole-foods diet including plenty of fruits and vegetables, and make sure they brush their teeth regularly and eat fruit after meals. As long ago as 1911, a survey in New Zealand of 1,500 schoolchildren found that if they ate alkaline, saliva-producing food after a meal, this food would neutralize the acidity of bacteria. This reduced the incidence of tooth decay enormously. One of the best alkaline saliva producers is fruit.

—V—

SURGERY

TEN

Standard Operating Procedure

Of all areas in medicine, surgery is probably the least scientific. Most decisions about operations have more to do with the personal taste of individual doctors, the arbitrary consensus of professional bodies, or just the fashion of the moment than with hard fact. For obvious ethical reasons, operations are almost never tested by controlled experiment, but are instead developed on an ad hoc basis and then taught to others—including trainees—more or less on the job. This means that many surgeons get enthused by new techniques before they know what they're doing or even whether the procedure is going to do any good at all.

Besides not knowing when to put down the knife, surgeons of all persuasions underestimate the simple risks involved in every type of surgery, no matter how "routine." A University of Oxford survey of some 225,000 operations in six nearby health districts found that one in ten emergency prostatectomies and more than one in five emergency hip replacements ended in death a year after the surgery. Although emergency procedures had far higher fatality rates, a number of elective procedures also carried high risks. For instance, people electing to have cataracts or their prostate removed had a one in twenty chance of dying up to a year after their operation due to complications during surgery.[1]

A high proportion of deaths occur because routine procedures aren't followed properly. According to one inquiry into deaths occurring around the time of surgery—information supplied voluntarily by over a thousand surgeons around Britain about postoperative deaths of patients in the month after an operation—many patients are needlessly dying after routine surgery. The inquiry found that deaths from deep vein thrombosis and blood clots in the lungs were commonplace, simply because drugs that would have counteracted the problem weren't administered. Many deaths were due to preoperative preparations or even the surgery itself being undertaken too hastily, or to too much fluid being given the patient during surgery, causing heart attacks. *A considerable number of deaths were caused by the surgeon's lack of familiarity with the operation.*[2]

Many treatments are faddish, adopted in a flurry of enthusiasm and soon discarded in favor of the next new possibility when evidence proves the original procedures don't work. Just consider the history of treatment for back pain. Earlier, in this century, sacroiliac joint disease was believed the culprit in many cases of back pain, leading to fusions (the joining of one vertebra to another) of the sacroiliac joints.

This was followed by such treatments as the removal of the coccyx, injections for slipped discs, lengthy bed rest, traction, and even nerve stimulation—all, in their turn, discarded.

The latest fad to be discredited is steroid injections in the facet joints (the cartilage covering of the bony junction between two vertebrae). Recent evidence finally revealed that injecting steroids is no-better than injecting salt water.[3]

Harvard Medical School once performed one of the few studies to see whether surgeons get it right when they recommend surgery. The Harvard researchers looked at the track record of over a hundred doctors in diagnosing one of the most common procedures—removal of nonmalignant moles. In all, the correct diagnosis was made in less than half the cases. Dermatologists—who should be able to do this with their eyes closed—got the diagnosis right only two-thirds of the time, while other types of doctors were only half as good as that. Like the diagnosis, the appropriate procedure was carried out only half of the time.

Standard Operating Procedure

Getting it wrong is nothing new with surgeons. In the United States some 6 million unnecessary operations and invasive tests get performed every year. Some 20,000 normal appendixes are mistakenly removed every year.[4]

In fact, with the vast bulk of surgery patients often go under the knife unnecessarily. Most children with chronic secretory middle ear infection undergo operations needlessly,[5] as do women undergoing a D and C (dilatation and curettage—scraping of the lining of the uterus) after complete miscarriage,[6] hysterectomy,[7] and even patients undergoing coronary bypass surgery. Bypass surgery might relieve symptoms in some patients, but there is no proof anywhere that this surgery actually prolongs life.[8] In one study involving researchers from fourteen major heart hospitals around the world, up to one-third of all bypass operations were found to be unnecessary and actually to hasten the death of the patient. One-third of the patients, considered low-risk cases, might have lived longer if they had received drug therapy rather than surgery.[9]

BYPASS SURGERY

Coronary bypass operations, in fact, are one of the most unnecessary operations of all. Heart surgeons have known this since the 1970s, when several major studies revealed that bypass surgery did not improve survival except among patients with severe coronary disease, particularly to the left ventricle. It did, however, appear to relieve severe angina.[10] The National Institutes of Health has estimated that 90 percent of American patients who undergo bypass surgery receive no benefits.

Bypass surgery may be the most appropriate choice only for

those with triple-vessel disease (when two-thirds of each artery is blocked). Although this covers just 10 percent of all heart condition sufferers, the bypass seems to be surviving better than its patients. (The death rate ranges from 3 to 23 percent in the United States.) This is not surprising when you consider that in America it is one of the best-paying of surgical procedures, earning surgeons some $40,000 per operation. This translates into an overall U.S. medical bill of $8 billion a year to treat just 200,000 people.

BACK PAIN

Treatment for back pain also aptly demonstrates how knife-happy many surgeons are without much in the way of evidence that operations will do any good. In most cases, medicine has shown a shocking ineptitude in diagnosing and treating back problems, often tending to make the problem worse.

Professor Gordon Waddell, orthopedic surgeon at Glasgow's Western Infirmary in Scotland, scathingly summed up this appalling track record: ". . . dramatic surgical successes, unfortunately, apply to only some 1 percent of patients with low back disorders. Our failure is in the remaining 99 percent of patients with simple backache, for whom, despite new investigations and all our treatments, the problem has become progressively worse."[11]

For back patients who undergo surgery, 15 to 20 percent will fall into the category of "the failed back"—the official name given to people with chronic, considerable back pain that doctors can't fix. Some 200,000 to 400,000 patients go under the knife in the United States every year. That translates into 30,000 to 80,000 Americans every year who will emerge from back surgery in considerably more pain than before they went to their doctor.

Many causes of disastrous residual pain are caused by inappropriate surgery for back pain. The most popular operations include: laminectomy, in which a disc and nearby bone are removed, to give the nerve branching off the central spinal cord more space to move without getting trapped or compressed by the spine; and fusion, in which one vertebra is surgically joined to another, in order to minimize what has usually been diagnosed as too much movement between the vertebrae. After fusion, this segment of the spine will be unable to move at all.

According to six studies of back operations, removing discs only relieves back pain in about half of all patients.[12] But of over a hundred cases of failed spinal surgery, primarily disc removal, surgery wasn't indicated for two-thirds of them.[13] Three out of four studies comparing operations with to those without lumbar (lower back) spinal fusion surgery found no advantage for fusion; complications, including chronic pain, were common.[14]

Another study of "failed back surgery syndrome" showed that in more than half of all such cases, the missed diagnosis or the surgery itself caused a condition called "lateral spinal stenosis," or narrowing of a portion of the spine, causing compression of the spinal cord or an abnormally tight fit.[15]

Even more fundamental are the sheer number of bad diagnoses. Of those patients referred to him at Gordon Waddell's clinic in Glasgow, "60 percent believe or have been told that they have a disc prolapse, although only 11 percent show any evidence of nerve root involvement," he says.[16]

Finally, postsurgical scarring ("epidural fibrosis") can itself cause failed surgery and chronic pain. Back specialist Henry La Rocca of Tulane University in Louisiana also found substantial evidence that surgeons cause nerve-root injury as the nerve is being separated from a herniated disc, causing scarring and therefore long-term pain and pressure on the nerve. "Damage to the dura or the cauda equina [membranes covering the spinal cord] from poor surgical technique yielding possibly catastrophic results completes the list," he writes.[17]

This is precisely what happened to Sarah. Her back problems developed after a hysterectomy, so she consented to surgery on her spine. The delicate layers of the spinal cord (meninges) became inflamed, and then thickened. This thickened membrane now presses constantly on her spine, incapacitating her with unbearable pain.

Gordon Waddell and others conclude that if there is a specific problem correctly identified—such as a spinal deformity or fracture or disc herniation—then surgery can help, but not for simple relief of unspecified back pain.[18]

SURGERY FOR BREAST CANCER

Besides being unnecessary, a large number of surgical procedures still widely used are clearly obsolete. The most obvious example is treatment for breast cancer. Despite a variety of surgical techniques, a host of back-up therapies, and many confident headlines about breast cancer breakthroughs, *the truth is that surgical treatment of breast cancer hasn't advanced one single step in the past century.* "Over a period of one hundred years," says Dr. Edward F. Scanlon of the Northwestern University Medical School in Illinois, who has studied breast cancer incidence in depth, "breast cancer treatment has evolved from no treatment to radical treatment and back again to more conservative management, without having affected mortality."[19]

Although governmental and most other official agencies recommend breast-conserving measures for breast cancer caught early, many surgeons persist in performing a mutilating operation developed in the nineteenth century and never really reviewed to see if it is still applicable to patients today—or indeed if it ever worked at all.

The standard procedure for breast cancer was developed by Dr. William Halsted a century ago. (Dr. Halsted is better known for advocating what was then a revolutionary notion: that surgeons should wear sterile gloves.) The operation he championed involves removing the breast, much of the skin, the chest wall, and the lymph nodes.

Shortly after the Second World War, a study at three hospitals in Illinois showed little difference in five- and ten-year survival rates between radical mastectomies, simple mastectomies, or simple removal of the tumor. Then, some twenty-five years later, *The Lancet* reviewed 8,000 cases and again found no difference in survival rates among the patients who had received any of these procedures.[20] Nevertheless, the Halsted procedure maintained a tight grip on the mind of the average surgeon over the next two decades. In some areas it was then replaced by "modified" radical surgery, which removed tissue and breast, but left the chest wall intact, or a simple mastectomy, which removed only the breast itself. But like its predecessor, the modified radical mastectomy was also put into place without any scientific studies proving its worth.

Like the earlier studies, new evidence in the 1980s showed that mastectomy provides no benefit in terms of cancer recurrence or survival over breast-conserving surgery (BCS) such as simple lumpectomy (removal of the tumor itself) or quadrantectomy (removal of a portion of the breast). In the most famous study, headed by Dr. Bernard Fisher and undertaken by the National Surgical Adjuvant Breast and Bowel Project in Pennsylvania, of nearly 2,000 women over nine years, there was no difference in survival rates among those who had undergone lumpectomy, those who had had lumpectomy plus irradiation, and those who had had a total mastectomy.[21]

Several years later, the Chicago Institute discovered that the Pennsylvania trial—which had been the largest in the United States on breast cancer—had been falsified. About 100 ineligible patients were included in the trial, which involved 5,000 patients in 485 academic and community hospitals. Once the fraud had been uncovered, two of the Pennsylvania teams pored over the research data again, excluding the ineligible patients, and nevertheless reached the same findings. After a second major U.S. cancer study also headed by Dr. Bernard Fisher was discredited, he resigned as research project chairman. In this second study, which tested the efficacy of tamoxifen to prevent breast cancer, Dr. Fisher was accused of withholding data about the association of tamoxifen and the development of endometrial cancer. Informed consent forms, which women have to read and sign before agreeing to join the trials, apparently did not include the latest data showing that four women had died after taking tamoxifen.[22]

Luckily, more recent research from the National Cancer Insti-

tute (NCI) in Bethesda, Maryland, confirms that lumpectomy
and radiation are just as effective as radical mastectomy in controlling early stage cancer. The NCI found that about three-
quarters of patients given lumpectomy and radiation survived,
which was comparable to the number of patients surviving after
a radical mastectomy.[23] And in Italy, researchers found that a
similar number of patients survived or had local recurrence of
cancer, whether they were given radical mastectomy or a breast-
conserving operation called a quadrantectomy (removal of only
a quarter of the breast), plus radiation.[24]

In 1990, the American National Institutes of Health recommended that surgeons opt for breast-conservation surgery over
mastectomy for the majority of women with stage I or stage II
breast cancer. By this they mean for tumors of less than 4 centimeters in diameter limited to the primary site (the single breast)
without involvement of the chest muscle or overlying skin. In
the past, doctors felt that cancer found in the axillary lymph
nodes was evidence of spread, and grounds for radical mastectomy. With the NIH's announcement, whether or not lymph
nodes are involved (so long as they are on the same side as the
tumor) is now considered immaterial.

Despite all the publicity about the safety of lumpectomies,
many doctors still think the more they cut out the better off a
woman is, and refuse to offer breast-conserving surgery to the
majority of women with early breast cancer. A Seattle study
examined cancer-registry information between 1983 and 1989.
Less than a third of women were offered BCS, even though
three-quarters of them clearly had early cancer. After 1985 (when
publicity about BCS had died down somewhat) the practice of
keeping breasts intact declined even further, and doctors returned
to modified radical mastectomies even though there was no evidence to support their choice.[25]

Doctors also failed to offer radiation therapy to women with
cancer who had already been through menopause, and were
more likely to sacrifice the breasts of older patients than younger
ones, even for the same stage of breast cancer. In fact, the more

affluent and well-educated the woman, the greater the chances of her breast being saved.[26]

Besides your education or ability to pay, where you live has a lot to do with whether you get to keep your breasts. Women are more likely to be offered BCS in the Northeast or Middle Atlantic States than in the South, in urban rather than rural areas, and in the larger hospitals with more facilities. Higher rates of conservation surgery also occur in those seventeen states with informed consent laws requiring doctors to offer breast-cancer patients information about their treatment options.[27]

The lack of information or support by doctors for BCS may account for the suspicion with which many women view breast-conserving measures. Many among the largely male fraternity of breast surgeons still believe that losing a breast isn't such a big deal. Several cancer specialists have attempted to demonstrate that women given mastectomies suffer no more psychological trauma than those undergoing BCS. As a batch of surgeons wrote: "Many view mastectomy as dealing with the problem immediately and completely, without postoperative radiotherapy. The acceptance, indeed preference, of mastectomy over breast-preserving surgery by the majority of our patients . . . implies that these patients adjust readily to the loss of the breast."[28]

Noted U.K. breast cancer specialist Michael Baum and others from London and Manchester studied the psychological outcome of women given mastectomies versus those given BCS. The study found that about a quarter of those given either operation were depressed or anxious. From this Baum and his colleagues concluded that there is no evidence to suggest that women with early breast cancer who undergo breast-conservation surgery are better off psychologically than those who undergo a mastectomy. Nevertheless, the key factor appeared to be control over the decision making; those patients who'd been allowed to choose their type of surgery were less likely to be depressed than those whose decision was made for them.[29]

HERNIA REPAIR

In the field of other types of surgery, often no one can agree on the best technique to sort out a problem. Although a good hernia repair is as difficult as the most complex abdominal surgery, senior surgeons leave this kind of surgery, which they consider routine and boring, to trainees to cut their professional teeth on. In some countries, interns are allowed to go it alone after only six hernia repairs.[30] This is perhaps one reason for its dismal success rate. It is four times more dangerous to have a hernia operation than to go without one if you're over sixty-five.[31] Up to one-fifth of operations have to be repeated within five years—a recurrence rate that rises to one in every two by the third operation.

There's also no professional consensus about the best procedure. In Britain, the Royal College of Surgeon's concluded that no clear-cut gold standard existed for hernia repair. The original Bassini technique, developed in 1887—a very effective operation that reinforced the ruptured abdominal wall by stitching through three layers after creating an "envelope of tissue"—has been corrupted into a simple "darning" of crisscross stitches, which any surgery student can readily do. The problem with the darn is that it can readily give way. Although the Bassini technique was resurrected in Toronto at the Shouldice Clinic, with excellent results (only 1 percent returned for repeat operations), only a fifth of surgeons in Britain currently practice it.[32]

PROSTATE CANCER

In too many instances, surgeons rush in with the scalpel too early, when simple watchful waiting—that is, monitoring the situation to see if it gets worse—is called for. This is the case with prostate cancer. The commonest form of cancer (and surgery) for men over forty concerns the prostate, the gland that lies just below the base of the bladder and produces some of the seminal fluid. Because it is so close to the bladder and urethra, problems in this area invariably cause problems with urination. Although the incidence of prostate cancer hasn't really gone up, the incidence of aggressive treatments such as radiation and surgery has— by a whopping 36 percent.

Nine cancer registries throughout America, plus data compiled by the National Center for Health Statistics, together showed only a modest increase in prostate cancer incidence between 1983 and 1989 (due mainly to increased attempts at detecting early-stage disease). There was no increase in the types of cancer that spread and that can be fatal. Nevertheless, the rates of prostatectomy (surgical removal of the prostate gland) increased by nearly 35 percent per year, and varied greatly from area to area.[33]

Nevertheless, all this aggressive cutting doesn't seem to make the slightest bit of difference to survival rates. Substantial evidence proves that conservative treatment of early prostate cancer—that is, maintaining a watchful wait-and-see attitude, and using other forms of therapy such as hormonal treatment rather than rushing into surgery—could be the best recourse, particularly in older men with a life expectancy of ten years or less.[34] This is largely because prostate cancer can be, in the main, a slow-growing form of cancer. According to autopsy reports, a third of men in the European Community have prostate cancer, but only 1 percent die of it.[35] Particularly in men over seventy, patients are more likely to die with their prostate cancer than of it.[36]

There is plenty of evidence that most prostate cancer doesn't spread. In two studies during a decade of observations, tumors had only undergone local growth and hadn't spread to other organs in two-third of the patients. In these patients, hormonal treatment was usually successful.[37]

Among men over seventy, radical prostatectomy not only isn't better than watchful waiting, but can also be downright harmful.[38] Thirty days after the operation, nearly 2 percent of men over seventy-five die. Survival rates can be higher in groups for whom nothing is done (other than watchful waiting), compared with groups undergoing surgery.[39] Many patients who undergo surgery die from a number of major heart-related complications within a month after they've had their operation.[40]

The reason for the sudden burgeoning of radical prostatectomies has to do with the introduction of the "nerve-sparing" technique. In this operation, both the inner gland and the capsule of the prostate gland are removed. However, nearly 100 percent of the nerves are spared, supposedly to maintain sexual potency.

Several studies have reported excellent survival rates with this technique—as high as 80 percent can enjoy a five- to ten-year survival rate.[41] However, the notion of the surgery "sparing" potency is largely fanciful. Half of all patients still lose potency, and around 5 percent become incontinent. The other downside is that it is major abdominal surgery, performed above the pubic bone, and you stand to suffer complications if your surgeon isn't very experienced.

Besides not improving survival, having any sort of medical treatment, whether with drugs or surgery, negatively affects your quality of life. Prostate cancer patients given surgery or drugs have been found to be significantly worse off in terms of sexual, urinary, and bowel function than those whose progress is simply monitored carefully. The incidence of complications with treatment are also much higher than generally thought.[42]

But the most important point is that radical surgery is indicated in only a very small number of cases: for those with a very early cancer (stage I), confined to the gland itself and not the capsule containing it or any lymph nodes. It is also only effective if the margins around the gland are free from cancer.[43]

If you were in your seventies, and had early cancer, the decision would be easy: to elect for watchful waiting. However, if you are younger than that, much depends on which stage the cancer is at and whether you meet the criteria for surgery. For those with a substantially longer age-related survival rate than ten years, the "watchful waiting" approach supposedly is associated with a higher probability of living with cancer that spreads, or dying from prostate cancer.[44]

However, most new evidence does show that conservative management can be a reasonable choice for men of all ages with stage I or II disease. It also admits that the benefit of aggressive treatment (as against conservative management) even for grade

III cancer is "less clear" and that new strategies for this stage of cancer are needed. Other research shows that even younger men—those who reach their sixties—with slow-growing prostate cancer are likely to live as long as men without tumors. In one University of Connecticut study, only 9 percent of patients with low-grade cancer had died, even after fifteen years. And only those with fast-growing—or higher-grade—tumors may die earlier, possibly losing between four and eight years off their life expectancy. Nevertheless, even those with higher-grade tumors may be better off without having radical surgery, as the years lost may not outweigh the significant problems associated with treatment.[45] This is as good as admitting that surgery for many patients may not be doing any good.

Aside from the fact that prostate surgery doesn't seem to improve survival, radical intervention and screening may simply bring to light many cancers that would otherwise remain dormant—and harmless—if left undetected. There is also some worry in certain medical circles that radical surgery to treat prostate cancer (and breast cancer) may only succeed in spreading the condition. Doctors have assumed that the poor survival rate had to do with the deadly ability of prostate cancer to spread. But it has now been discovered that surgeons are accidentally spreading cancer cells to other parts of the body while performing the surgery. In one study, among fourteen monitored operations, prostate cancer cells were discovered in the blood of twelve patients afterward. Only three had had such cell circulation before they'd been operated on.[46] Similar concerns have arisen over whether breast surgery causes tumor cells to spread,[47] particularly as surgery appears to increase the risk of relapse or death within three years of the procedure.[48]

HYSTERECTOMY

The hysterectomy is second only to cesarean section on the list of most common operations in the United States. If you are a woman in America, you've got a one in three chance of losing your uterus by the time you're sixty.

But hysterectomy outranks all others when it comes to the most unnecessary of surgical procedures. Three-quarters of all hysterectomies are performed on women under fifty for highly dubious reasons. Although the only viable reasons for performing a hysterectomy are uterine or endometrial cancer or uncontrollable bleeding after childbirth, these account for only about 10 percent of all procedures performed.[49]

The remaining 90 percent of hysterectomies are carried out for a number of questionable purposes: fibroids, endometriosis, bladder prolapse, tipped wombs, heavy periods or unexplained period troubles, which are often given the fanciful gynecological appellation "pelvic congestion." One measure of how little treatment rests on solid evidence or a strict criteria for recommending the operation is the enormous variation in the rates of hysterectomy between individual doctors or areas of the country, with the highest rates often among black or poor American women.[50]

Hysterectomy is often used to "prevent" ovarian cancer in women who have had uterine cancer even though only 2 in every 1,000 women who've had a hysterectomy will go on to develop ovarian cancer,[51] and the disease itself is rare. Besides just-in-case removal of ovaries, hysterectomy for other sorts of cancer prevention is equally unjustified. Less than 2 of every 1,000 fibroids, and less than 3 percent of abnormal endometrial cells, will progress to cancer.[52] Since hysterectomy carries a mortality rate of 1 per every 1,000 procedures—a risk that increases with age—and serious complications occur fifteen times more frequently than that, the risk of contracting cancer is far less than the risk of dying or being seriously injured from the operation. In fact, in abdominal hysterectomies, side effects can occur in more than 40 percent of operations.[53]

These side effects can include bowel problems,[54] urinary retention or incontinence,[55] and the risk of a fatal blood clot, particularly in women after menopause,[56] which can occur in one in every 6,000 operations. One-third to nearly one-half of all women undergoing hysterectomy or removal of ovaries report a decrease in sexual response.[57] If a woman's ovaries are removed at the same time, she will experience severe menopausal symptoms.[58] Even if the ovaries are left in, hysterectomy may lead to early ovarian failure, bringing on menopause far earlier than usual.[59]

Other than the true indications for hysterectomy, virtually every other indication for hysterectomy can be treated with conservative surgery, medication, diet, nutritional supplementation, alternative medicine or, in the case of fibroids, waiting until you reach menopause, when they will automatically shrink.[60]

TRANSCERVICAL RESECTION OF THE UTERUS

Surgeons are great enthusiasts of new procedures that haven't stood the test of time. In May 1991, doctors were enthusing about a supposed gynecological breakthrough, transcervical resection of the endometrium (TCRE), or removal of the lining of the uterus, for women with abnormally heavy periods. This new procedure was meant to replace the more radical former treatment of choice: hysterectomy. Medical magazines proclaimed that 18,000 women a year could substitute outpatient TCRE surgery for hysterectomy. After one study—the source of all the fanfare—doctors noted that over 90 percent of the patients enjoyed improved menstrual symptoms during the two and a half years of follow-up. There were a number of warning signals— out of 234 patients, up to forty-two of the women stopped having periods, sixteen needed repeat TCREs, two reported severe cyclical pain, ten went on to have hysterectomies, and a majority were left with a severely shrunken uterus that had developed fibroids.[61]

Just two months later, journals that had been enthusing about the new breakthrough procedures were now issuing warnings following the deaths of five women who had undergone the procedure. In two other cases, a patient lost a leg and another suffered a hole in the aorta as a result of the procedure, even though she was in the care of very experienced surgeons. Uterine perforation is one of the main severe complications; endometrial resection can stimulate a particular nerve, causing violent closing of the patient's thighs and thus causing the surgeon to "miss" and perforate the uterus.[62] One patient whose uterus was perforated nearly died, and since then she has suffered from chronic pelvic pain and diarrhea. In one study, one in twenty of the women with resections went on to have hysterectomies.

Two years after the procedure, four healthy women who'd had the treatment for heavy periods went on to develop encephalopathy, or inflammation of the brain, and one died after suffering seizures. These conditions were caused by the "irrigating solution," which is continuously infused into the uterus to wash away debris and tissue during the laser treatment. In the case of these four women, enough of the solution was apparently absorbed to cause encephalopathy.[63]

For all the hoopla, the procedure has made no dent in the number of hysterectomies being performed, as a number of government reports demonstrate. In Britain, Oxford Regional Health Authority, which studied surgery rates in six local districts, discovered that endometrial ablation has simply created a new niche for surgeons. The number of hysterectomies performed has remained constant since before the procedure was introduced.[64] In fact, most women who have the lining of their uterus removed by endometrial resection will end up having a full hysterectomy anyway. About 87 percent complain afterward of continual vaginal bleeding and in some cases quite heavy loss of blood—one of the problems the technique is supposed to treat. Women who have the procedure are also more likely to suffer pain after surgery—in 11 percent of cases, worse pain than before the operation, and about a fifth of women also experience worse premenstrual symptoms.[65]

BLOOD TRANSFUSIONS

Perhaps the biggest risk you face when you have an operation has nothing to do with the scalpel. The U.S. Red Cross now admits that even in the most dire of emergencies, blood transfusions oftentimes only add to complications or increase a patient's chances of dying. Although the specter of AIDS- and HIV virus-contaminated blood has curtailed blood donation and transfusions (both the United States and the United Kingdom have critically low supplies of blood at the time of writing), the latter is still routine in most surgical procedures and emergencies—in many cases without any medical justification whatsoever for its use or any guidelines as to when it is necessary.

Like so many other practices in medicine, the guidelines doctors follow when deciding whether or not to give a transfusion have been adopted with very little in the way of scientific evidence. An estimated one-third to three-quarters of those given blood are transfused inappropriately to treat a diminished volume of blood or a low nutritional status (that is, anemia). Anthony Britten of the Red Cross Blood Services has admitted that there is "gross overuse of blood products like albumin and plasma and also whole blood or red blood cells. Usage patterns vary so widely from place to place that it is clear that common standards do not exist for their use."[66]

In 1989, an Office of Technology Assessment Task Force report estimated that as much as 20 to 25 percent of red blood cells, 90 percent of albumin, and 95 percent of fresh-frozen plasma transfused into patients is not needed. Indeed, a common "transfusion trigger" is the measurement of hemoglobin (a compound in red blood cells transporting oxygen to the cells). Medicine uses the same "trigger" level for men and women, even though women naturally have lower red blood cell counts than do men. "Iron deficiency anemia continues to be among the leading reasons for transfusions, even though it rarely warrants [them]," said the report.[67]

Many in medicine have begun to question some of the most established practices for administering blood before and during surgery. A survey of 1,000 American anesthesiologists concluded that there were "wide variations in transfusions practices" among anesthesiologists, based on "habit rather than scientific data."[68] One such habit is the automatic administration of blood before operations in patients whose hemoglobin level is below 10 grams per 100 milliliters of blood. The practice apparently arose from a misreading by a hematologist of a study performed on dogs, which was accepted as gospel and preached to an entire generation of anesthesiology students.[69]

Premature infants probably get more transfusions than any other body of patients in hospitals (apart from hemophiliacs).[70] Transfusion is automatic if a baby is under 1,500 grams (3 pounds), a practice that has little in the way of evidence.[71] Blood components are also routinely irradiated, supposedly to reduce the risk of patients with immune-system problems rejecting the foreign blood. It has always been assumed that irradiation is harmless to red cells and has little effect on the function of the various components in the blood. But this irradiated blood may have too high a concentration of potassium, which could be especially hazardous to babies and pregnant mothers.

Besides giving blood for the wrong reasons, doctors often give out the wrong blood. In an informal questionnaire sent to 4,000 hospital hematology laboratories in Britain, one-third of the 245 labs that responded reported multiple incidents in which their patients received the wrong blood. In most cases, the patient was given the wrong blood while on the ward or in the operating room. Of some 111 such errors, 6 people died and 23 got ill.[72] And, since the question about handing out the wrong blood wasn't even asked on the questionnaire (but was volunteered by the labs), even the study had to admit that this was probably a gross underestimate of transfusion mistakes.

This questionnaire represented the first time that blood transfusions had ever been monitored in Britain, even though they have been practiced for fifty years. However, this error rate corresponds with that of the United States, which is supposed to have the tightest strictures on blood usage in the world.

After tallying the questionnaires, the study concluded that the wrong blood is given in one of every 6,000 red cell units given. In other research most errors have been found to arise when blood samples are inadequately documented or when information about which blood to be given to which patient is incorrect;

two London teaching hospitals recently studied were shown to have inadequate information on the blood of a quarter of its patients.[73]

A recent conference announced that transfusions have never been subjected to proper scientific study—that is, a randomized, double-blind trial—to see if indeed there are any benefits. *Like much of modern medicine, what probably is a useful court of last resort has been introduced and adopted as a first-line standard practice on the a priori assumption of benefit without one shred of scientific proof.*

Even if you believe that giving and getting blood is warranted, the number of blood-borne diseases you can contract from other people might well change your mind. The arrival of AIDS has given blood transfusion the quality of Russian roulette.

Because we really don't understand what causes AIDS or whether there needs to be another cofactor to convert HIV to AIDS (as Luc Montagnier, the codiscoverer of the AIDS virus, now maintains), we also don't understand how long the HIV virus (if indeed it is the cause of AIDS) incubates before transforming into the full-blown disease.[74] What we do know about is the considerable risk of contracting hepatitis from donated blood. Hepatitis from transfusions develops in an estimated 7 to 10 percent of blood recipients from unpaid donors in the United States.[75] This incidence multiplies three to four times among recipients of blood from paid donors. This translates to up to 230,000 new cases of hepatitis in the United States every year. The reason for the epidemic of cases is that there is, to date, no test reliable or sensitive enough to detect the agents that cause the disease. In fact, most cases of hepatitis C are due to blood transfusions or needle sharing among drug users. The Irish government has attempted to trace some 100,000 rhesus-negative mothers given blood transfusions in 1977 to see if they have developed hepatitis C, following an outbreak of hepatitis C among people who received transfusions in that year.[76]

Although the Centers for Disease Control and Prevention claim the Irish outbreak is the first of its kind, some among the medical community believe that anyone who received a blood transfusion before 1991 could be at risk of hepatitis C infection.

Indeed, in Britain, some 3,000 hemophiliacs were recently found to have contracted hepatitis C. Doctors now wonder whether intravenous immunoglobulin, a protein given to stimulate the immune system, can actually trigger hepatitis C. More than one hundred cases were recorded in the United States last year, and a new group of twenty victims has been reported in Norway.

Since 1991, a screening test has been developed for the hepatitis C virus, showing that one in 2,000 blood donors supposedly is positive for hepatitis C antibodies.[77] However, even this screening test isn't necessarily going to protect you. A number of doctors recently wrote to the British Medical Journal to complain about the inaccuracy of the test.[78] These doctors, from the virology departments of City Hospital in Edinburgh, Scotland, and John Radcliffe Hospital in Oxford, said that in the first eight months of screening for hepatitis C virus in the Oxford region, some 83,000 units of blood (from some 70,000 donors) were subjected to a second-generation enzyme-linked immunoassay (ELISA) test, the test most often used to detect hepatitis C.

In the sample, 358 donors showed up repeatedly as positive. When all those tested as positive were tested again by two other, more recently developed tests, the second-generation recombinant immunoblot assay (RIBA-2) or the Murex BCJ11 ELISA, the ELISA test was proved wrong more than three-quarters of the time.

Besides hepatitis, the risk of contracting human T-cell leukemia (HTLV-1) from blood is ten times higher than the risk of contracting HIV.[79] This risk skyrockets when you consider that many blood recipients, including premature babies, are given the blood components from what can be, on average, as many as nine donors.

The medical literature is awash with studies about patients undergoing operations who have fared worse on foreign transfused blood than on autotransfusion (receiving their own stored or recovered blood). Blood transfusion has been linked with organ system failure, recurrence of cancer, a high risk of postoperative infection, and graft-versus-host disease—a condition affecting the joints, heart, and blood cells in which the recipient rejects the transfused blood.

Besides the various diseases you can contract from someone else's blood, if you're a cancer patient a blood transfusion may depress your immune system, causing or in some way aiding a recurrence. In one study, the recurrence rate for patients with cancer of the larynx was 14 percent among those who didn't receive blood transfusions, and more than four times as great among those who did. Of those with cancer of the oral cavity, pharynx, and nose, the recurrence rate was 31 percent without transfusions and more than double that with them.[80]

A poorer outcome was also experienced in patients receiving blood transfusions after surgery for lung cancer[81] as well as for those with colonic, rectal, cervical, and prostate cancers.[82] There also seemed to be a higher incidence of recurrence if a patient received whole blood rather than simply red blood cells alone.

Having a transfusion during an operation also increases your chances of infection.[83]

In patients undergoing major abdominal surgery, blood transfusion has been the most significant contributor to organ system failure.[84]

Besides lowering your chances of surviving, you can suffer side effects from blood that are every bit as severe as the worst reaction to a drug. Although the usual reactions include hives, fever, or chills, some patients experience a severe reaction in the lungs, sometimes fatal, with some kinds of plasma, a risk that is higher than previously thought.[85] There are also substantial risks of general infection and life-threatening allergic reactions, as well as of contracting a sexually transmitted disease such as cytomegalovirus (CMV). It may well be, as one study concluded, that blood, like fingerprints, is uniquely—untransferably—individual: "The unavoidable, biological (and now legally recognized) fact is that each person's blood contains a multiplicity of antibodies, antigens, and infectious agents, many of which have yet to be identified by scientists and cannot presently be detected. 'Pure blood' . . . is finally understood by courts to be imaginary."[86]

JUST A MINUTE, SURGEON

Before you go in for surgery, it's important, in effect, to interview your surgeon, not least about his batting average. It is not
automatically the case that surgery will make you feel better or
that your surgeon is incapable of making a horrendous mistake.
Ask your surgeon how many of these operations he's done and
which procedure he follows. If he's just cutting his teeth himself
and hasn't done more than ten or fifteen, find a more experienced hand. It's also essential that you know exactly who is
doing the operating. In many cases, particularly routine surgery,
experienced surgeons supervise juniors, who get to practice routine procedures. Insist that the experienced surgeon does the job,
or find one who will. And, most important, make sure you feel
comfortable and confident with the surgeon; after all, you are
going to be completely in his hands.

You can also help to make up your mind about risks and
benefits by finding out about the complication rate for a procedure. Discuss the other treatment options with a variety of specialists. Ask about the scientific evidence supporting their claimed
results. Carefully weigh the risks of refusing surgery against the
risks of the procedure itself on your future quality of life.

If you have any doubt concerning the surgeon's candor about
treatment options or his ability to consider you an equal partner
in any treatment decisions, reach for your hat, walk out the door,
and find yourself a surgeon who will.

As for transfusions, bear in mind that doctors have successfully
transfused patients with their own blood, donated ahead of time,
for all sorts of major surgery, including coronary bypasses, congenital heart surgery, or cancer. Thirteen-year-old Lucy Buxton
of England made the news in early 1994 for donating her own
blood to have on hand before having her tonsils out. This technique can even be used during emergencies such as hemorrhage
and trauma.

Doctors can also use hemodilution, a procedure that maintains
the amount of fluid circulating around the body through artificial
fluid-volume expanders. One study of some 10,000 surgery pa-

tients concluded that adult patients can undergo rapid loss of a third of the total volume of blood and not go into irreversible shock if hemodilution is adequate.[87] During emergencies, contaminated blood (which has been exposed to, say, intestinal contents) can be safely cleaned and recycled with a cell-washing system. Circulating blood volume can also be kept up with fluid replacements. Six thousand patients undergoing open heart operations demonstrated that they had improved outcomes once blood transfusion was stopped and volume expanders substituted.[88]

ELEVEN

Gee-Whiz Technology: The Video-Games Wizard and Blocked Drains Mechanic

Twenty years since the first successful heart transplant, with the arrival of the computer chip and many highly specialized drugs, Western medicine is without parallel in offering miraculous solutions to what used to be considered the hopeless case. These days, medicine can give you a new heart or liver, install a new, artificial hip or knee, clear your arteries without the slightest incision, and even make babies in women well past menopause. The wheelchair-bound believe they are an operation away from walking; the infertile, a test tube away from a new baby. But like the rest of surgery (and most of these techniques *are* operations of a sort), every last one of these glamorous new technologies has been adopted incautiously, given the official seal of approval and employed on millions before the slightest shred of evidence exists that they work, especially over the long term, let alone whether they truly represent advances over any techniques they replace. It is only after millions of desperate patients rush to try the new miracle solutions that we begin to find out what the potential problems are.

The most insidious part of "miracle-breakthrough" technology concerns the gushing public relations exercise surrounding it. The press often uncritically portray a new procedure as a miraculous breakthrough without reservation, before it has stood the test of time. On February 4, 1990, one newspaper proclaimed in banner headlines about fetal surgery: "Unborn baby wanted by doctors for Miracle Op." A week later, once the appropriate candidate had been found, the same newspaper published, with slightly less fanfare, the chilling results: "Womb Operation Baby Dies in Mother's Arms."[1]

There is no doubt that for many individuals with no alternatives, fetal surgery, joint replacement operations, or organ transplants can prove lifesaving. But in too many instances the idea of the "miracle cure" captures the imagination of both doctor and patient and the new technique becomes the first (rather than the last) port of call for everyone, regardless of whether they are the right candidate. In the rush to embrace this new technique, and the doctor's eagerness to try his hand at the latest space-age gadgetry, the downside of the various techniques get played down, if not entirely ignored. We hear about the fact that heart, liver, pancreas, lung, and intestinal transplants are now routine. We hear a good deal less about the fact that a third of these transplants get rejected, or about the dilemma facing many patients in choosing between the possibility that their body may reject the transplanted organ and the side effects of powerful immunosuppressive drugs such as cyclosporine (which must be taken to prevent the body from rejecting a new organ as "foreign"). Many patients who remain on cyclosporine keep the transplant, but at the expense of their own kidneys, which may develop chronic and progressive (and permanent) disease, and eventually fail, even after the immunosuppressive drugs are withdrawn.[2]

KEYHOLE SURGERY

At the moment, the surgical fad *du jour* that has taken the operating theater by storm is minimally invasive, or keyhole, surgery. This form of surgery has been hailed as one of the great medical innovations of the century, and there's no doubt that the technology is impressive. Using the latest microtechnology, surgeons can perform major operations without the trauma (and cutting) of conventional open surgery. In theory, at least, the patient should be able to leave the hospital quickly—often, that same day—and enjoy a far less painful and far more speedy recovery, sometimes months sooner than he would after a conventional operation.

One of the fastest-growing techniques in the entire health field, keyhole surgery is already being used in one in five of all abdominal operations, and is likely to be used in 70 percent of all operations by the end of this century.

Video-Games Playing

Minimally invasive surgery (also known as MIS) involves making four or five minor incisions—usually only 5 to 7 centimeters (2 to 3 inches) long—through one of which a device called a laparoscope is threaded. The laparoscope works as the surgeon's "eyes"; a minute lens on its tip transmits pictures of the internal organs onto a video screen.

Once other tubular instruments are threaded down the other incisions, the operation takes place via the video screen. If a tumor or part of an organ has to be removed, it is first cut away, then compressed and squeezed through the incisions. The technique also involves the use of xenon light beams and lasers.

Although the laparoscope has been used for over twenty years by gynecologists, only recently has the technology developed sufficiently to allow instruments to be fitted and used for investigative procedures (say, to check the state of a woman's ovaries) or to cut and perform ligatures (such as tying up arteries or cutting out tumors). The entire procedure can take up to seven times as long as conventional open surgery.

While keyhole techniques have been used most frequently to date for gallbladder surgery, hernias, and a variety of abdominal operations, it is now being tried out on other types of surgery.

The first operation on cancer using laparoscopic equipment was carried out in 1991; the first kidney was removed using the procedure a year earlier.

The biggest problem with this most sensational of surgical techniques is that most surgeons have gone at it with inadequate training. This was the tacit admission of a clinic in London where a woman died after receiving keyhole bowel exploratory surgery. Although the surgeon's name was cleared, the clinic where the operation was performed banned all laparoscopic procedures until independent experts could confirm that surgeons were qualified to perform the operations.

"It was merely the surgeons' enthusiasm for something new and the worry of being left behind if they did not master the technique that led to the explosion in popularity of this minimally invasive surgery." Dr. David Lomax wrote in a letter to *The Lancet,*[3] commenting about the sudden explosion of this technique for any and all surgery, often inappropriately.

It is widely accepted that the general level of skill is low, sometimes dangerously so. In Britain, the government has set aside $6.6 million to train surgeons specifically in keyhole techniques. This training program came about as a result of a report by a working party of surgeons headed by keyhole-surgery pioneer Professor Alfred Cushieri. The British government has refused to publish the findings of this report—which can only lead to speculation that the findings are far more alarming than the currently known facts.

"Adverse Incidents"

These facts include 158 reported "adverse incidents" involving keyhole surgery between August 1990 and May 1992 in New York State alone. Twenty-four of these were "permanent or life threatening," and more than two-thirds required further surgery to repair injuries.[4] In the first twenty-six kidney laparoscopic operations done at Washington University, nearly a third of patients suffered complications. Those with major complications had to be operated on again, using open surgery.

With laparoscopic cholecystectomy—the removal of the gall-bladder by keyhole surgery—the number of complications and hospital readmissions has risen sharply with the increased use of keyhole surgery techniques. The number of bile duct injuries has increased by 305 percent in three years, now that keyhole surgery is used in 86 percent of such gallbladder operations. Although the problem was always blamed on lack of skill, researchers now believe the dangers are inherent in the procedure itself, and that even after doctors become familiar with the procedures, the number of injuries don't go down.[5]

Serious complications arise in 15 out of every 1,000 procedures in gynecological operations, a favored area for laparoscopic surgery, according to figures from the American Association of Gynecologic Laparoscopists; 3 out of every 100,000 patients die as a result. Even the favorite of laparoscopic techniques, a gallbladder operation, is not without a high error rate, considering the number of procedures now being performed. In a recent U.S. survey of 77,604 of these operations, over half of the deaths due to the surgery were attributed to complications of the laparoscopic technique.[6] In Britain, the first legal compensation has been awarded to a woman who may need a liver transplant after a routine gallbladder operation went wrong when the surgeon accidentally cut her bile duct, which leaked and caused jaundice.

Lucy underwent a gallbladder operation by keyhole surgery in August 1991:

> Shortly afterward I experienced pain on walking. After various investigations I was diagnosed as having avascular necrosis of the head of the left thigh. [That means death of some of the cells in a tissue, not involving blood vessels but possibly caused by inadequate blood supply to the tissue, or injury.] The surgeon who carried out the cholecystectomy stands by his opinion that there is no connection, even though he can offer no explanation as to why I should have contracted avascular necrosis—a condition usually associated with deep-sea divers, chronic alcoholics, and people who fracture their hip.

Lucy is now permanently disabled. Because the condition is so new, it has not been recognized by the Royal College of Surgeons as being caused by the operation. Nor is there any compensation scheme available to recompense patients who suffer this sort of injury.

Up until now, so long as a surgeon passed his general training he was allowed to have a go at this new technique, even if he hadn't a clue about how to do it. In many cases, surgeons were virtually experimenting with their patients, for fear of being seen to be old-fashioned.

Gynecologists, in particular, as one surgeon put it, were particularly prone to rushing in too early as "kamikaze surgeons," and either "push the bounds of this surgery to the outer limits" or are clumsy at it—"as maladroit as a beetle on its back."[7]

Instead of the usual "hands-on" experience the surgeon is used to, he has to have the skills of a video-games player. Rather than being able to see the organ in front of him, he has to judge three dimensions by using a scope, and then has to manipulate his instruments to do the work ordinarily done by his hands. It means that he is, in effect, operating without the sense of touch, and must get used to different way of seeing—with a microtechnology that doesn't afford even the most experienced surgeon the normal full range of vision.[8]

A common complication is the puncturing of organs with the microscopic equipment, which accounted for 3 out of 10,000 complications in gynecological surgery done in the United States, and 0.05 percent of laparoscopic cholecystectomies. Of these, two patients died as a result of their injury. A case in Australia also showed up the inadequacy of some of the microtechnology being used. One charge of negligence has been filed because the surgeon in question did not fully appreciate that the field of vision provided through a laparoscope is limited.[9] Because the surgeon could not see what he was doing properly, a needle entered the patient's colon during the procedure (the surgeon was later found not to be negligent).

Another complication—usually among the elderly or those with a heart condition—can be triggered by the carbon dioxide used to inflate the abdomen, a standard procedure in order to give the laparoscope room to "see." After carbon dioxide is introduced, sudden irregular heartbeat is reported in 17 percent of patients, according to one British study. A third of patients in another study suffered a slowing heart rate.[10]

In the United States, some states do not allow surgeons to perform minimally invasive surgery unless they have been properly trained. In other countries, such as the United Kingdom, surgeons with little or no experience have been able to carry out the procedure. The Society of American Gastrointestinal Endoscopic Surgeons has suggested that surgeons should first carry out procedures on animals before being allowed to operate on people.

In early 1994, the senate of the Royal Surgical Colleges of Great Britain and Ireland introduced new quality assurance levels and a certificate of competence, which established surgeons now have to work for before they can practice keyhole surgery. Training, assessment, and certification will become mandatory, and those trainees not found up to scratch will not receive certification or be able to carry out the procedures.

Even open surgery for treating cancer carries a high risk of spreading diseased cells to healthy ones. But this risk multiplies with keyhole surgery, because the surgeon does not have full visibility or control, and also because cancerous organs and cells have to be squeezed through small incisions, thus increasing the likelihood that the diseased cells will drop off and "plant" themselves within healthy organs. This problem was highlighted recently in Cardiff, where two women who underwent keyhole surgery for gallbladder cancer both went on to die from cancer. In both cases, as the surgeons pulled the malignant tissue through the small hole in the wall of the abdomen, cancer cells broke off and planted themselves in the abdomen.

Longer and More Dangerous

Some of the risks associated with keyhole surgery might be worth it, if this technique definitely could be shown to offer real benefits to patients—such as a genuinely far speedier recovery rate than after conventional surgery. But the studies finally being done show that keyhole is not always best. One of the first major randomized studies comparing removal of the appendix with laparoscopic techniques and conventional open appendectomy showed there was no difference in postoperative pain and recovery rate among patients. This devastating finding kicks away one of the platforms on which laparoscopic procedures have been championed.

The study, by the Prince of Wales Hospital in Hong Kong, was based on a comparison of seventy patients who underwent open appendectomy and seventy on whom laparoscopic procedures were performed. Each study group was similar in age, sex ratio, and duration of symptoms. There were no major complications in either group, although 20 percent of the laparoscopic group had to convert to an open operation during their keyhole surgery.

The Hong Kong research team found no difference between the groups in terms of severity of pain, need for painkilling drugs, timetable for reintroducing a normal diet, or hospital stay. Similar numbers from both groups attended follow-up examinations three weeks after surgery, and similar proportions—79 percent of laparoscopic patients versus 74 percent of open-surgery patients—had returned to work by that time.[11]

In fairness, it should be noted that open appendectomy is no longer the major invasive technique it once was, but can now be performed by making a small, muscle-splitting incision. Hence the difference between keyhole and open surgery in this particular operation may be slight, compared to, say, gallbladder surgery.

Another study, setting laparoscopic hysterectomy against the standard vaginal procedure, concluded that keyhole surgery took nearly twice as long. A study team from the Royal Free Hospital in London found that the traditional method was not only much faster, but that recovery rates were similar for both groups.[12] A study done by the Indian Council of Medical Research revealed that the complication rate of keyhole sterilization surgery was seven times that of minilaparotomy (the usual open "Band-Aid" approach).[13] Hernia operations are known to result in a high prevalence of internal scar tissue and salpingitis (inflammation of the fallopian tubes in women).[14]

Obviously what is needed are wholesale studies setting keyhole surgery against its conventional counterpart, to gauge the type of operations for which MIS is most appropriate. It may well become the procedure favored for operations such as cholecystectomy, but may prove inappropriate for appendectomy and cancer.[15]

Surgeons eager to try their hand at the new technique also need to be reined in when the surgery isn't needed. A recent study found that gallbladder operations had increased by a fifth since the advent of keyhole surgery.[16]

JOINT-REPLACEMENT SURGERY

The new joint-replacement surgical technique is another example of a faddish procedure embraced without proper testing. Joint replacement entails replacing the cartilage of hip or knee joints, worn away by osteoarthritis, with an artificial joint made of a mix of metal and polyethylene. Undoubtedly this procedure, which has transformed the lives of many older people, restoring the wheelchair-bound to normal activity, is justifiably regarded as miracle surgery. But largely because of the heady experience of making the lame walk, doctors are too quick to order up an operation without considering the consequences or any alternatives, particularly in young people. It's estimated that 10 percent of people over sixty-five have a hip replacement, making it the most common form of surgery in the United Kingdom (more than 45,000 were performed in 1991). In the United States, some 141,000 patients had total knee replacement surgery in 1990.[17]

Old and New Technologies

Both knee replacement and hip replacement have a relatively good track record when performed with the older types of equipment. When artificial knee joints are cemented into place, an analysis of 130 studies shows that 89 percent are successful and the knee remains functional for more than four years.[18] The Royal Orthopaedic Hospital in Birmingham, Great Britain, showed that the Charnley hip replacement—the original design that has been tested over time more than any other type of material—has a 91 percent survival record after ten years and 82 percent survival over twenty years.[19]

Because even the most tried-and-tested design has a limited life span (ten years in the case of knee replacements), medical technology firms have been trying since the 1980s to fix artificial joints biologically to bone via little metal beads or mesh. These products, called "uncemented porous-coated" knee replacements, proved disastrous, resulting in a far greater need for "revision"— that is, replacement of the joint replacement. This is a much more formidable operation, with far more bone loss and removal of tissue—and a far lower success rate. As Mike Wroblewski of the Wrightington Hospital in Wigan, the British hospital that pioneered the operation over thirty years ago, puts it, "First time is the best time. After that it's salvage."[20]

In just one of the many studies demonstrating the high failure rate of knee replacement, of about one hundred procedures roughly one-fifth failed due to problems with the lower leg component. After seven years, more than half the replacements were recommended for revision.[21] As for hip replacements, a Swedish study found that after ten years, only about a quarter of the two new devices studied survived.[22]

If uncemented varieties of hip replacement have been found wanting, the other cemented versions don't fare much better. One study following a group of patients under fifty for fifteen years found that a little less than a third needed revision because the parts had loosened and become infected.[23] In fact, in the last decade first-time failures requiring revision tripled, to 12 percent.[24]

Complications

Among the spectacular successes, there looms a high potential mortality rate. Among more than 11,000 cases of total hip replacement (THR) between 1976 and 1985, 11 out of every 1,000 THR patients died within three months of the operation, and 28 out of every 1,000 had to have emergency readmissions. This translates into 1 in every 91 patients dying and 1 in every 36 returning for an emergency readmission within a month of the operation. Most deaths had to do with heart attacks, most emergencies with strokes.[25]

As for knee replacements, a U.S. analysis found an overall complication rate of 18 percent, with the most common complications including infection, blockage in the lung (pulmonary embolism), or a blood clot in a vein.[26] Stroke from a blood clot in the lung remains the most common cause of death.[27]

George, a seventy-five-year-old, tells this story:

> I had two total knee replacements, which have become infected with staphylococcus as a result of mismanagement during a minor throat infection. After a long period of treatment with antibiotics I am told I shall have to continue with this for life.

His alternative to taking antibiotics forever is to have the joints replaced yet again and to face potential failure, a prospect, at his age, he is loath to consider.

George's experience isn't as rare as it might be hoped. Associations have been made between oral infection and subsequent blood infection after total joint replacement operations, particularly if the patient has gum disease in his mouth. Nevertheless, few doctors take the precautions with hip replacement patients that they do with heart valve patients, who receive antibiotic treatment with dental surgery.[28]

New and Improved?

Most new "designer hips" are put on the market without any sort of testing, as a stream of new, supposedly improved models with all manner of unproven claims are continually introduced and quietly withdrawn, a few hundred hapless patients later. In

1971 the only artificial hip was the Charnley design; twenty years later, thirty-four varieties flooded the market.

As one orthopedic surgeon put it: "You can design a hip replacement in your garden shed today and be putting it in patients tomorrow."[29] One particular problem is the use of titanium, or a mix of titanium, vanadium, and aluminum in most new artificial joints. These materials have been shown to break down and send particles into the body, the long-term effect of which nobody knows. Emerging evidence shows that high levels of these microscopic metallic debris—all potential carcinogens—generated by constant contact between the artificial parts of the joint or by simple corrosion migrate to major organs of the body.

In Britain, a group called the Bristol Wear Debris Analysis Team did a comparison study of patients who'd died with and without metal implants as used in joint replacement. The analysis team found high levels of debris in the liver, lymph glands, bone marrow, and spleen of patients who'd had stainless steel and cobalt-chrome implants. But the highest number of particles migrated in people whose joint replacements were considered loose and worn. The main source of the debris was the matte coating of the joint. In one patient, the level of cobalt found in his bone marrow was *several thousand times* that considered normal.[30]

Although the Bristol researchers have not yet proved a link between this metal debris and disease, they believe that an accumulation of metallic particles such as these is associated with chronic inflammation, lymph node disease, destruction of bone marrow, bone loss, and implant loosening. "There is concern" they wrote guardedly, "that metals used in prostheses may cause [cancer] since they are potentially carcinogenic in other situations."[31] Although only twenty-four tumors developing near implants had been reported in the scientific literature up until 1992, two studies suggest an association between cancer of the lymph nodes or leukemia and hip replacement.[32] This is quite worrying when you consider the increasing tendency to do joint replacements on young people, a situation given further endorsement as celebrities such as Liza Minnelli have replacement surgery. And this shot-in-the-dark nature of joint replacement is likely to continue, since no one is keeping track of who develops cancer after replacement surgery. There is no adequate reporting system for implant-related tumors, despite appeals among researchers for an international register dating back to 1989.[33] Possibly because of the specter of future litigation, several chemical companies have ceased selling polymers (used for coating the joints) to medical implant manufacturers.[34]

ANGIOPLASTY: UNBLOCKING THE PLUMBING

In just a few short years, coronary balloon angioplasty—or percutaneous transluminal coronary angioplasty (PTCA), to give it its proper name—has grown to be the major method of treating heart problems, particularly angina. This has been largely in response to an epidemic: In 1989, 1 million people died of heart disease in the United States. Medicine has focused on it as a preventive measure because in the overwhelming majority of cases, the first heart attack is often the last. Of the 1.5 million people who suffer a heart attack in the United States each year, just 350,000 live to tell the tale.

Coronary balloon angioplasty has been in the ascendant since 1978, and involves threading a tiny balloon through blocked arteries and expanding it to clear them—usually by pressing the atheromatous (fatty) plaques against the coronary artery wall.

When angioplasty first arrived on the scene, the wonder solution to arterial disease of the time was coronary bypass surgery. As angioplasty became more sophisticated it gained ground on heart surgery, representing as it did the cheaper, easier, and less-traumatic alternative. Before long it came to be regarded as a virtual cure-all for heart disease, offered to angina sufferers, those recovering from a heart attack, and even as a "just-in-case" remedy for those concerned about the state of their arteries.

By 1990, twelve years after its first mention in the scientific literature, 200,000 people in the United States were treated with the procedure, and a further 100,000 in Europe, even though only a smattering of scientific prospective trials had thus far assessed its efficacy.[35] The extraordinary success rate of initial tests—some ranging above 90 percent, with complications in fewer than 10 percent of cases—tended to support the enthusiasts. Even Mother Teresa, who received the treatment in her eighty-first year, gave it a further endorsement.

One of the most comprehensive surveys to date seemed to vindicate the initial fanfare. Of 5,827 patients treated with angioplasty between January and June 1991 in the state of New York, 88 percent were reported successful, although postdischarge complications were never studied.[36]

It wasn't until 1991 that *The Lancet*—the very journal that first applauded the wonder treatment—was in the vanguard of those voicing concerns. A delegate from the journal attended an angioplasty course in 1991 and wrote that, based on his own observations, he tended to take a less favorable view of the outcome than the clinician doing the procedure. "In general the results of coronary angioplasty seemed inferior to those reported in journals."[37]

In the United States an even more damning statement was issued by the American College of Cardiologists: "Observations raise the question of whether cardiology has focused too much on doing coronary angioplasty procedures rather than on addressing who needs it, what are the criteria, and what are the results. Is angioplasty being done for cardiologists or for patients?"

As the experience of nearly twenty years of use now demonstrates, far from being an instant miracle cure-all, the truth about angioplasty is much more complicated. First off, it is more effective for simple cases. A study in Boston discovered that angioplasty patients with two to three risk factors had a survival rate over five years of just 13 percent.[38]

Stenosis (narrowing of the artery) has been found to recur within six months after angioplasty; the diameter of the blood vessels treated were only 16 percent larger than before treatment, according to the American College of Cardiologists. In one Italian study, restenosis occurred in three-quarters of cases.[39]

Because of the need for continual retreatment and monitoring, the real costs of angioplasty may be much higher than those for medical therapy in cases of mild angina and single-vessel disease. Hospital charges have doubled in the ten years that angioplasty has been used, one study done in Maryland estimated.[40]

Angioplasty doesn't fare very well with patients who have triple-vessel disease—that is, where all the main arteries of the heart are clogged. An Italian study reported only a 52 percent success rate in these cases. Angioplasty was also unsuccessful in more than two-thirds of cases of total blockage of the artery.[41]

Angioplasty also has a very poor success rate when used to treat blocked arteries in the lower part of the body. If those types of blockages aren't treated, the patient can end up having a leg amputated. Despite a twenty-four-fold increase in the use of the treatment for lower-body blockages from 1979 to 1989 in Maryland, the numbers of leg amputations remained constant, at 30 per 100,000.[42]

There is also strong evidence that many angioplasty operations may be unnecessary. A damning American study looked at patients who had been referred for angioplasty; the study concluded that, for half of them, the operation wasn't needed or could safely be deferred. And although coronary angioplasty was originally expected to replace bypass surgery, in fact both techniques have grown in tandem, neither of them reducing the frequency of the other. "Evident over the past decade is the ever lowering threshold for carrying out bypass as well as angioplasty . . . even asymptomatic patients are not exempt," they wrote.[43]

In fact, new evidence shows that bypass surgery may be the more successful treatment for angina than angioplasty. In one study, nearly four times as many angioplasty patients needed repeat treatment or surgery as those who had had bypass surgery; angina was almost three times as common in angioplasty patients as in bypass patients within six months of the treatment.[44]

In other studies, the two procedures have shown that neither one makes a substantial difference in terms of saving lives, preventing heart attacks, or increasing arterial blood flow after three years.[45] Actually both procedures have serious downsides: One scientific study found that those treated with angioplasty are more likely to need further intervention and drugs, whereas the bypass group were more likely to have an acute heart attack during the operation. And the latest research, which examined more than 1,000 patients from twenty-six heart centers around Europe, shows that the survival rate among patients in the first year after angioplasty is lower than among those who have major bypass surgery. Angioplasty patients also need to be on more medication than those given a bypass, and are more likely to need a repeat operation within the first year.[46]

Atherectomy

Atherectomy is a new technique for unclogging blocked heart vessels meant to be an improvement over angioplasty by solving the thorny problem of restenosis. Nevertheless, so far it compares poorly with the technique it was supposed to supersede. In one study, the heart vessels of those having atherectomy were less blocked after treatment than those given angioplasty, but this success rate was undermined by the fact that the probability of death or heart attack within six months was found to be higher among the atherectomy group—in fact, nearly double.[47] Two other important trials showed little or no difference between the two techniques in terms of the subsequent rate of reclogging arteries.[48]

ASSISTED CONCEPTION

Louise Brown—the world's first "test tube baby"—is eighteen years old at this writing—and so is test-tube-baby technology. In that time the media has largely painted a pretty picture of "assisted conception," as it is known in medical circles, as a brilliant breakthrough for the infertile. As the percentage of infertile couples increases—the latest estimates are that one out of every seven couples of childbearing age has trouble conceiving—infertility drugs or techniques are becoming the first port of call for the childless.

Most doctors helping a couple investigate infertility are quick to rush into piecemeal investigations without a systematic overview to determine where the problem really lies. Mystifyingly, they also tend to look automatically to the woman as the source of the couple's infertility problem, even if the man is found to have a low sperm count.

There are three main ways that medical science plays at being stork:

- In vitro fertilization (IVF), or embryo transfer, is supposed to be used when a woman has blocked tubes, when the sperm cannot manage to get through the cervical mucus, or in other cases where for some reason sperm cannot unite with egg. This technique involves removing one or more eggs from the woman, fertilizing the eggs with her partner's sperm outside the body in a petrie (shallow) laboratory dish, and reinserting the embryos (fertilized eggs) into the woman's uterus,

- GIFT (gamete intrafallopian transfer) is a means of giving nature a gentle nudge. Although eggs are removed from the woman, and sperm is taken from her partner, they are placed separately at the outer edges of the woman's fallopian tubes. In this way, goes the theory, sperm of low motility won't have as far to go as they would if they had to travel the long and precarious journey through a woman's reproductive canal in order to make it to their target.

- Fertility drugs, now used for some twenty years, are supposed to be offered only to women who have trouble ovulating. Drugs such as clomiphene citrate (trade name Clomid or Serophene) work by blocking the production of estrogen and fooling the brain into thinking the body is not ovulating. The brain then produces larger amounts of Follicle Stimulating Hormone (FSH), causing the ovaries to "superovulate"— often producing two, three, or more eggs.

Although Louise Brown resulted from the reimplantation of a single fertilized egg, test-tube pioneers Patrick Steptoe and Professor Bob Edwards then came up with the idea of improving what was ordinarily a low success rate. It stood to reason that a woman's chances of having a pregnancy "take" would improve if they put back more than one egg. (It would also save the cost and trouble of going through multiple treatments.) They then began offering women fertility drugs to make them "superovulate" and produce more than one egg at a go, which they would return all at once. Drugs such as Pergonal and Metrodin, which are even more potent than Clomid, can make the ovaries produce anywhere from three to thirty eggs at a time.

In practice, many of these more potent drugs are employed as a matter of course at the first sign that a couple is having a problem, and even before the nature of the fertility problem is investigated. This is despite the fact that fertility drugs such as Clomid don't have a very good success rate other than with those clear-cut cases in which the problem is the fact that the woman isn't ovulating. Indeed, even the manufacturers of Serophene, one of these drugs, says that it is less effective after three goes and should not be used indefinitely.[49]

Fertility drugs are also often given to men with low sperm counts, even though most studies have shown these drugs do very little good.

Fertility drugs are known to have substantial side effects—many of which will affect your pregnancy or baby if you do get pregnant while taking them. Doctors underplay the side effects of the fertility drugs as limited to hot flashes or abdominal discomfort, but one of the manufacturers, Swiss-based pharmaceutical firm Serono, warns that Serophene causes ovarian enlargement (in about 14 percent of patients) and blurred vision (for reasons they don't understand). This has particular repercussions if you have endometriosis or ovarian cysts, as it will make the problem worse and possibly permanently affect your fertility. In addition, these problems cannot be detected immediately: "Maximum enlargement of the ovary . . . does not occur until several days" after discontinuation of the drug.

Besides ovarian enlargement, superovulation drugs such as Metrodin also cause Ovarian Hyperstimulation syndrome (OHSS), a serious medical problem causing a rapid accumulation of fluid in the abdominal cavity, the thorax, and even the sac surrounding the heart, requiring immediate hospitalization. This situation can worsen if the patient is also pregnant. "With OHSS there is an increased risk of injury to the ovary," says Serono in the U.S. drugs bible, the *Physicians' Desk Reference.* "Pelvic examination may cause rupture of an ovarian cyst." If this does occur, it may be necessary to remove the ovary surgically.

Seven years after more than two million women in the United States alone had taken some sort of fertility drug, the first complete study to examine all the data was finally tallied. Its chilling findings were that fertility drugs such as clomiphene can double or even triple the risk of developing ovarian cancer if taken for longer than a year. The study, which looked at the records of nearly 4,000 infertile American women in Seattle, Washington, between 1974 and 1985, discovered that eleven in the group reported an invasive or borderline malignant ovarian tumor, against an expected average of 4.4. Of these, nine were taking clomiphene, five of these for longer than a year.[50]

The American Collaborative Ovarian Cancer Group, of Stanford University in California, which analyzed twelve studies, also concluded that infertile women taking fertility drugs face three times the risk of ovarian cancer as infertile women who haven't taken the drugs.[51] These findings have prompted the FDA to now require that manufacturers of fertility drugs add the risk of ovarian cancer to the list of possible adverse reactions published about the drugs.

If that isn't enough to make you think twice before taking one of these drugs, Serono also warns of pulmonary and vascular complications such as thrombosis in the veins or arteries that could result in a heart attack, stroke, or the loss of a limb. There's also the risk of an ectopic (tubal) pregnancy, which of course results in the removal of an ovary, thereby lowering your fertility even more.

The media has published lots of photos of boisterous triplets with cheery captions about how fertility drugs have increased the incidence of twins, triplets and quads, and that formerly childless couples are suddenly having to cope with a houseful of children. And there's no doubt that these drugs increase your chances of having anything from twins to quints. In clinical trials with Metrodin, Serono reported multiple births in 17 percent of pregnancies; with Serophene, 10 percent were twins, less than 1 percent triplets or more. This percentage increases, depending upon the number of eggs replaced into the woman. In 1988 the overall multiple pregnancy rate was 24 percent for IVF and 19.9 percent for GIFT. The multiple pregnancy rate for GIFT increases to 31.2 percent when five or more eggs are replaced.

The problem isn't so much coping with a houseful of children, however, as making sure any of them survive in the first place. According to a ten-year British study published in 1990, multiple births of all kinds, whether natural or assisted, carry greater risks than singleton births. Of about 1,000 babies born as part of a multiple birth, 25 percent were premature (compared with a usual rate in ordinary deliveries of 6 percent) and nearly 33 percent weighed less than 5.5 pounds/2.2 kilograms (compared with only 7 percent of all deliveries born at that weight). More than twenty-five of the 1,000 IVF babies in the study died, at around birth, compared with the 9.8 per 1,000 national average).[52]

The working party claims that when allowances are made for the women's ages and multiple births, this death rate is similar to ordinary infant mortality rates, which isn't a very compensatory thought if they happened to be your babies. If born alive, IVF babies also have a higher incidence of birth defects.

Fertility drugs can increase the chances of birth defects such as spina bifida by nearly six times (although other reports claim the risk is only doubled, still others that it is nonexistent).[53] One study found the risk was lower with clomiphene, which is only about three-quarters as risky as stronger fertility drugs. After examining all multiple births in Australia in the 1980s, one study concluded that triplet pregnancies produced a child with cerebral palsy eight times more often than twin pregnancies, and forty-seven times more often than singleton pregnancies. Some 86 percent of the cases of cerebral palsy among the babies born in multiple births occurred in twins. Even when twins were of normal birthweight, they were still at a greater risk of developing cerebral palsy than singletons.[54] IVF babies also risk being born with anencephaly (a defect in the development of the brain and skull, which results in brain hemispheres that are small or missing altogether).

A multiple pregnancy also introduces a Solomon-like decision for a mother—killing off one or more of the fetuses so that the other(s) may live. Because of the increased risk in multiple births, particularly for three or more embryos, some centers in Europe quietly engage in what is euphemistically described as "embryo reduction" or, the even more clinically neutral, "reducing the products of conception." What this amounts to is "selective termination" of one or more of the healthy embryos through an injection of saline in order to decrease the risk of all of them dying.

This dilemma becomes more likely the higher the number of eggs replaced inside the woman's body.

There's also recent evidence that embryo reduction may harm those fetuses left behind. "The obstetric outcome after pregnancy reduction in the first trimester is often complicated," said the British report, which cited a case of triplet embryos "reduced" by one. An ultrasound scan revealed that one of the remaining twins had developed an anencephaly-like malformation, after which he got the needle, too. The remaining baby was born healthy and normal at thirty-nine weeks. The same occurred with a quadruplet pregnancy which was "reduced" to twins— or, as the report put it, after "a twin pregnancy was achieved as in the first case." (Note the strict avoidance of emotive language.) One of these surviving twins was found to have an anencephaly-like malformation; he was then "reduced," after which the only survivor was delivered premature at thirty-two weeks.[55] An Australian study also found that if one half of a set of twins dies in the uterus, the survivor is at higher risk of cerebral palsy.

Considering that GIFT and IVF still carry a low success rate (only about 20 percent), are only indicated for about 20 percent of infertile couples, and carry such high risks, anyone faced with a fertility problem should consider it the court of last resort. Furthermore, organizations such as Foresight: The Association for Preconceptual Care and the doctors they work with claim that a large number of "unexplained" fertility problems and even blockages or low sperm counts, thought to be untreatable, can be resolved if a couple improve their nutritional status and resolve any allergies. Over 80 percent of couples with previous histories of miscarriage or infertility went on to give birth to healthy babies, after following the Foresight diet and supplement program.[56]

LITHOTRIPSY

Besides test tubes, doctors have been experimenting with waves of all sorts derived from light and sound. The latest surgical toy of the past decade is a high-tech invention with the unwieldy name of "extracorporeal shockwave lithotripsy" (ESWL), which has revolutionized the medical management of kidney stones. In ESWL, the lithotriptor creates shockwaves which, guided by X rays, are aimed at the kidney stone, causing it to disintegrate. By use of sound, the lithotriptor is theoretically able to distinguish between the body's own tissues and those of the kidney stone.

Urologists all over the world rushed to embrace lithotripsy without subjecting it to proper clinical trials because it seemed, on the face of it, an improvement over surgery (the conventional method of handling stones). Plus, all the initial reports didn't show any short- or long-term damage to the kidney or its surrounding tissues. Lithotripsy is now recommended for three-quarters of all stone problems.

A number of the studies (which are only now being done) cast a few shadows over the initial rosy assumptions. It now seems evident that lithotripsy definitely causes damage to the kidney in a good percentage of cases. Most patients experience internal bleeding, ranging from a tiny hemorrhage to major bleeding requiring transfusion.

This bleeding also seems to change the dynamics of the blood in the kidney, causing kidney hypertension (abnormally high blood pressure in the kidneys) in up to 8 percent of patients.[57] Other studies show irreversible kidney failure,[58] a one-quarter reduction in the rate at which the kidney filters out impurities,[59] and a rise in blood pressure[60] and heartbeat.[61] Rarely, it can even rupture the kidney.[62] The extent of damage appears to depend upon the intensity of shock waves used, but in any case nearly a fifth of patients may sustain damage as a result of ESWL.[63]

A computed tomography (CT) scan performed two years after a group of French patients had undergone lithotripsy showed that 40 percent had a recurrence of stones; 25 percent had scarring.[64] Some patients followed over time suffered chronic changes to their kidney.[65] Apart from the risk of septic shock,[66] another worry concerns the bacteria within the stones, which is released when they are broken up and which can cause inflammation.[67]

Shock waves may also damage male sperm. In experiments on male rats, using ESWL, after five weeks the treated rat testes appeared to have atrophied and could no longer produce sperm. In human cells, sperm movement became frenetic and the percentage of abnormal sperm increased.[68] The procedure has also been known to cause hemorrhage in the scrotum.[69]

The problem with disintegrating kidney stones with shock waves is that it doesn't address the reasons why the body produced the stones in the first place. One major cause is prescription drugs: Stones have now been linked to carbonic anhydrase inhibitors (acetazolamide or methazolamide), used to treat glaucoma;[70] to furosemide in infants, used for congenital heart failure;[71] to some antiepileptic drugs;[72] to triamterene (used to combat hypertension);[73] to trisilicate-containing antacids (used for gastric discomfort and heartburn);[74] to ceftriaxone (which prevents the body from rejecting transplants);[75] and even to thiazide diuretics in patients with high blood pressure.[76]

Numerous studies have made the connection between kidney stones and the use of sulfasalazine, particularly in AIDS patients given drugs such as Septrin over the long term as a "just-in-case" measure against *pneumocystis carinii* pneumonia.[77] Laxative abuse can also bring on kidney stones.

INJECT-AND-GO CONTRACEPTION

Even after the disastrous outcome of silicone breast implants, which resulted in one of the biggest successful class-action suits of all time, medicine, undaunted, continues to play around with new types of silicone implants. Norplant, manufactured by Roussel, was supposed to be the new "inject-and-go" contraception. One small implant operation with this progestogen-only contraceptive, made up of six soft matchstick-sized rods of silicone, and you could forget about contraception for up to four years. The implant would be inserted in a fan shape in the upper arm under local anesthetic. It would then provide a gradual release of levonorgestrel, the main drug in the mini-Pill, over two or five years, depending on the strength chosen.

Launched in the United Kingdom in October 1995, Norplant has had some three million users worldwide. It has been used in the United States since 1990, when it gained the seal of approval from the FDA. The implant got some unexpected publicity when the media discovered it was being used as a form of involuntary contraception on teenage mothers as a condition of their continuing to receive benefits. Nevertheless, Norplant was hailed as such a miracle improvement over the contraceptive pill that demand was far outstripping supply.[78]

Because of the sustained-release action, lower levels of hormone were needed than those found in the standard Pill. Doctors extolling Norplant claimed that the trials among 55,000 women showed it to be as effective as sterilization and "four times" more effective than the Pill. They also claimed that there was less risk of deep-vein thrombosis or blood clots in the lungs than that posed by the Pill because the drug never passed through the liver.

After what promised to be a bright start, however, things seem to be going disastrously wrong for Roussel and for Wyeth-Ayerst Laboratories, the American suppliers of Norplant. At least 400

American women are suing Wyeth-Ayerst after suffering permanent injury when doctors tried to remove the silicone rods. Jewel Klein, a Chicago lawyer representing some of these women, has said these actions are merely the beginning, and that many more suits will follow when other women try to have Norplant taken out: The women, she says, have suffered lengthy and repeated procedures to remove the rods, and have experienced excruciating pain.

In the United Kingdom, 475 women have sought legal advice on possible compensation claims, after suffering a variety of side effects, mainly heavy bleeding or problems having Norplant inserted or removed. At this writing, no writs have been issued.[79]

About three million women around the world have the six rods fitted under their skin, including 900,000 in the United States alone. Wyeth-Ayerst believed that removal is a simple, half-hour procedure. It's now reckoned that up to half of women could suffer complications on removal; this translates into some 180,000 women who might suffer permanent injury.

Some of the women now suing wanted the rods removed because they wished to conceive; others were suffering serious side effects. Virtually all women who have been fitted with Norplant have complained of some side effect.[80] In another group of nearly 200, almost half were considering having the implants removed because of adverse reactions. Side effects affecting up to 10 percent of women have included irregular bleeding, weight gain, breast tenderness, acne, nausea or dizziness; hair growth or loss, and mood swings. In one study, nearly all women experienced at least one adverse reaction. The most common side effect is irregular bleeding, experienced by between 50 and 80 percent of women. A quarter to a half of all women complain of headaches. Disrupting ovulation can also cause ovarian cysts.[81]

Although pregnancy is rare while a woman is on Norplant, among those that occur there is a high incidence of tubal pregnancies, which can entail removing the impregnated fallopian tube, thus affecting a woman's future fertility.

The greatest damage can be done when the rods are taken out, it appears. The rods are usually removed under local anesthetic, although some of the American women filing lawsuits had to have general anesthesia before all the rods could be removed. They have complained of permanent scarring after repeated attempts by doctors to remove the rods. Lawyers fear that doctors have not gained enough experience of removing Norplant, but at this point it's too early to assess the damage. So far, only 15 percent of users have had the implants removed.

These experiences are contrary to other research findings, which claim Norplant is far safer than the contraceptive Pill because it releases much lower levels of hormone.

The latest concern is that a revised version containing a change in formulation was introduced with relatively little in the way of data.[82] Nor is there any data on the long-term effects of inserting silicone into the arm, although 5 percent of women have experienced irritation and some 1 percent had the implant removed because of arm pain. Some women have reported darkening of the skin around the tubes, or the buildup of fibrous tissue, which remains for some time after the tubes are removed.

Janet from Nottingham in Britain decided to have a Norplant fitted under the skin of her arm by her family doctor, once she and her husband decided not to have any more children. They were impressed by the patient guide put out by the manufacturer, assuring them that Norplant could be removed at any time during the five years. "Just make an appointment with your doctor or clinic."

As soon as the Norplant rods were implanted, however, Janet began suffering increasingly heavy periods, sometimes bleeding for up to thirty days with only a four-day break. At one stage, her blood loss was so excessive that she fainted and had to be taken to the hospital. There, a specialist took one look at her and recommended that the Norplant be removed immediately by her doctor.

"But when my doctor tried to remove the Norplant, he couldn't find it," says Janet. When they contacted Roussel, a representative admitted to Janet's doctor that if he wasn't able to remove it, no one from the drug company could, either. The representative recommended a Dr. Walling in Boston, who'd been specially trained to remove the device. Subsequently, Roussel paid for Dr. Walling's transport to England to remove Janet's Norplant, and indicated to Janet that they were also shipping him over to show others how it's done.

> At my doctor's surgery, Dr. Walling gave me a local anesthetic and managed to extract four of the capsules [the rods], but a fifth one broke and only half could be removed. The [sixth rod] couldn't be found. By this time, I had four small incisions and a two-inch scar along my arm.

It now appears likely that Janet is going to have to undergo a major operation under general anesthetic to locate and remove the missing capsules, plus plastic surgery to attempt to conceal the scarring. And all this some six months *after* several doctors insisted that she have the Norplant removed "immediately."

The future of Norplant now appears bleak. Prescriptions for the contraceptive have plummeted from a high of 5,000 a month in its first year to about twenty per month as a result of the legal actions and media attention. Hoechst Roussel, the European manufacturer, says that prescriptions for the device are 100 percent down on those of the same period a year ago. A spokesman said that the product, which was "well received by the medical profession and by the vast majority of users," was being "killed off by an unholy alliance of the media, lawyers, and government bureaucracy." Problems were being "blown out of all proportion," and women were being "left with the feeling that there is something 'dodgy' about this," he said.[83]

— VI —

TAKING CONTROL

TWELVE

Taking Control

My maternal grandmother, Stella, who emigrated to the United States from Italy at the age of fifteen, had both her babies at home. This was not because she advocated home birth so much as because she had been taught to regard medical progress with a fair degree of suspicion. *"Don't go to hospital; they change your baby!"* her own mother had admonished her in broken English. My grandmother, being the good daughter she was, duly complied, for it would have been unthinkable not to: In all regards, in her native culture, mothers knew best.

As it turned out, not even home proved to be the safe haven Stella and her mother had anticipated. Stella's husband—my grandfather—agreed to go along with these "female superstitions" only so long as a bona fide doctor was present at both deliveries. Many years later, on more than one occasion my grandmother would lament her second and final birth. "The doctor—he *ruin* me!" she'd invariably exclaim. The force of her anger over the incident even a half-century later rendered the details too terrible for me ever to probe into, but I assumed that she was talking about a botched episiotomy.

During my childhood, the reason for my mother's birth at

home was always recounted and held up to me with ridicule—an example of pig-ignorant hocus-pocus. *Imagine thinking that professionals like doctors could send you home with the wrong baby!* However, the more I reflect upon it over time, the more I realize the wisdom inherent in my great-grandmother's cautionary tale. Birth at home has since been proven to be safer than hospital births for low-risk deliveries,[1] and babies born in the hospital have not only been mixed up but snatched on more than a few occasions. Furthermore, behind that terse pronouncement was a rather sophisticated philosophy about medicine in general: View any newfangled medical progress with the most profound suspicion; don't go anywhere near a hospital if you aren't really ill; trust that your own healthy body doesn't need much help; assume that doctors are capable of making the most basic and calamitous mistakes.

As it turned out, my grandmother's wariness about hospitals proved prescient on the single night of her life that she did spend any time in one. At the age of ninety she was rushed to the emergency room in the mistaken notion that she was having a heart attack, and kept overnight for "observation." Her problem turned out to be indigestion, but she was so utterly alarmed by the entire experience, was so moved to resist the parade of strangers poking at her and invading her privacy, that when we came to collect her the following morning we found her tied up in a straitjacket—the only means by which the hospital staff had managed to gain her compliance.

My Italian forebears correctly deduced what by now should be clear to you: that your doctors often doesn't know what they're doing—not because they aren't good people with good intentions, but because the equipment inside their black bags doesn't work particularly well. In fact, most of the time, your body can manage things better than any doctor can.

Besides their decidedly inferior set of tools, there is something fundamentally wrong with doctors' perception of the material they work with. As sophisticated as it is in many regards, medical science utterly lacks any understanding whatsoever of the extraordinary dynamics of the human body. With its emphasis on interrupting and often opposing your body's own processes, medicine never takes into account the exquisite mechanism of the organism it is trying to fix or the body's extraordinary potential to operate beyond the empirical. This includes the power of faith, hope, and the will to live—what medicine now refers to as "psychoneuroimmunology"—all long-proven elements of so-called "miracle" cures or spontaneous healing.[2] By reducing your body's own response to a stress—by lowering a fever, your body's best defense against outside agents—the doctor often ends up permanently weakening your body's ability to fight back.

Without a true appreciation of this wondrous ability, medicine is a blunt and clumsy instrument, a pointless meddler, a caveman being called upon to fix a mainframe computer, whose solution is to bash it with a club. And even this metaphor is crudely inexact, because even the most complex computer system cannot begin to approximate the body's mysterious ability to move from total disarray to order—in short, to heal itself.

Every medical solution appears clumsy and primitive beside some of the body's own highly sophisticated and shrewd mechanisms: the ability of a mother's breast milk to create antibodies to fight her *baby's* infections. We also know that a component of breast milk helps to complete brain growth, affecting areas such as visual acuity, for the entire first year of life.[3] Then there are the hormones in the brain that are produced whenever necessary to reduce anxiety. And new evidence shows that a woman's risk of developing high blood pressure during pregnancy decreases the longer she's been with her partner.[4] This may mean there is something in her partner's sperm that keeps her and the pregnancy healthy. The most complex drug in the world cannot begin to match this subtlety.

Vitamin K

Medicine often operates on the premise that nature is imperfect. Figuring that all that's required is a little tweak here or there, it clumsily upsets an exquisite balance, thereby causing a load of new problems far worse than what it set out to resolve in the first place. This may be the case with vitamin K injections, which are meant to prevent children from dying from a rare hemorrhagic disease of the newborn. Recently, a British study found that this practice could increase by 2.5 times the risk of a child developing cancer.[5] Although these results haven't been replicated anywhere else, there is a private consensus that medicine doesn't really know what it is doing in this area.[6] When the practice first started in the 1950s, vitamin K3 was administered to babies—until it was discovered that K3 leads to high levels of blood bilirubin, damaging the brain and causing deafness, mental retardation, and involuntary movement. It is also associated with hemolysis—where red blood cells are destroyed. Medicine then quickly changed to K1, which appears not to pose these risks.[7] Nevertheless, both the injected and oral varieties don't appear to last very long, and many babies with low vitamin-K stores appear to self-correct the problem.[8]

Another area where researchers have discovered that nature didn't make a big mistake after all is low iron stores during pregnancy. New evidence shows that this is not a sign of illness but of health, signifying good expansion in blood volume and resulting in bigger babies. All those iron pills and transfusions given to anemic pregnant women all these years may have contributed to many premature births and small-for-dates babies.[9]

A Faulty Paradigm

Modern medicine doesn't work because the very paradigm on which it is based is faulty—that germs or genes alone are responsible for illness and that our bodies are akin to complicated machines. Medicine is largely based upon the "germ theory," which holds that most illness depends entirely on the invasion of bacteria and viruses. According to this theory, disease is a random, stealthy entity that can strike down anyone at any moment, regardless of his nutritional, physical, emotional, and environmental condition. This means that an undernourished child of the ghetto would have the same odds of dying from measles as a well-fed middle-class one.

This legacy from Louis Pasteur persists even though scientists are well aware that several pounds' worth of bacteria exist in a healthy body, providing either a positive service or there as the result, rather than as the cause of, disease. There is also growing evidence that the body's susceptibility to disease—its emotions, physical state, and response to its environment—determines whether a patient succumbs to illness.

Blaming outside agents for every modern illness encourages a blinkered approach, which tends to justify the most basic solutions. When researchers discovered that babies in day care were more likely to have earaches and respiratory diseases than those breast-feeding and at home with their mothers, they came up with a drug with eight species of bacterial extracts to prevent these recurrent respiratory infections among day-care children. The researchers centered on the notion that the bugs worked in isolation. They didn't consider such possible factors as lack of breast-feeding, the toddlers' lack of proximity to their moms, or the effects of placement in an institutional setting too early. Not surprisingly, vaccinating children against institutionalization didn't work.[10]

It's as well to keep in mind that what we think of as a long and distinguished tradition in medicine is only fifty years old. The flowering of drug therapy as we know it has mainly occurred in the wake of the big discoveries of the 1940s. Much as it gives the impression of being space-age, medical science, alone among the other scientific disciplines, is some four centuries out of date. In physics, for instance, the Cartesian view that everything works in predictable, reliable, and hence measurable fashion, which still forms the basis of modern medicine, was long discarded in favor of relativity and, more recently, quantum theories, which hold that the universe and the way it works aren't quite as mechanical and bit-part as we used to think. Nevertheless, medical science still adheres to the notion of a static, clockwork universe, with human beings looked upon essentially as machines and the mind operating as a separate entity from the body.

Gene therapy is very much the new frontier in medicine. Scientists throughout the world working on the Human Genome

Project reckon that, by the year 2005, they will have cracked the three-billion letter code that constitutes our genetic makeup; by getting a handle on this genetic blueprint, medical researchers believe they will be able to conquer many diseases more easily. In fact, the current vogue is to blame most illness on your genes—the idea being that one day doctors will be able to cut out your "bad" DNA and paste in some better genetic instructions. Researchers are investigating interventions that would alter the DNA of your body in order to diagnose, prevent, or treat genetic disorders.

One area where this is being tested is Parkinson's disease using an unlikely solution: the herpes virus. Since the herpes virus lives in the body of victims forever, often quietly hibernating in nerve cells, scientists from King's College reasoned that if they could tinker with the genetic coding of the virus and get it to make dopamine, perhaps it could carry this genetic message to the brain cells of its host.

All they needed to do was to chop out a few chunks of the virus' "bad" DNA, having to do with all the harmful bits like reproduction and infection, insert some new chunks with genetic instructions for making dopamine, and there you'd have it: Frankenstein's monster gets turned into the fairy prince in Snow White.

In practice, however, scientists have had to return to the drawing board since they discovered that the engineered virus is potentially fatal. Medicine's intention of "editing" you and me to engineer all disease out of us has thus far proved elusive.

The biggest weakness with modern medical theory is that it assumes that we all get ill in the same way—that all illness stems from the same cause, all illnesses act alike, and there is only a single method of curing them. But as Dr. Leon Eisenberg of the Department of Social Medicine, Harvard Medical School, argued in a lecture to doctors:

> The premise is that as we go down the scale of magnitude from organisms to organs to tissues to cells to organelles to molecules, the understanding becomes ever deeper. The person whose body

*houses the collection of aberrant molecules is transformed into
an incidental host, deserving of the physician's sympathy, of
course, but essentially irrelevant. What "really" matters is disease pathophysiology.*

*How absurd! Between genotype and phenotype, a lifetime of
individual experience has fashioned what began as an envelope
of stochastic probabilities into a singular personal embodiment:
the patient who faces us. In clinical practice, it is the particulari-
ties and the idiosyncrasies of the individual patient that challenge
the physician. The same disease never presents in quite the
same way in successive patients. Complaints vary; severity varies; response to treatment varies . . . Medicine includes but
cannot be reduced to molecular biology.*[11]

This theory that all illnesses (and therefore all patients) are alike
also requires that every disease has a label. To hide their ignorance (and consequent fear), doctors need to turn what they
don't understand into a "syndrome," which makes it sound like
something that they've managed to get under control. Recently,
a phenomenon obviously due to bowel problems became "tight
pants syndrome," infants being improperly fed by their parents
were suffering from "soda-drinking syndrome," and even itching
whose source had not yet been identified became "scratch-itch
syndrome." As for anything that doesn't fit a recognizable pattern, it is deemed "all in the patient's mind."

Food as Prevention

If much of the drugs-and-surgery interventionist approach to
healing has proved useless or dangerous, except in emergencies,
the most impressive and promising research at the moment concerns methods of providing the body with the appropriate tools
to heal itself, particularly the role of food and nutrients in preventing or creating disease. Although they aren't publicized every
day, studies showing the protective value of the antioxidant vitamins and minerals (vitamin A and beta-carotene, B_2 [riboflavin],
B_3 [nicotinic acid], vitamin C, E, and selenium) against cancer

and a host of other illnesses now fill the medical literature. Antioxidants protect the body from damage caused by harmful molecules called free radicals, from oxygen. Besides respiration, the body's cells use oxygen to metabolize (and literally "burn") food for its energy, and also for immune activity, to burn away germs and toxins. Free radicals are created from many sources—ultraviolet radiation, smoke pollution, heavy metals, or overheating of oils, such as in fast-food restaurants. They wreak havoc by destroying cell membranes, causing genetic damage, depressing immune function, hardening the arteries, disrupting hormone regulation, contributing to diabetes and other systemic disorders, and, of course, causing the growth and spread of cancer.

But we're now learning that damage from free radicals can be prevented and even reversed if there are sufficient concentrations in the body of free-radical scavengers, the antioxidants.

The largest and most recent study of cancer prevention, an investigation of 30,000 Chinese people in an area of historically high risk for a certain type of cancer, proved that certain antioxidants could protect people from developing cancer by as much as one-fifth. The same study found a 38 percent reduction in mortality from stroke among people following the recommended diet.[12]

Antioxidants have been shown to prevent eye disease such as macular degeneration, the leading cause of irreversible blindness in adults, and heart disease.[13] People suffering from angina have been shown to have significantly lower levels of vitamins C, E, and beta-carotene than healthy individuals.

Besides the antioxidant vitamins, the vegetables containing them may have even more powerful protective effects. One study from Dartmouth Medical School in New Hampshire showed that vegetables are better than supplements in lowering the risks of developing cancer of the colon.[14] It may be that other factors we have yet to identify are at play in a diet high in vegetables and fruits.

While a high-fat diet may increase the risks of several types of cancer, olive oil is apparently not one of the offenders. In fact, certain populations which consume great quantities of olive oil appear to have low levels of cancer. In Greece, where the average consumption of olive oil is 80 grams a day, there is a very low rate of breast cancer. It may be that the components of olive oil have a protective effect.

Many of what are now seen as healthy elements to a diet—meat as a "condiment" rather than the centerpiece of meals, so as to cut down on saturated fats, large helpings of fruits and vegetables, olive oil, and fish—are present in the Mediterranean diet. Researchers have discovered that two populations with some of the lowest incidence of heart attacks are those on Crete and on Kohama Island in Japan. The people of these islands have high intakes of essential fatty acids, a fish-oriented diet, and a high intake of the natural antioxidants. In the Lyon Diet Heart Study, researchers found that a Mediterranean diet could protect you from a second heart attack if you'd suffered one already. Only eight of the 302 patients on the Mediterranean regime died from a second attack, against twenty in a similar-sized group on a traditional, low-fat diet. Levels of vitamins E and C were also found to be higher in the group on the Mediterranean diet.[15] The Mediterranean diet has also been shown to prevent stroke, as have the omega-3 essential fatty acids.[16] Clearly, this is where medicine should be directing more of its research efforts.

Despite this growing evidence, very little has filtered down to the rank and file. The average doctor still regards food and nutritional supplements with suspicion and doubt, or at best as an adjunct to the "real" treatment—drugs and surgery. Although many now allow that pregnant women need folic acid, which has been proven to prevent spina bifida, so far few obstetricians have made the lateral mental leap that healthy living may prevent many other birth defects as well.

Government agencies even regard nutritional medicine as something virtually criminal. In May 1993, fifteen FDA agents with flak jackets, backed up by a batch of county policemen with guns at the ready, surrounded the clinic of noted nutritional therapist Dr. Jonathan Wright in Kent, Washington. Instead of knocking, they kicked in the door commando-style and forcibly picked the locks of the three additional back and side door entrances so that armed police and agents could pour into the clinic from all sides. While pointing guns at some of Dr. Wright's terrified staff, this SWAT team filled a police van with nearly every important element of Dr. Wright's practice.

Dr. Wright's crime, it seems, was using injectable vitamins. A medical doctor with a Harvard degree, Wright now uses naturopathic methods. He imports pure vitamins from Germany because he can no longer get them in America; their U.S. counterparts have preservatives that cause allergic reactions in his patients. In the eyes of the FDA, Dr. Wright was guilty of smuggling.[17]

Besides the role of vitamins and food as prevention, there is also growing evidence about the role of food in *creating* illness. A number of pioneers in medicine are discovering that allergies to food or modern-day chemicals are behind many of our chronic, so-called "incurable" illnesses, such as arthritis, eczema, asthma, hyperactivity, and even epilepsy and mental diseases such as schizophrenia. Copious research already exists in respected medical journals supporting the role of allergies or nutritional deficiencies in causing disease.[18] A respectable body of opinion among orthodox medicine, for instance, believes that gluten sensitivity may be one of the major causes of epilepsy. The largest study of this to date, performed in Italy, found that three-quarters of a group of epileptics passed the test for celiac disease—a biopsy of the small bowel found the characteristic atrophy of the villi (the tiny hairs of the gut).[19]

Sharon, whose husband, Gary, prints our newsletter, is just one of many patients who've been helped by this approach. A young woman in her twenties, she was virtually crippled with rheumatoid arthritis and consigned to a lifetime of drugs. She'd also had no luck conceiving. When Gary mentioned her to us, we suggested that she see one of our panel members who has spent years investigating the role of allergies in illness, particularly migraine and arthritis. Sharon did go along to see him, and he isolated her problem as an allergy to potatoes, a common situation among arthritics. As soon as she eliminated potatoes from her diet, Sharon's arthritis disappeared. Several months after that, she became pregnant.

And of course "hostile foods" aren't the only problem. We also need to look to some 25,000 chemicals—pesticides, plastics, byproducts—now in common use in Britain alone, most of which humans have only been exposed to since the Second World War. Scientific evidence is mounting about the role of pesticides in infertility and cancer.[20] Some scientists are pioneering important research into the more subtle effects of these chemicals on our bodies and their ability to cause many chronic, puzzling diseases such as arthritis.

One Swiss woman, called Irene, suffered from multiple joint pains and swelling that required cortisone treatments. Once she'd identified and eliminated certain foods from her diet, she improved somewhat but she was still left with residual pain—until she went to visit her mother in Zurich, where her pain and swelling disappeared completely. As soon as Irene returned home, however, she was dismayed to find that many of her joint pains returned. When she sought out a doctor highly skilled in food and chemical sensitivity, he suspected that she might be reacting to household gas; her mother's apartment in Zurich was all electric, while her home had a gas stove and gas central heating. Irene underwent a trial period of turning off her gas, and in a few days her joints were as good as they'd been in Switzerland. The gas central heating boiler was removed to an outhouse, and five years later Irene remains free of any arthritic symptoms.[21]

We are also only beginning to understand the precise role of exercise in preventing disease of all varieties. The latest report from the Harvard Alumni Society, which was set up in the early 1960s to follow more than 17,000 graduates (of an average age of forty-six when first recruited), reported that deaths from all causes were reduced by physical exercise. The amount of protection offered by vigorous exercise, as compared with not exercising, was the equivalent to the difference in the mortality rate between nonsmokers and those who smoke twenty cigarettes a day.[22]

Many doctors have come to believe that the future of medicine depends upon a better understanding of how to boost the tools our bodies have for fighting disease. Michael Baum, one of the world's foremost breast cancer specialists, bravely went on record in a letter to the newspapers to argue that the way forward in cancer was no longer high-dose chemotherapy and bone-marrow transplants, which, in his view, "echoes the death throes of the conventional belief systems." He continued:

> Many of us believe that the future lies not in a blunderbuss attack attempting to eradicate all cancer cells present at the time of diagnosis, but a more sophisticated attempt to maintain a dynamic equilibrium controlling the disease by modulation of the body's natural defence systems.[23]

Medicine desperately needs to take a fresh, objective approach to many illnesses and discard any treatment that has no basis in fact. Lately, articles have abounded about "evidence-based medicine"—which simply means looking up what has been proven in medical research before using it on patients.[24] The Cochrane Collaboration—named after epidemiologist Archie Cochrane, who spent most of his life pointing out the weakness of the evidence supporting much conventional medical evidence—has been set up to create and maintain a register of all randomized, controlled trials in biomedical research. But at the moment, this fresh approach—which might seem the obvious way forward to you and me—is only the subject of debate or thoughtful review in the medical literature. Whether the rank and file ever adopt it remains to be seen.

Suspicious of Alternatives

Doctors also need to suspend their preconceptions about other systems of medicine. Orthodox medicine has always taken a high-handed position against alternative medicine, denouncing it as experimental and unproven.[25] If alternative or complementary approaches are acknowledged at all, they are so only as adjuncts to the "real" thing—as a feel-good practice akin to having a facial.

Actually, many so-called scientific treatments have far less proof than many medical systems such as homeopathy or acupuncture that defy empirical logic. These treatments, along with herbalism and even arcane practices such as Romany medicine—have been proven by proper scientific trials to work for many ailments.[26] This doesn't take into account the evidence of clinical use over centuries, as compared with a paltry few years or decades of use in the case of most "orthodox" drugs. Many alternative systems also have the superior advantage of diagnosing and treating people as individuals, creating remedies unique to the individual, and viewing the body, mind, emotions, and environment as inextricable.

Not long ago, a doctor attempting to discredit alternative medicine proposed that he and a practitioner of acupuncture convene over a body on the operating table about to undergo surgery. Once the body in question was cut open, if it revealed the existence of meridians and physical evidence of the theories upon which Chinese medicine is based, the medical man would concede defeat and take the acupuncturist out to dinner. If, on the other hand, the work of the scalpel revealed a collection of organs such as a heart, liver, and kidneys, concluded the doctor, with high-minded relish, then the acupuncturist should pick up the tab for the meal.

Actually, empirical evidence does prove the existence of meridians, but not in the strictly visual sense that this doctor required. Research has shown that many acupuncture points on the body demonstrate electrical resistance, which is dramatically decreased compared with points on the skin surrounding them (10 kiloohms at the center of a point compared with 3 megaohms in the surrounding skin).[27] It's also been shown that slight stimulation of these points releases painkilling endorphins and the steroid cortisol, while more intense stimulation releases important mood-regulating neurotransmitters such as serotonin and norepinephrine. The same doesn't occur when the skin surrounding these points is stimulated.[28] We also know that acupuncture can dilate the circulatory system and increase blood flow to even distant organs in the body.[29]

Nine times out of ten—with ordinary fever, colds, and flu, common earache, or childhood illnesses—the body can sort itself out if you only wait before rushing to the doctor. In many instances of infection, chicken soup—so-called Jewish penicillin—is better for you than the real thing.

Of course, no matter how clever and self-healing your body is, there are times when it may need professional assistance. But if your doctor doesn't always know what he's doing, and you're never told what he's doing, where does this leave you? Because so little in orthodox medicine is really proven, taking control of your health requires that each of us view all medicines as both helpful and potentially dangerous, and do a good deal of detective work before consenting to treatment. It requires that we suspend our own preconceptions about how our bodies work and heal, and embrace other proven systems when they offer more help than we can get from a more conventional approach.

For some reason, the notion persists that there is something wrong with a patient knowing exactly what is being done to him. All of us hold doctors in such high regard that we view questioning them as something akin to treasonous disloyalty or extreme rudeness, a tactic that will undermine this special relationship. If anyone you knew were to avoid questioning a builder or plumber about to do work on his house because he thought it was rude, you would think him embarrassingly naïve. But the most assertive individual can turn into Jell-O when faced with asking for a simple clarification on a life-or-death procedure proposed by his doctor.

A Medical Consumer

No matter whether you are on a managed care program or paying for the Mayo Clinic, you have an absolute right to know everything you can about any medical treatments being proposed. Certainly you would never buy a car or a camcorder without painstakingly investigating the pros and cons. Why should something as vital as your health or that of your loved ones be any different? It's vital that you view yourself as a paying consumer and your doctor's advice as *services that you are purchasing*. Far from eroding trust, asking questions will cement the relationship between you and your doctor (if he's a good one, that is) to one of shared responsibility between two intelligent adults (rather than that of all-knowing adult and awestruck child). Even though medicine, like most professions, protects its own through the use of convoluted language, all medical procedures can be explained in terms that you can understand. At one time, that fellow with all those complicated initials after his name was a lay person learning this gobbledygook from scratch.

This same vigilance applies to alternative medicine. Although in the main, tried-and-tested alternative medicine practiced by experienced, qualified individuals can be more benign than orthodox medicine, it can also kill if in the wrong hands. Several years ago a short course of Chinese herbs screwed up my menstrual cycle for an entire year. When I had the herbs analyzed by a poison control unit, they discovered that they contained *eleven different estrogens—enough to rival HRT*. Another alternative heart treatment—beloved of Hollywood film stars—has been responsible for at least five deaths. In the wrong hands, acupuncture can bring on migraines and even stroke. Many alternative practitioners are given a license to practice after a few weekend courses, even with highly potent substances such as Chinese herbs. Natural does not always equal better. It's vital that you grill your alternative therapist, as you would your doctor, about his experience, track record, and knowledge of your condition, and to exit immediately if you don't like his answers.

Although it is more difficult to obtain, scientific data does exist about many treatments in alternative medicine. Explore information about your treatment with your practitioner, or call the official registry or body regulating that therapy to see where they can direct you. Do a Medline computer search or visit a medical library. Virtually nothing apart from a genuine medical emergency cannot wait a day or two while you do your homework.

There's also no reason why you have to take one set of answers as gospel. Get a second opinion (or a third or fourth) until you're confident and satisfied about the suggested treatment, but view all your healers as technicians and remain in control of all decisions.

Above all, refuse to accept a death sentence. These days it is fashionable for doctors to level with patients about whether or not they have a terminal illness. In fact, this would appear to be the will of the people: A Harris Poll in 1982 found that 96 percent of Americans said they would want to be told if they had cancer, and 85 percent wanted a "realistic estimate" of how long they would live if their type of cancer was one that usually led to death in less than a year.[30]

However, as many cases demonstrate, being straight with patients may only hasten their death. One fellow in his mid-fifties was referred to the department of hematology at his local hospital with a history of a highly benign form of leukemia, for which he only occasionally required small doses of drugs such as steroids. He had never been told the true nature of his condition, and over the next couple of years remained well, with his blood profile stable. Although he was ordinarily quite punctilious about attending his outpatient clinics, one day he never showed up, and only later turned up on a surgical ward in a highly neglected state. It turned out that he'd looked over his doctor's shoulder at his case notes and seen the word "leukemia." From there he went rapidly downhill and in three weeks he was dead, even though his blood count was unchanged. None of his doctors or even the pathologists conducting his autopsy could find any biological cause for his rapid decline.[31]

This particular issue is especially close to home. Six years ago, my eighty-one-year-old English mother-in-law, Edie, was diagnosed as having end-stage breast cancer. Privately her doctor told us, "If I were you, I'd get her affairs in order." When he'd examined her, he'd been shocked; her breast, he told me, looked like raw meat. In fact, so advanced was the cancer that it was too late to try chemotherapy or any other intervention. She had three months to live, at the very outside, we were told.

Her doctor then wrote her a prescription for two drugs: ta-moxifen, to slow the cancer, and metronidazole (Flagyl), to heal the open sores on her breast.

Two days later we heard from my father-in-law that Edie had nearly collapsed in town.

Her doctor then started Edie on morphine, since, he told us, she'd asked if she could have something for the pain. "To be honest," he added, "I'd be looking into nursing home care as soon as possible."

Two days later, Edie was unable to get out of her bathtub and was vomiting so violently that she couldn't eat.

One of the side effects of metronidazole is a sudden drop in blood pressure, particularly in the elderly, which could have accounted for Edie's loss of consciousness and falls. Tamoxifen can cause pain, and both Flagyl and morphine cause nausea. In other words, every symptom she was displaying—besides the breast lumps themselves—appeared to be due mainly to the drugs—and also perhaps to the word "terminal" on the various forms we were asked to fill in.

We told her to throw her drugs in the trash. Before long we'd managed to get the drugs out of her system, but not her doctor's gloomy prognosis.

Fortunately, because of our work we knew of Dr. Patrick Kingsley, a medical pioneer in Leicestershire in Britain who helped people with a variety of conditions. We didn't know how successful he would be with a case of terminal cancer, but were encouraged to hear that he had a local cancer group consisting of many other no-hopers who were apparently out-living the odds.

We contacted him and he examined Edie. I was in the room with them and he didn't flinch when he saw her breast, "I think we can handle that," he said with offhand confidence.

His regime consisted mainly of designing a modified healthy diet and vitamin supplement program, tailored to the pocketbook and tastes of someone reared on standard British fare, cutting out foods he'd found her to be allergic to and administering large doses of intravenous vitamin C twice a week. Several months later, Edie's doctor, who'd delivered the death sentence on her in the first place, came to examine her. He was rendered utterly speechless. The cancer that had ravaged her breast, which he was so sure was beyond hope or treatment, *had completely receded*.

At this writing, little ninety-eight-pound Edie is still beating cancer, and we're not sure what exactly in her treatment was responsible. To a great degree, it may have had to do with my mother-in-law's optimism that Patrick would cure her, which in turn had something to do with his imperturbability during that first consultation, his refusal to be discouraged by cancer or to betray any doubt. Or perhaps it was the close rallying of her family around her and the courage of this ordinary senior in deciding (for we left it to her) to explore what must have appeared a bizarre and radical course. Some practitioners consider family support and personal commitment key elements in recovery from illness.

Although there is some good scientific evidence for Patrick's treatment (particularly with high-dose vitamin C), I tend to believe that the success of his approach also had to do with the fact that my husband endorsed this treatment option. Edie's youngest son had told her it was going to work, and that was proof enough for her.

Another essential factor was Patrick's steadfast refusal to characterize the likely path of Edie's illness—to make a judgment call about "how long" the illness would linger or how long she would live. Whatever the method, it had the single vital ingredient conspicuously left out of every potion dispensed by most doctors today: hope. Hope is the most important medicine there is. Everyone's confidence gave Edie hope, and hope is what saved her life.

Hope is what doctors used to provide before they presumed to have the knowledge to determine exactly how many months anybody's got left. Very few doctors have the humility to realize that no scientist, no matter how learned, can predict how a given patient will respond to the challenge of illness and healing, or say with certainty who will live and who will die.

REFERENCES

CHAPTER I

1   *British Medical Journal,* 1980; 280: 1–2.

2   *Times,* November 1, 1994.

3   'Cancer at a Crossroads,' National Cancer Advisory Board, 1994; which notes that rates of cancer have increased 18 percent since 1991 and the mortality rate grown by 7 percent. See also *Journal of the American Medical Association,* 1990; 264 (24): 3178–83.

4   Dr. Vernon Coleman, 'The Betrayal of Trust,' *European Medical Journal,* 1994: 4.

5   Figures on the world's first study into hospital safety, carried out by the Australian Department of Health, June 1995.

6   *Journal of the American Medical Association,* 1995; 274 (1): 29–34.

7   Edgar A. Suter, correspondence, *The Lancet,* 1993; 342: 112.

8   *New Scientist,* September 17, 1994: 23.

9   *What Doctors Don't Tell You,* 1992; 3 (12): 4.

10 Robert S. Mendelsohn, MD, *Confessions of a Medical Heretic* (Chicago: Contemporary Books, 1979): xiii–xiv.

11 See I. Chalmer, M. Enkin and M. Keirse (eds), *Effective Care in Pregnancy and Childbirth* (Oxford: Oxford University Press, 1989).

12 *New England Journal of Medicine*, 1995; 332 (5): 328–29.

13 *New England Journal of Medicine*, 1992; 326: 501–6; also 560–1. See also *Adverse Drug Reaction Bulletin*, June 1992 and *The Lancet*, 1993; 342: 818–19.

14 *The Lancet*, 1994; 344: 844–51.

15 *The Daily Telegraph*, September 23, 1994.

16 *Journal of the American Medical Association*, 1993; 269: 873–77, 878–82.

17 Interview with Norman Begg, December 1989.

18 *The Lancet*, 1993; 341: 343–45.

19 *The Lancet*, 1994; 344: 1601–6.

20 *The Lancet*, 1994; 344: 1585.

CHAPTER 2

1 Stephen Fulder, *How to Be a Healthy Patient* (Hodder and Stoughton, 1991): 26.

2 *The Lancet*, 1989; ii: 1190–91.

3 *The Lancet*, 1994; 344: 1339–43.

4 *The Lancet*, 1994; 344: 1309–11.

5 Mark Brown *et al.*, correspondence, *British Medical Journal*, 1991; 303: 120–21.

6 *British Medical Journal*, 1992; 305: 1062–66.

7 *Journal of Hypertension*, 1994; 12: 857–66.

8 Barnabus N. Panayiotou, correspondence, *Journal of the American Medical Association*, 1995; 274 (17): 1343.

9   M. J. Quinn, correspondence, *The Lancet*, 1991; 338: 130.

10 *The Lancet*, 1996; 347: 139–42.

11 Robert S. Mendelsohn, MD, *Confessions of a Medical Heretic* (Chicago: Contemporary Books, 1979): 2.

12 Dr. Edward D. Folland, correspondence, *New England Journal of Medicine*, 1992; 327 (25): 1819; *New England Journal of Medicine*, 1992; 327: 458–62.

13 Mendelsohn, *Confessions*: 3.

14 Fulder, *Healthy Patient*: 26.

15 *The Lancet*, 1994; 344: 1190–92.

16 *Journal of the American Medical Association*, 1992; 268: 2537–40.

17 J. Isner, *Circulation*, 1981; 63 (5), as quoted in S. Fulder, *How to Survive Medical Treatment* (Century Hutchinson, 1987): 24, 27.

18 R. Wootton, ed., *Radiation Protection of Patients* (Cambridge: Cambridge University Press, 1993): 16.

19 Ibid.

20 As quoted in *Which?*, January 1991: 41.

21 *Journal of the American Medical Association*, 1991; 265 (10): 1290.

22 R. Wootton, op cit.

23 *Journal of the American Medical Association*, 1991; 265 (10): 1290.

24 *International Journal of Cancer*, 1990; 46: 362–65.

25 *British Journal of Cancer*, 1990; 62 (1): 152–68.

26 *New Scientist*, 1979; 82: 18, as reported in Fulder, *Medical Treatment*: 35.

27 *New England Journal of Medicine*, 1993; 328 (2): 87–94.

28 *Journal of the American Medical Association*, 1994; 272 (15): 1160.

29 Fulder, *Medical Treatment*: 29.

30 *British Medical Journal*, 1991; 303: 813–15.

31 *The Lancet*, 1989; ii: 1190–1.

32 *FDA Consumer,* January 1980, as cited in Fulder, *Medical Treatment*: 30.

33 *British Medical Journal,* 1991; 303: 811–12.

34 *British Medical Journal,* 1991; 303: 813–15.

35 Royal College of Radiologists and National Radiological Protection Board, 'Patient dose reduction in diagnostic radiology' (HMSO, 1990), as reported in *British Medical Journal,* 1991; 303: 812.

36 *Journal of the American Medical Association,* 1991; 265(10): 1290.

37 J.G.B. Russell, consultant radiologist, position paper, 'Reactions to the Recommendations from the Royal College of Radiologists': 1.

38 Russell, 'Reactions': 2.

39 *British Medical Journal,* 1991; 303: 809–12.

40 *Which?,* op cit.

41 *British Medical Journal,* 1992; 304: 1411.

42 *British Journal of Cancer,* 1990; 62 (1): 152–68.

43 As reported in *The Independent,* April 27, 1990.

44 *British Medical Journal,* 1991; 303: 1497.

45 *Radiology,* 1977; 123: 523–7.

46 *New England Journal of Medicine,* 1994; 331 (21): 1449–50.

47 *Mount Sinai Journal of Medicine,* 1991; 58 (2): 183–87.

48 Charles V. Burton, 'Lumbo-Sacral Adhesive Arachnoiditis: The Modern New Guinea Syndrome.' Position paper: 9.

49 P.G. Bain and A.C.F. Colchester, correspondence, *The Lancet,* 1991; 338: 252–53.

50 K. Noda *et al.,* correspondence, *The Lancet,* 1994; 337: 681.

51 *Mount Sinai Journal of Medicine,* 1991; 58 (2):185–86.

52 Susan M. Ott, editorial, *British Medical Journal,* 1991; 308: 931–32.

53 Ibid.

54 David M. Reid *et al.*, correspondence, *British Medical Journal*, 1994; 308: 1567.

55 *British Medical Journal*, 1996; 312: 296–97.

56 Angela Raffle and Cyrus Cooper, correspondence, *The Lancet*, 1990; 336: 242; Albert M. Van Hemert, correspondence, *The Lancet*, 1990; 336: 818.

57 *British Medical Journal*, 1996; 312: 1254–58.

58 Wootton, *Radiation Protection:* 2; also *The Lancet*, 1992; 340: 299.

59 *The Lancet*, 1992; 340: 299.

60 *The Lancet*, 1976; i: 847–48. See also Joseph K. Lee (ed.), *Computed Body Tomography with MRI Correlation* (New York: Raven Press, 1989): 1117–18.

61 *British Medical Journal*, 1993; 306: 953–55.

62 *British Medical Journal*, 1994; 309: 986–89.

63 *New England Journal of Medicine*, 1994; 330: 25–30.

64 *American Journal of Public Health*, 1993; 83 (4): 588–90.

65 *Rofo Fortschr Geb Rontgenstr Neuen Bildgeb Verfahr*, 1992; 156 (2): 189–92.

66 *Radiology*, 1991; 178: 447–51.

67 Joseph Lee, *Computed Body:* 1119.

68 *New England Journal of Medicine*, 1993; 328 (12): 879–80.

69 *New England Journal of Medicine*, 1990; 323 (10): 621–26.

70 *British Medical Journal*, 1991; 303: 205.

71 *Chicago Tribune*, May 13, 1984, as reported in *The People's Doctor*, 10 (11).

72 *Oral Surgery, Oral Medicine and Oral Pathology*, 1993; 76 (5): 655–60.

73 *Acta Oto-Laryngologica*, 1993; 113 (4): 483–88.

74 *British Medical Journal,* 1991; 303: 205.

75 Karl Dantendorfer *et al.,* correspondence, *The Lancet,* 1991; 338; 761–62.

76 *IEEE Transactions on Biomedical Engineering,* 1993; 40 (12): 1324–27; *American Journal of Physical Medicine & Rehabilitation,* 1993; 72 (3): 166–67.

77 *American Journal of Roentgenology,* 1994; 162 (1): 189–94.

78 *American Journal of Roentgenology,* 1990; 154 (6): 1229–32.

79 *Journal of Magnetic Resonance Imaging,* 1992; 2 (6): 721–28.

80 *American Journal of Roentgenology,* 1990; 154 (6): 1229–32.

81 Stephen Fulder, *Medical Treatment*: 24.

82 *The Lancet,* 1989; ii: 1190–91.

83 *British Medical Journal,* 1979; ii: 21–24.

84 *British Medical Journal,* 1994; 309: 983–86.

85 *Medical Hypotheses,* 1988; 25: 151–62.

86 *Nature,* 1985; 317: 395–403; *The Lancet,* 1989; ii: 1023–25.

87 *New England Journal of Medicine,* 1988; 318: 448–49.

88 Abstracts VII International Conference on AIDS; Florence, Italy, 1991; 1: 326.

89 As reported in the *Sunday Times,* May 22, 1994.

90 *New England Journal of Medicine,* 1986; 314: 647.

91 *The Lancet,* 1986; i: 1090–92.

92 *AIDS,* 1988; 2: 405–06.

93 *Gut,* 1995; 36: 462–67.

94 *What Doctors Don't Tell You,* 1991; 2 (10): 4.

95 Charles Williams and Norman Frost, correspondence, *The Lancet,* 1994; 344: 1086–87.

96 *British Medical Journal,* 1993; 306: 953–55.

Chapter 3

1   Dr. Christopher R. B. Merritt, editorial, *Radiology*, 1989; 173 (2): 304–06.

2   *Journal of the American Medical Association*, 1982; 247 (16): 2196.

3   *Mother & Baby*, May 1990: 20–22.

4   Ibid.

5   American College of Obstetricians and Gynecologists, Tech. Bull No. 63, October 1981, as quoted in *Journal of Nurse-Midwifery*, 1984; 29 (4): 241–44.

6   Statement, Doris Haire, Chairman, Committee on Maternal and Child Health, National Women's Health Network, Diagnostic Ultrasound Education Workshop, April 26–28, 1990, Baltimore, Maryland.

7   *British Medical Journal*, 1993; 307: 13–17.

8   *New England Journal of Medicine*, 1993; 329 (12): 821–27.

9   Dr. Richard Berkowitz, editorial, *New England Journal of Medicine*, 1993; 329 (12): 874–75.

10 *The Lancet*, 1992; 340: 1299–1303.

11 *British Medical Journal*, 1993; 307: 159–64.

12 *The Lancet*, 1993; 342: 887–91.

13 *Canadian Medical Association Journal*, 1993; 149 (10): 1435–40.

14 Marc J.N.C. Keirse, editorial, *The Lancet*, 1993; 342: 878–79.

15 International Childbirth Education Association (ICEA) position paper: Diagnostic Ultrasound in Obstetrics, International Childbirth Education Association, March 1983.

16 Ibid.

17 *Obstetrics and Gynecology*, 1984; 63: 194–200.

18 *British Medical Journal*, 1975; 2: 62–64.

19 *Journal of Nurse-Midwifery*, 1984; 29 (4): 241–46.

20 Robert Bases, correspondence, *British Journal of Obstetrics and Gynaecology*, 1988; 95: 730.

21 *Journal of the American Medical Association*, 1982; 247 (16): 2195–97.

22 Ibid.

23 ICEA position paper, op cit.

24 *British Journal of Obstetrics and Gynaecology*, 1982; 89: 694–700.

25 *Obstetrics and Gynecology*, 1983; 62: 7–10.

26 HHS Publication FDA 82-8190, July 1982, Bureau of Radiological Health, Food and Drug Administration, as cited in ICEA position paper, op cit.

27 *Obstetrics and Gynecology*, 1984; 64 (1): 101–07.

28 *The People's Doctor* 11 (1): 7.

29 *British Medical Journal*, 1993; 307: 13–17.

30 *Daily Mirror*, June 3, 1994.

31 *Radiology*, 1989; 173: 304–06.

32 *Contemporary Obstetrics and Gynecology*, 1980; 6: 75–80.

33 *New England Journal of Medicine*, 1990: 322: 588–93.

34 *New England Journal of Medicine*, 1996; 334 (10): 613–18.

35 See *British Journal of Obstetrics and Gynaecology*, 1982; 89: 716–22; *British Journal of Obstetrics and Gynaeology*, 1982; 84: 427–33 and *British Journal of Obstetrics and Gynaecology*, 1983; 90: 1018–26 and *British Journal of Obstetrics and Gynaecology*, 1985; 92: 1156–59.

36 *What Doctors Don't Tell You*, 1990; 1 (6): 6.

37 Mr. Chalmers recommends that readers consult the *Journal of Perinatal Medicine*, 1984; 12: 227–33 and P. Mohide and M. Keirse, 'Biophysical assessment of fetal wellbeing,' in I. Chalmers *et al.*, *Effective Care in Pregnancy and Childbirth* (Oxford: Oxford University Press, 1989).

38 Helen Klein Ross,. *Mothering Magazine*, Summer 1990.

39 *British Medical Journal*, 1981; 282: 1416–18 as cited in Belinda Barnes and Suzanne Gail Bradley, *Planning for a Healthy Baby* (Vermilion, 1990): 164.

40 Roger Williams *et al.,* correspondence, *The Lancet,* 1986; ii: 757, as cited in *The People's Doctor,* 11 (1): 3.

41 Ross, op cit.

42 Leaflet handed out by obstetric unit, St. John's & St. Elizabeth's Hospital, London, 1993.

43 *The Lancet,* 1991; 337: 1491–99.

44 Froas J. Los *et al.,* correspondence, *The Lancet,* 1993; 342: 1559.

45 *The Lancet,* 1991; 337: 1491–99.

46 Karin Sundberg and Steen Smidt-Jensen, correspondence, *The Lancet,* 1991; 337: 1233–34.

47 M. J. Le Bris, correspondence, *The Lancet,* 1994; 344: 556.

48 *The Lancet,* 1991; 337: 762–63.

49 *The Lancet,* 1991; 337: 1091.

50 *The Lancet,* 1994; 343: 1069–71.

51 Ibid.

52 *The Lancet,* 1994; 344: 435–39.

53 F.P.H.A. Vandenbussche, *et al.,* correspondence, *The Lancet,* 1994; 344: 1032.

54 *The Lancet,* 1994; 344: 1134–36.

55 Name withheld, Barking, Essex, *The Spectator,* July 8, 1995.

56 Robert S. Mendelsohn, MD, *Male Practice: How Doctors Manipulate Women* (Chicago: Contemporary Books, 1981): 54.

57 *British Medical Journal,* 1994; 309: 158–62.

58 *Journal of Epidemiology and Community Health,* 1995; 49: 164–70.

59 *The Lancet,* 1990; 353: 7467–50.

60 *Mortality and Morbidity Weekly Report,* 1994; 43: 617–22.

61 Janet Carr, *Down's Syndrome* (Cambridge: Cambridge University Press, 1995).

62 See Barnes and Bradley, op cit.

CHAPTER 4

1   *British Medical Journal,* 1992; 304: 4632.

2   *The Lancet,* 1993; 341: 343.

3   Johannes Schmidt, correspondence, *The Lancet,* 1992; 339: 810.

4   *American Journal of Obstetrics and Gynecology,* 1941; 42: 193–205.

5   J. McCormick and P. Skrabanek, *Follies and Fallacies in Medicine* (Glasgow: The Tarragon Press, 1989): 103–04.

6   J. McCormick, 'Dogma Disputed,' *The Lancet,* 1989; ii: 207–09.

7   *The Lancet,* 1990; 335: 97–99.

8   J. McCormick, op cit.

9   Vernon Coleman, *The Health Scandal: Your Health in Crisis* (Sidgwick & Jackson, 1988): 171.

10 *The Lancet,* 1993; 342: 91–96.

11 A.B. Miller, 'Evaluation of Screening for Carcinoma of the Cervix,' *Modern Medicine Canada,* 1973; 28: 1067–69.

12 McCormick and Skrabanek, *Follies:* 104.

13 Ibid.

14 Tom Bell, correspondence, *The Lancet,* 1990; 336: 1260–61.

15 *British Medical Journal,* 1990; 301: 907–10. *British Medical Journal,* 1994; 308: 357–58.

16 *British Medical Journal,* 1990; 301: 907–10.

17 Ibid.

18 *British Medical Journal,* 1994; 308: 357–58.

19 *The Lancet,* 1995; 345: 1469–73.

20 Ibid.

21 McCormick, op cit.: 208.

22 *British Medical Journal,* 1988; 297: 18–21.

23 *The Lancet,* 1992; 339: 828.

24 *British Medical Journal*, 1993; 306: 1173.

25 *British Medical Journal*, 1986; 293: 659–63, as cited in *The Lancet*, 1990; 335: 97–99.

26 McCormick, op cit.

27 National Audit Office report, Cervical and Breast Screening in England, 1992.

28 *Daily Telegraph*, April 29, 1993.

29 Coleman, *The Health Scandal*: 172.

30 Robert S. Mendelsohn, MD, *Male Practice: How Doctors Manipulate Women* (Chicago: Contemporary Books, 1981): 42–43.

31 National Audit Office report, op cit.

32 *The Lancet*, 1993; 342: 91–96.

33 *British Medical Journal*, 1994; 308: 79.

34 *Journal of the American Medical Association*, 1994; 271 (10): 733–34.

35 *British Medical Journal*, 1995; 311: 1391–95.

36 M. Baum, correspondence, *The Lancet*, 1995; 346: 436; see also correspondence, *New England Journal of Medicine*, 1994; 331: 402–03.

37 *The Lancet*, 1993; 341: 1509–11.

38 Ibid.

39 *Journal of the American Medical Association*, 1994; 2;71 (2): 96.

40 *The Lancet*, 1994; 343: 1091.

41 *British Medical Journal*, 1993; 336: 1481–83.

42 *Journal of the American Medical Association*, 1994; 271 (2): 96.

43 *The Lancet*, 1995; 345: 1629.

44 Minerva, *British Medical Journal*, 1993; 306; 1280.

45 J.A. Muir Gray *et al.*, correspondence, *British Medical Journal*, 1991; 302; 1084.

46 Petr Skrabanek and James McCormick, correspondence, *British Medical Journal*, 1991; 302: 1401.

47   N. Wald *et al.*, correspondence, *British Medical Journal*, 1991; 302: 845.

48   Skrabanek and McCormick, op cit.

49   *The Lancet*, 1995; 346: 29–32.

50   Ibid.

51   Ibid.

52   *British Medical Journal*, 1996; 312: 273–76.

53   Johannes G. Schmidt, correspondence, *The Lancet*, 1992; 339: 810.

54   *Canadian Journal of Public Health*, 1993; 84: 14–16.

55   Michael Swift, correspondence, *The Lancet*, 1992; 340: 1538.

56   J. Mark Elwood, Brian Cox and Ann K. Richardson, correspondence, *The Lancet*, 1993; 341: 1531.

57   *British Medical Journal*, 1988; 297: 943–98.

58   Rob Boer *et al.*, correspondence, *The Lancet*, 1994; 343: 979.

59   Schmidt, op cit.

60   *Journal of the American Medical Association*, 1990; 263: 2341–43.

61   *Journal of the American Medical Association*, 1996; 275: 913–18. See also Cecily Quinn and Julian Ostrowski, correspondence, *The Lancet*, 1996; 347: 1259.

62   Personal interview with Dr. James McCormick, June 12, 1996; see also *The Lancet*, 1994; 343: 969.

63   Mendelsohn, *Male Practice*: 110.

64   The Royal College of Radiologists, 'Making the Best Use of a Department of Clinical Radiology,' London 1993: 33–37.

65   *Glamour*, October 1992; see also *Daily Telegraph*, December 28, 1991.

66   D.J. Watmough and K.M. Quan, correspondence, *The Lancet*, 1992; 340: 122.

67   E.J. Roebuck, correspondence, *The Lancet*, 1992; 340: 366.

68 J. P van Netten *et al.*, correspondence, *The Lancet*, 1994; 343: 978–79.

69 *Ultrasound Med Biol*, 1979; 5: 45–49.

70 J. Michael Dixon and T.G. John, correspondence, *The Lancet*, 1992; 339: 128.

71 J. Stevenson, correspondence, *British Medical Journal*, 1991; 303: 924.

72 Nicholas E. Day and Stephen W. Duffy, correspondence, *The Lancet*, 1991; 338: 113–14.

73 *What Doctors Don't Tell You*, 1990; 1 (2): 4.

74 *British Medical Journal*, 1994; 308: 79.

75 D. Sienko *et al.*, correspondence, *New England Journal of Medicine*, 1989; 320: 941.

76 *Journal of the American Medical Association*, 1993; 269 (20): 2616–17.

77 Graham Curtis Jenkins, correspondence, *British Medical Journal*, 1992; 305: 718.

78 *British Medical Journal*, 1994; 308.

79 Ibid.

80 Syed Bilgramia and Bernard Greenberg, commentary, *The Lancet*, 1994; 344: 700–1.

81 *Journal of the American Medical Association*, 1995; 273: 289–94.

82 *Urology*, 1996; 47: 511–16.

83 *British Medical Journal*, 1992; 304: 534.

84 Dr. Joan Austoker, adviser to Britain's Chief Medical Officer, as quoted in the *Sunday Times*, October 6, 1991.

85 Daniel Kopans, correspondence, *The Lancet*, 1991; 338: 447.

86 *Radiation Medicine*, 1994; 12 (5): 201–08.

87 *Anticancer Research*, 1994; 14 (5B): 2249–51.

88 *Geburt und Frau*, 1994; 54 (8): 432–36.

89 *Geburt und Frau*, 1994; 54 (10): 539–44.

90 *Ultraschall in der Medizin,* 1994; 15 (1): 20–23.

91 *Journal of Clinical Pathology,* 1949; 2: 197–208, as cited in *The Lancet,* 1993; 341: 91.

CHAPTER 5

1 Newman and Hulley, correspondence, *Journal of the American Medical Association;* 1996; 275: 1481–82; *British Medical Journal,* 1993; 306: 1367–73.

2 *British Medical Journal,* 1994; 309: 11–15.

3 *The Lancet,* 1994; 344: 1182–86.

4 *Journal of the American Medical Association,* 1995; 274 (2): 131–36.

5 *The Lancet,* 1994; 344: 963–64.

6 *The Lancet,* 1995; 345: 882.

7 *The Lancet,* 1995; 345: 1408.

8 *Journal of the American Medical Association,* 1995; 273 (24): 1926–32.

9 *Journal of the American Medical Association,* 1994; 272 (17): 1335–40.

10 *Daily Telegraph,* April 16, 1993.

11 Ibid.

12 *The Lancet,* 1994; 344: 633–38.

13 Michael F. Oliver, editorial, *British Medical Journal,* 1992; 304: 393–94; also Drs. George Davey Smith and Julia Pekkanen, debate, 304: 431–34.

14 *The Lancet,* 1994; 344: 1383–89.

15 *Monitor Weekly,* November 30, 1994: 17.

16 *New England Journal of Medicine,* 1995; 333: 1301–07.

17 *Circulation,* 1995; 92: 2419–25; also *Journal of the American College of Cardiology,* 1995; 26: 1133–39.

18 Jan P. Vandenbroucke, Rudi G. J. Westendorp, correspondence, *The Lancet,* 1996; 347: 1267–68.

19 Robert J. MacFadyen *et al.*, correspondence, *The Lancet*, 1996; 347: 551–52.

20 R. Fey and N. Pearson, essay, *The Lancet*, 1996; 347: 1389–90.

21 William E. Stehbens, correspondence, *The Lancet*, 1995; 345: 264.

22 Vandenbroucke and Westendorp, op cit.

23 *Journal Watch*, 1995; 15 (24): 190, and 15 (23): 181–82.

24 Dr. Nilesh J. Samani and David P. De Bono, correspondence, *New England Journal of Medicione*, 1996; 334 (20): 1333–34.

25 *New England Journal of Medicine*, 1996; 335: 1001–09.

26 Fey and Pearson, op cit.

27 *Journal Watch*, 1996; 16 (10): 83–84.

28 Donald R. Davis, Ph.D., correspondence, *New England Journal of Medicine*, 1996; 334 (20): 1334.

29 *Journal of the American Medical Association*, 1995; 274 (14): 1152–58.

30 Rodney Jackson and Robert Beaglehole, commentary, *The Lancet*, 1995; 346: 1440–41.

31 *British Medical Journal*, 1994; 308: 373–79.

32 All calculations performed by Dr. Stewart Rogers, correspondence, *New England Journal of Medicine*, 1996; 334 (20): 1333.

33 Vandenbroucke and Westendorp, op cit.

34 Drs. George Davey Smith and Julia Pekkanen, debate, *British Medical Journal*, 1992; 304: 431–33.

35 *British Medical Journal*, 1995; 310: 1632–36.

36 *British Medical Journal*, 1996; 313: 649–64.

37 *The Lancet*, 1993; 341: 75–79.

38 Bruno Bertozzi *et al.*, correspondence, *British Medical Journal*, 1996; 312: 1298–99.

39 *The Lancet*, 1993; 341: 75–79.

40 *Psychology of Medicine* 1990; 20: 785–91.

41 Dr. Melvyn Werbach, *Nutritional Influences on Mental Illness* (Tarzana, CA: Third Line Press, 1991): 145–49.

42 *Arch. Intern. Med.,* 1995; 155: 695–700.

43 M.R. Law and N.J. Wald, correspondence, *British Medical Journal,* 1995; 311: 807.

44 *Am J. Clin. Nutri.,* 1995; 62: 1–9. See also *What Doctors Don't Tell You,* 1995; 6 (6): 1–3.

45 *British Heart Journal,* 1978; 40: 1069–1118.

46 *Physicians' Desk Reference* (Montvale, NJ: Medical Economics Data Production Company, 1995): 710–12.

47 *Physicians' Desk Reference:* 1851–54.

48 *British Medical Journal,* 1997; 314: 1584.

49 *Journal of the American Medical Association,* 1996; 275: 55. See also *Journal Watch,* 1996; 16 (10): 83–84.

50 Newman and Hulley, op cit.

51 *The Lancet,* 1994; 344: 1195–96.

52 Petr Skrabanek and James McCormick, *Follies and Fallacies in Medicine* (Glasgow: Tarragon Press, 1990): 95.

53 *The Lancet,* 1990; 336: 129–33.

54 *Journal of the American Medical Association,* 1995; 274: 894–901.

55 *The Lancet,* 1992; 339: 563–69.

56 *New England Journal of Medicine,* 1996; 334 (20): 1298–1303.

57 *Circulation,* 1996; 93: 1346–53.

58 Drs. Edward Siguel *et al.* and K. Lance Gould, correspondence, *Journal of the American Medical Association,* 1996; 275 (18): 1402–03.

59 Drs. K. Lance Gould and Dean Ornish, correspondence, *Journal of the American Medical Association,* 1996; 275 (18): 1402–03.

60 Drs. Edward Siguel *et al.,* correspondence, *Journal of the American Medical Association,* 1996; 275 (10): 759.

61 *The Lancet,* 1994; 343: 1268–71.

62 Ibid.

63 *J. Lipid. Res.*, 1992; 33: 399–410.

64 *Br. J. Preven. Soc. Med.*, 1975; 29: 82–90.

65 *The Lancet*, 1993; 341: 581–85.

66 *Townsend Letter for Doctors*, 1995; 139/40: 68–70.

67 *The Lancet*, 1995; 345: 273–78.

68 *Journal of Nutritional Medicine*, 1991; 2: 227–47.

69 *New England Journal of Medicine*, 1985; 312 (5): 283–89, as quoted in *Journal of Nutritional Medicine*, 1991; 2: 227–47.

70 *Journal of Nutritional Medicine*, 1991; 2: 227–47.

CHAPTER 6

1 National Vaccine Information Center News, August 1994, as quoted in *Campaign Against Fradulent Medical Research Newsletter*, Spring/Summer 1994; 2 (2): 10.

2 Correspondence, February 1994 between DOH and National Immunization Program, confirmed by interview with Mark Papania of the U.S. National Immunization Program, October 1994.

3 *The Lancet*, 1995; 345: 567–69.

4 Gordon Stewart, *World Medicine*, September 1994: 17–20.

5 Personal interview with Dr. J. Anthony Morris, December 1989.

6 *Journal of Pediatrics*, 1973; 82: 798–801.

7 *The Lancet*, 1995; 345: 963–65.

8 *Campaign Against Fradulent Medical Research Newsletter*, 1995; 2 (3): 5–13, quoting statistics from the London Bills of Mortality 1760–1834 and Reports of the Registrar General 1838–96, as compiled in Alfred Wallace, *The Wonderful Century*, 1898.

9 *Bulletin of the World Health Organization*, 1975; 52: 209–22.

10 Derrick Baxby, correspondence, *British Medical Journal*, 1995; 310: 62.

11 Walene James, *Immunization: The Reality Behind the Myth* (Massachusetts: Bergin & Garvey, 1988): 26–27.

12 Neil Z. Miller, *Vaccines: Are They Really Safe and Effective?* (Santa Fe, NM: New Atlantean Press, 1992): 20.

13 James, *Immunization*: 27–28.

14 James, *Immunization*: 32.

15 *Health Freedom News*, January 1983: 26, as quoted in James, *Immunization*: 28.

16 *The Herbalist New Health*, July 1981: 61, as quoted in James, *Immunization*: 28.

17 Richard Moskowitz, 'Immunization: The Other Side,' in *Vaccinations: The Rest of the Story* (Santa Fe, NM: *Mothering*, 1992): 89.

18 *Science*, 1978; 200: 905, as quoted in Miller, *Vaccines*: 32.

19 Miller, *Vaccines*: 24, 33.

20 Michael Alderson, *International Mortality Statistics: Facts on File* (Washington, D.C., 1981): 182–83, as quoted in Miller, *Vaccines*: 25.

21 Report from the Office of Population Censuses and Surveys, 1993, as reported in *The Independent*, August 10, 1993.

22 *Journal of the American Medical Association*, 1993; 269 (2): 227–31; also 269 (2): 264–66.

23 Personal interview with Norman Begg, Deember 1989.

24 *Journal of the American Medical Association*, 1972; 220: 959–62.

25 *American Journal of Epidemiology*, 1980; iii (4): 415–24.

26 *The Lancet*, 1986; i: 1169–73; *British Medical Journal*, 1932; 2: 708–11, as reported in *Townsend Letter for Doctors*, January 1996: 29. Also, *New England Journal of Medicine*, 1990; 323: 160–64.

27 *World Medicine*, September 1984: 20.

28 Ibid.

29 Moskowitz, *Vaccinations*: 92.

30 *The Lancet*, 1977; i: 234–37.

31 *World Medicine*, September 1984: 20.

32 Gordon Stewart, correspondence, *British Medical Journal*, 1983; 287: 287–88.

33 *New England Journal of Medicine*, 1994; 331: 16–21.

34 Personal interview with Dr. J. Anthony Morris, April 1992.

35 *World Medicine*, September 1984: 19.

36 Dr. J. Anthony Morris, testimony before the Subcommittee on Investigations and General Oversight, May 1982.

37 *Journal of the American Medical Association*, 1995; 274 (6); 446–47.

38 *New England Journal of Medicine*, 1995; 333: 1045–50.

39 *The Lancet*, 1996; 347: 209–10.

40 November 20–21, 1975 minutes of the fifteenth meeting of the Panel of Review of Bacterial Vaccines and Toxoids with Standards and Potency (Bureau of Biologics and Food and Drug Administration), as quoted in Robert S. Mendelsohn, MD, *But Doctor . . . About That Shot* (Evanston, IL: The People's Doctor, Inc., 1988): 6.

41 *The Lancet*, 1995; 345: 963–65.

42 Zhurnel Mikrobiologii, *Epidemiologii i Immunobiologii*, 1994; 3: 57–61.

43 Mendelsohn, op cit.

44 *African Journal of Medicine and Medical Sciences*, 1994; 23: 19–22.

45 *Developmental Medicine and Child Neurology*, 1993; 35: 351–55.

46 *The Lancet*, 1996; 348: 1185–86.

47 *Journal of Gerontology*, 1993; 48: M19–25.

48 *Centers for Disease Control Mortality and Morbidity Weekly Report*, June 6, 1986, as reported in Mendelsohn, *But Doctor*: 81.

49 *Annals of Internal Medicine*, 1979; 90 (6): 978–80.

50 *New England Journal of Medicine*, 1987; 316: 771–74.

51 *Centers for Disease Control Mortality and Morbidity Weekly Report*, June 6, 1986, as reported in Mendelsohn, *But Doctor*: 81.

52 *New England Journal of Medicine*, 1989; 320 (2): 75–81.

53 *Pediatric Infectious Disease Journal*, 1994; 13: 34–38.

54 Dr. Stanley Plotkin, professor of Pediatrics, University of Pennsylvania School of Medicine, as quoted in Mendelsohn, *But Doctor*: 12.

55 M. G. Cusi *et al.*, correspondence, *The Lancet*, 1990; 336: 1071.

56 Minnesota epidemiologist Michael Ostenholm, as reported in *St. Paul Pioneer Press Despatch*, quoted in Mendelsohn, *But Doctor*: 87.

57 Kathleen Stratton *et al.*, *Adverse Events Associated with Childhood Vaccine: Evidence Bearing on Causality* (Washington, D.C.: National Academy Press, 1993): 261.

58 *New England Journal of Medicine*, 1986; 315: 1584–90.

59 *The Lancet*, 1991; 338: 395–98.

60 *New England Journal of Medicine*, 1991; 324 (25): 1767–72.

61 *Journal of the American Medical Association*, 1993; 269 (19): 2491.

62 *The Lancet*, 1991; 338: 395–98.

63 *The Lancet*, 1997; 349: 1197–1201.

64 *Journal of the American Medical Association*, 1995; 273: 888–89; figures supplied by the U.S. Centers for Disease Control and Prevention.

65 *AJDC*, 1991; 145: 742.

66 *The Lancet*, 1994; 344: 630–31.

67 Ibid.

68 James, op cit.

69 *The Lancet*, December 8, 1984.

70 *The Lancet*, 1990; 1192–98.

71 *Vaccine*, 1993; 11: 75–81.

72 *Israeli Journal of Medical Science*, 1995; 31: 49–53.

73 *Journal of Infectious Diseases,* 1997; 175: 545–53 and 1995; 171: 1097–106.

74 *Journal of Infectious Diseases,* 1993: 168: 452–54.

75 S. O. Cameron, *et al.,* correspondence, *British Medical Journal,* 1992; 304: 52.

76 *British Medical Journal,* 1992; 302: 495–98.

77 *Medical Monitor,* June 5, 1992.

78 *The Lancet,* 1992; 339: 636–39.

79 *The Lancet,* 1995; 346: 1339–45.

80 Professor David Baum and Dr. Susanna Graham-Jones, *Child Health: The Complete Guide* (Penguin: 1991): 89.

81 Dr. Bob Chen and Dr. John Glasser, Vaccine Safety Datalink, the National Immunization Program's Large-Linked Databased Study, Advisory Commission on Childhood Vaccines, presented on September 28, 1994.

82 *The Lancet,* 1995; 345: 567–69.

83 *Acta Paediatrica,* 1993; 82 (3): 267–70.

84 Information supplied by the National Vaccination Information Center in Vienna, Virginia.

85 Harris L. Coulter and Barbara Loe Fisher, *A Shot in the Dark* (New York: Avery Publishing Group, 1985): 8–9.

86 *World Medicine,* September 1984: 17.

87 *The Lancet,* 1996; 347: 209–10.

88 Coulter and Fisher, *A Shot in the Dark*: 13–14.

89 Stratton *et al., Adverse Events*: 309–19.

90 Coulter and Fisher, *A Shot in the Dark*: 32.

91 Stratton *et al.,* op cit.

92 Kathleen Stratton *et al.,* 'DPT vaccine and chronic nervous system dysfunction: a new analysis,' Division of Health Promotion and Disease Prevention, Institute of Medicine (Washington, D.C.: National Academy Press, 1994).

93   Gordon Stewart and John Wilson, correspondence, *British Medical Journal,* 1981; 282: 1968–69.

94   Gordon Stewart, correspondence, *British Medical Journal,* 1983; 287: 287–88.

95   House of Commons, Hansard, 1980; December 3: col. 262, as reported in Stewart and Wilson, correspondence, *British Medical Journal* 1981; 282: 1968–69.

96   Mendelsohn, *But Doctor:* 19.

97   *Pediatric Infectious Disease Journal,* January 1983, as reported in Mendelsohn, *But Doctor:* 42.

98   Ibid.

99   A. Kalokerinos, *Every Second Child* (New Canaan, CT: Keats, 1981), as cited in Coulter and Fisher, *A Shot in the Dark:* 131.

100   Stratton *et al., Adverse Events:* 67–117.

101   *New England Journal of Medicine,* 1981; 305: 1307–13.

102   *Physicians' Desk Reference* (Montvale, NJ: Medical Economics Data Production Company, 1995): 1288.

103   Department of Health Press Release, October 3, 1988.

104   Interview with the National Vaccine Information Center, August 1994.

105   *International Symposium on Immunization: Benefit Versus Risk Factors,* Brussels, 1978. *Developmental Biology Standard,* 432: 259–64 (S. Kurger, Basel, 1979).

106   *The Lancet,* 1989; ii: 1015–16.

107   *Annals of Internal Medicine,* 1979; 90 (6): 978–80.

108   *The Lancet,* 1995; 345: 1071–73; *The Lancet,* 1995; 345: 1062–63.

109   *The Lancet,* 1994; 343: 105; also Kohji Heda *et al.,* correspondence, *The Lancet,* 1995; 346: 701–02.

110   Stratton *et al., Adverse Events:* 118–86.

111   *American Diseases of Childhood,* 1965; 109: 232–37.

112   *The Lancet,* 1985; i: 1–5.

113 W. Ehrengut, correspondence, *The Lancet*, 1989; ii: 751.

114 *Pediatric Infectious Disease Journal*, 1989; 8 (11): 751–55.

115 *Can. Dis. Weekly Report*, 1987; 13–35: 156–57, as reported in *The Lancet*, 1989; ii: 1015–16.

116 *Pediatric Infectious Disease Journal*, 1989; 8 (5): 302–08.

117 *Pediatric Infectious Disease Journal*, March 1991.

118 *The Lancet*, 1993; 341: 979–82.

119 Ibid.

120 *The Lancet*, 1993; 341: 46.

121 *Physicians' Desk Reference*: 1575.

122 *The WDDTY Vaccination Handbook: A Guide to the Dangers of Child-hood Immunization* (The Wallace Press, 1991): 7.

123 *MacLean's*, February 8, 1982, as reported in Mendelsohn, *But Doctor*: 30.

124 *The Washington Star*, February 12, 1981.

125 *ASM News*, 1988; 54 (10): 560–62.

126 *Journal of the American Medical Association*, 1995; 274 (1): 12–13.

127 *British Medical Journal*, 1992; 305: 79–81.

128 T. Mertens and H. Eggers, correspondence, *The Lancet*, 1984; ii: 1390.

129 *American Journal of Clinical Nutrition*, 1977; 30: 592–98.

130 Yan Shen and Guohua Xia, correspondence, *The Lancet*, 1994; 344: 1026

131 M. Uhari *et al.*, correspondence, *The Lancet*, 1989; ii: 440–41.

132 A. D. Langmuir, 'The Safety and Efficiency of Vaccines for the Prevention of Poliomyelitis,' paper presented for Committee to Study the Poliomyelitis Vaccine at the Institute of Medicine, National Academy of Sciences, March 14–15, 1977.

133 Interview with Dr. J. Anthony Morris, April 1991.

134 *Danish Medical Bulletin*, 1960; 7: 142–44.

135 *U.S. Medicine,* April 1983, as reported in Mendelsohn, *But Doctor.* 60.

136 *The Lancet,* 1992; 339: 1060.

137 All information about the New Zealand experience with the HB vaccine from a report authored by Dr. Anthony Morris and Hilary Butler, 'Nature and Frequency of Adverse Reactions following Hepatitis B Vaccine Injection in Children in New Zealand, 1985–1988.' Submitted May 4, 1992 to the Vaccine Safety Committee, Institute of Medicine of the National Academy of Sciences, Washington, D.C.

138 *Journal of Infectious Diseases,* 1992; 165: 777–78.

139 Ohio Parents for Vaccine Safety, *Vaccine News,* Summer 1995.

140 *The Lancet,* 1990; 336: 325–29.

141 Ibid.

142 *Gastroenterology,* 1992; 102: 538–43.

143 A. J. Zuckerman, *et al.,* correspondence, *The Lancet,* 1994; 343: 737–38.

144 *Pediatric Infectious Disease Journal,* 1992; 18: 6.

145 *The Lancet,* 1993; 341: 851–54.

146 See Harold S. Ginsberg, *The Adenoviruses* (New York: Plenum Press).

147 *Transactions of the Royal Society of Tropical Medicine and Hygiene,* 1985; 79: 355–58 and 1989; 83: 545–49.

148 Mertens and Eggens, op cit.

149 *Transactions of the Royal Society of Tropical Medicine and Hygiene,* 1985; 79: 355–58 and 1989; 83: 545–49.

150 *New England Journal of Medicine,* 1995; 332 (8): 500–07.

151 *What Doctors Don't Tell You,* 1994; 5 (9): 12.

152 Ibid.

153 Michel Odent, *Journal of the American Medical Association,* 1994; 272 (8): 592–93.

154 *J. Pediatrics,* 1986; 108 (1): 671–76.

155 *Pediatric Infectious Disease Journal,* 1992; 11: 955–59, as reported in *Journal of the American Medical Association,* 1994; 271 (1): 13.

156 *American Dis. Child,* 1992; 146: 182–86.

157 *The Lancet,* 1986; i: 1169–73.

158 *New England Journal of Medicine,* 1990; 323: 160–64.

159 *British Medical Journal,* 1987; 294: 294–96.

160 *What Doctors Don't Tell You,* 1996; 7 (2): 8.

161 *Pediatrics* (Supplement), June 1986; 963.

162 *American Journal of Public Health,* 1990: 80.

163 See 'Alternatives' by Harald Gaier, *What Doctors Don't Tell You,* 1995; 5 (11): 9.

164 *British Medical Journal,* 1987; 294: 294–96.

Chapter 7

1 *Journal of the Royal Society of Medicine,* 1992; 85: 376–79.

2 *Times,* November 11, 1994.

3 *New England Journal of Medicine,* 1993; 329 (16): 1141–46.

4 *New England Journal of Medicine,* 1993; 329 (16): 1192–93.

5 *American Journal of Medicine,* 1988; 85: 847–50.

6 *Annals of Internal Medicine,* 1995; 122: 9–16.

7 Anne Szarewski *et al., British Medical Journal,* 1994; 308: 717.

8 See Kitty Little, *Bone Behaviour* (Academic Press, 1973); also Dr. Ellen Grant, *Sexual Chemistry* (Cedar, 1994).

9 Dr. John McLaren Howard, *Current Research in Osteoporosis and Bone Mineral Measurement II,* proceedings of the third Bath Conference on Osteoporosis Bone Mineral Measurement, Bath, June 23–26, 1992 (British Institute of Radiology, 1992).

10 *New England Journal of Medicine*, 1993; 328 (15): 1069–75.

11 *British Medical Journal*, 1994; 308: 1268–69.

12 *New England Journal of Medicine*, 1993; 328 (15): 1115–17.

13 *The Lancet*, 1991; 337: 833–34.

14 *British Medical Journal*, 1994; 308: 1268–69.

15 *The Lancet*, 1991; 337: 833–34.

16 F. M. Ward Posthuma *et al.*, correspondence, *British Medical Journal*, 1994; 309: 191–92.

17 *New England Journal of Medicine*, 1985; 313: 1038–43.

18 *New England Journal of Medicine*, 1985, 313: 1044–49, as cited in *The Lancet*, 1991, 337: 833–34.

19 *Ann. J. Epidemiol*, 1988; 128: 606–14; *Circulation*, 1987; 79: 1102–09, as cited in *The Lancet*, 1991; 337: 833–34.

20 *American Journal of Medicine*, 1991; 90: 584–89; *New England Journal of Medicine*, 1993; 328 (15): 1115–17.

21 *New England Journal of Medicine*, 1991; 325 (11): 800–02.

22 Ibid.

23 *Journal of the American Medical Association*, 1995; 273 (3): 199–208.

24 *British Medical Journal*, 1996; 313: 687.

25 *Journal of the American Medical Association*, 1995; 273: 199–208.

26 M. Riedel and A. Mugge, correspondence, *The Lancet*, 1993; 342: 871–72.

27 *British Medical Journal*, 1995; 311: 1193–96.

28 P. Y. Scarabin *et al*, correpsondence, *The Lancet*, 1996; 347: 122.

29 *Journal of Clinical Epidemiology*, 1997; 50: 275–81.

30 *New England Journal of Medicine*, 1985; 313: 1038–43; and 1991; 325: 756–62.

31 *Journal of the American Medical Association*, 1993; 269 (20): 2637–41.

32 *British Journal of Obstetrics and Gynaecology*, 1990; 97: 917–21.

33 *The Lancet*, 1992; 339: 290–91.

34 *The Lancet*, 1992; 339: 506.

35 *Times*, February 1, 1992.

36 *British Medical Journal*, 1992; 305: 1403–08.

37 See Dr. Ellen Grant, *The Bitter Pill* (Corgi Books, 1985) and *Sexual Chemistry* (Cedar, 1994).

38 *British Medical Journal*, 1990; 300: 436–38.

39 *Journal of the Royal Society of Medicine*, 1992; 85: 376–79.

40 *Obstetrics and Gynecology*, 1992; 79 (2): 286–94.

41 *Journal of the American Medical Association*, 1991; 265 (15): 1985–90.

42 *New England Journal of Medicine*, 1989; 321: 293–97.

43 *The Lancet*, 1991; 338: 274–77.

44 *New England Journal of Medicine*, 1995; 332 (24): 1589–93.

45 *Obstetrics and Gynecology*, 1993; 81 (2): 265–71; *Annals of Internal Medicine*, 1992; 177 (12): 1016–37.

46 *The Lancet*, 1997; 349; 458–61.

47 Interview with Klim McPherson, February 1995.

48 *American Journal of Epidemiology*, May 1995.

49 *British Medical Journal*, 1992; 305: 1403–08.

50 *Obstetrics and Gynecology*, 1991; 78: 1008–10.

51 *British Medical Journal*, 1992; 305: 1403–08.

52 *British Journal of Obstetrics and Gynaecology*, 1990; 97: 939–44.

53 *The Lancet*, 1996; 348: 977–80 and 981–83.

54 *The Lancet*, 1996; 348: 1668.

55 *Clinical Therapeutics*, 1990; 12 (5): 447–55.

56 *Journal of the American Geriatrics Society*, 1992; 40 (8): 817–20.

57 *Australian and New Zealand Journal of Obstetrics and Gynaecology*, 1992; 32 (4): 384–85.

58 *Journal of Neurology*, 1993; 240 (3): 195–96.

59 *The Lancet*, 1979; i: 581–82.

60 *Obstetrics and Gynecology*, 1994; 83: 5–11.

61 Ellen Grant, *Sexual Chemistry* (Cedar, 1994): 144–45.

62 *American Journal of Clinical Nutrition*, 1991; 54: 1093–1100.

63 Gillian Walker (ed.), *ABPI Data Sheet Compendium*, 1993–94 (Data-pharm Publications Ltd., 1993.) See also *What Doctors Don't Tell You*, 1995; 6 (8): 8–9 and 6 (11): 8–9.

64 Klim McPherson *et al.*, correspondence, *British Medical Journal*, 1995; 310: 598. See also Dr. David Grimes, editorial, *Fertility and Sterility*, 1992; 57 (3): 492–93.

65 De Boever *et al.*, 'Variation of Progesterone, 200 alpha-Dihydro-progesterone and Oestradiol Concentrations in Human Mammary Tissue and Blood after Topical Administration of Progesterone,' in P. Mauvais-Jarvis *et al.*, *Percutaneous Absorption of Steroids* (Academic Press, 1980): 259–65.

66 Melvyn Werbach, *Nutritional Influences on Illness* (Tarzana, CA: Third Line Press, 1993).

67 McLaren Howard, op cit.

68 *Journal of Nutritional Medicine*, 1991; 2: 165–78.

69 *British Medical Journal*, December 5, 1992. See also *Journal of the American Medical Association*, 1994; 272 (24): 1909–14.

70 Ibid.

71 *Here's Health*, March 1991: 13.

72 See Harald Gaier, 'Alternatives,' *What Doctors Don't Tell You*, 1995; 6 (9): 9.

CHAPTER 8

1 John Mansfield and David Freed, 'Choking on Medicine,' *What Doctors Don't Tell You*, 1993; 4 (6): 12.

2   Dr. Sidney M. Wolfe and Rose Ellen Hope, *Worse Pills, Best Pills, II* (Washington, D.C.: Public Citizens' Health Research Group, 1993): 10.

3   *The Lancet,* 1994; 343: 871–81.

4   *Science,* 1994; 264: 1538–41, as reported in Minerva, *British Medical Journal,* 1994; 308: 1726.

5   *British Medical Journal,* 1994; 308: 283–84.

6   Ibid.

7   See *Journal of the American Medical Association,* 1994; 271 (15): 1205–07; *The Lancet,* 1994; 343: 784; *British Medical Journal,* 1994; 308: 809–10.

8   Both examples taken from The Honorable John D. Dingell. Shattuck Lecture—Misconduct in Medical Research, *New England Journal of Medicine,* 1993; 328: 1610–15.

9   *Science,* 1994; 263: 317–18, as reported in Minerva, *British Medical Journal,* 1994; 308: 484.

10 *What Doctors Don't Tell You,* 1994; 5 (2): 3.

11 Charles Medawar, *The Wrong Kind of Medicine?* (Consumers' Association and Hodder & Stoughton, 1984): 79.

12 Personal interview with Geoffrey Cannon, January 1991.

13 *The Lancet,* 1981; 2: 883–87; *Archives of Otolanryngology:* 1974; 100: 226–32; *Clinical Otolaryntology,* 1981; 6: 5–13, as reported in Harald Gaier, 'Alternatives,' *What Doctors Don't Tell You,* 1994; 5 (12): 9.

14 T. T. K. Jung *et al.,* in D. J. Lim *et al.* (eds), *Recent Advances in Otitis Media with Effusion* (Philadelphia: B. C. Decker, 1984), as reported in Harald Gaier, 'Alternatives,' *What Doctors Don't Tell You,* 1994; 5 (12): 9.

15 *Mims,* 1991; 18 (3): 32.

16 Personal interview with Professor Ian Phillips, January 1991.

17 See William Crook, *Solving the Puzzle of Your Hard-to-Raise Child* (New York: Random House, 1981).

18 *Townsend Letter for Doctors,* October 1995: 9.

19 *British Medical Journal*, 1996; 313: 648.

20 See Dr. Lisa Landymore-Lim, *Poisonous Prescriptions* (Subiaco, Western Australia: PODD, 1994).

21 *Journal of Hospital Infections*, February 1988.

22 *Mortality and Morbidity Weekly Report*, 1995; 43: 952–53, as reported in *Journal of the American Medical Association*, 1995; 273 (6): 451.

23 *New England Journal of Medicine*, 1992; 326 (8): 501–06.

24 *Adverse Drug Reaction Bulletin*, June 1992.

25 *The Lancet*, 1995; 345: 2–3.

26 *Journal of Allergy and Clinical Immunology*, 1987; 80: 415–16, as reported in Mansfield and Freed, op cit.

27 *Adverse Drug Reaction Bulletin*, June 1992.

28 *The Lancet*, 1990; 336: 1391–96.

29 *British Medical Journal*, 1991; 303: 1426–31.

30 Gillian Walker (ed), *ABPI Data Sheet Compendium*, 1993–4 (Datapharm Publications Ltd., 1993): 45–46.

31 See *The Lancet*, 1990; 336: 436–37.

32 *American Journal of Respiratory and Critical Care Medicine*, March 1994.

33 *Annals of Internal Medicine*, 1993; 15: 963–68.

34 S. Teelucksingh, correspondence, *The Lancet*, 1991; 338: 60–61.

35 *Archives Disease in Childhood*, 1982; 57: 204–07.

36 *Acta Pediatrician*, 1993; 82: 636–40.

37 *Science*, 1990; 250: 1196–98.

38 V. D. Ramirez, commentary, *The Lancet*, 1996; 347: 630–31.

39 *European Respiratory Journal Supplement*, 1989; 6: 566s–67s.

40 *British Medical Journal*, 1996; 312: 542–43.

41 J. K. H. Wales, correspondence, *The Lancet*, 1991; 338: 1535.

42 *The Lancet*, 1966; ii: 569–72.

43 *Clinical and Experimental Rheumatology,* 1991; 9 Suppl. 6: 37–40.

44 J.K.H. Wales, *et al.,* correspondence, *The Lancet,* 1991; 338: 1535.

45 *J. Asthma,* 1986; 23 (6): 291–96.

46 Faruque Ghanchi, correspondence, *The Lancet,* 1993; 342: 1306–07.

47 *Pediatric Nephr,* 1994: 8 (6): 667–70.

48 *Clinical Pharma,* 1993; 25 (2): 126–35.

49 *Arthro,* 1985; 1 (1): 68–72.

50 *Journal of Rheumatology,* 1994; 21: 1207–13.

51 *British Journal of Dermatology,* 1993; 129: 431–36; *New England Journal of Medicine,* 1990; 322: 1093–97.

52 *Journal of Dermatology,* 1991; 18 (8): 454–64. *Skin Pharmacology,* 1992; 5 (2): 77–80.

53 *Dermatological Clinics,* 1992; 10 (3): 505–12; *Graefes Archive for Clinical Experimental Ophthalmology,* 1988; 226 (4): 337–40; C. J. McLean *et al.,* correspondence, *The Lancet,* 1995; 345: 330.

54 *Zeitschrift fur Hautkrankheiten,* 1988; 63 (4): 302–08.

55 *Archives of Disease in Childhood,* 1982; 57: 204–07.

56 *Archives of Disease in Childhood,* 1987; 62 (9): 876–78; J.K.H. Wales, op cit.

57 *Journal of the American Medical Association,* 1980; 244: 813–14.

58 C.J. McLean *et al.,* correspondence, *The Lancet,* 1995; 345: 330; *British Dermatology,* 1989; 120: 472–73; *Eye,* 1993; 7: 664–66; Dr. Evan Benjamin Dreyer, correspondence, *New England Journal of Medicine,* 1993; 329: 1822.

59 R.H. Meyboom, correspondence, *Annals of Internal Medicine,* 1988; 109 (8): 683.

60 Drs. Peter M. Brooks and Richard O. Day, *New England Journal of Medicine,* 1992; 327 (ii): 749–54; *The Lancet,* 1984; ii: 1171–74.

61 Drs. Peter M. Brooks and Richard O. Day, *New England Journal of Medicine,* 1991; 324 (24): 1716–25.

62 See *Physicians' Desk Reference* (Montvale, NJ: Medical Economics Data Production Company, 1995).

63 J. Hollingworth, correspondence, *British Medical Journal*, 1991; 302: 51; *British Journal of Rheumatism*, 1987; 26: 103–07.

64 *Journal of the American Medical Association*, November 28, 1990.

65 L. Theilmann *et al.*, correspondence, *The Lancet*, 1990; 335: 1346.

66 *Journal of the American Medical Association*, September 14, 1994.

67 Michael Gleeson, *et al.*, correspondence, *The Lancet*, 1994; 344: 1028.

68 *New England Journal of Medicine*, 1991; 325: 87–91.

69 *Drugs and Therapeutics Bulletin*, 1993; 31: 18.

70 *Journal of Clinical Epidemiology*, 1993; 46 (3): 315–21.

71 *Drugs and Therapeutics Bulletin*, 1993; 31: 18.

72 *Arthritis Rheumatol*, 1990; 33: 1449–61.

73 *Annals of Rheumatism Disease*, 1986; 45: 705–11.

74 *Arthritis Rheumatol*, 1990; 33: 1449–61.

75 *New England Journal of Medicine*, 1994; 330: 1368–75.

76 *Physicians' Desk Reference* (Montvale, NJ: Medical Economics Data Production Company, 1995): 1165–69.

77 *European Journal of Rheumatology Inflammation*, 1991; 11: 148–61.

78 *Annals of Rheumatism Disease*, 1990; 49: 25–27.

79 *Drugs and Therapeutics Bulletin*, 1993; 31: 18.

80 See G. W. Cannon and J. R. Ward, *Arthritis and Allied Conditions* (Philadelphia: Lea & Febiger, 1989).

81 *Archives of Internal Medicine*, 1993; 153: 154–83.

82 P. Sever, correspondence, *The Lancet*, 1994; 344: 1019–20.

83 *Blood Pressure*, 1993; 2 (suppl.): 5–9.

84 Wolfe and Hope, op cit.

85 Peter T. Sawick, correspondence, *British Medical Journal*, 1994; 308: 855.

86 *British Medical Journal*, 1993; 306: 609–11.

87 *Journal of Internal Medicine*, 1992; 232: 493–98, as reported in *Journal of the American Medical Association*, 1993: 269 (13): 1692.

88 *New England Journal of Medicine*, 1992; 327: 678–84.

89 *The Lancet*, 1993; 341: 967.

90 *British Medical Journal*, 1992; 304: 946–49.

91 *Journal of the American Medical Association*, May 20, 1992.

92 Larry Cahill *et al.*, correspondence, *Nature*, 1994; 371: 702–04.

93 *New England Journal of Medicine*, 1989; 320: 709–18.

94 Ibid.

95 *The Lancet*, 1995; 346: 767–70 and 346: 586.

96 *The Observer*, December 1992.

97 *British Medical Journal*, 1994; 310: 177–78.

98 *Epilepsia*, 1988; 29: 590–600.

99 *British Medical Journal*, 1993; 307: 483.

100 *The Lancet*, 1991; 337: 406–09; *Epilepsy Research*, 1993; 14: 237–44.

101 *Neurology*, 1996; 46: 41–44.

102 *New England Journal of Medicine*, 1990; 323: 497–502.

103 *Neurology*, 1993; 43: 478–83.

104 *Journal of Neurolology Neurosurgery and Psychiatry*, 1995; 58: 44–50.

105 *The Lancet*, 1996; 347: 709–13.

106 *Townsend Letter for Doctors*, October 1995: 100.

107 *British Medical Journal*, 1995; 310: 215–18.

108 Harold Silverman, *The Pill Book: A Guide to Safe Drug Use* (New York: Bantam Books, 1989): 278.

109 Ibid.

110 *Journal of Clinical Psychiatry*, 1995; 56:3.

111 *New England Journal of Medicine*, 1991; 325: 316–21; *Journal of the American Medical Association*, 1991; 265: 2831–35.

112 *The Lancet*, 1994; 344: 985–86.

113 S. Hood *et al.*, correspondence, *The Lancet*, 1994; 344: 1500–01.

114 *New England Journal of Medicine*, 1993; 329: 1476–83.

115 *The Lancet*, 1993; 341: 1564–65.

116 *British Medical Journal*, 1993; 307: 1185.

117 *The Lancet*, 1993; 341: 861–62.

118 Theresa Curtin, *et al*, correspondence, *British Medical Journal*, 1992; 305: 713–14.

119 *New England Journal of Medicine*, 1993; 329: 1476–83.

120 Carl Dahlof, correspondence, *The Lancet*, 1992; 340: 909.

121 *British Medical Journal*, 1994; 308: 113.

122 *The Lancet*, 1993; 341: 221–24.

123 *British Medical Journal*, 1996; 312: 657.

124 *Physicians' Desk Reference*, op cit: 897–98.

125 As cited in Peter Breggin, *Toxic Psychiatry* (New York: HarperCollins, 1991): 384–85.

126 *Journal of American Acad. Child Adol. Psych.*, 1987; 26 (1): 56–64.

127 Breggin, *Toxic Psychiatry*: 380.

128 Breggin, *Toxic Psychiatry*: 382.

129 Dr. Gerald B. Dermer, *The Immortal Cell* (Garden City Park, NY: Avery Publishing Group, 1994): 107.

130 See Ralph Moss, *Questioning Chemotherapy* (New York: Equinox Press, 1995).

131 Ibid. See also Dr. Urich Abel, *Der Spiegel*, 1990; 33: 174–76.

132 *New England Journal of Medicine*, 1992; 326 (8): 563.

133 *The Lancet*, 1996; 347: 1066–71.

134 *Current Opinion in Oncology*, 1995; 7 (5): 457–65.

135 Moss, *Questioning Chemotherapy*: 104.

136 See Moss, op cit.

137 *Physicians' Desk Reference* (1995): 673.

138 *British Medical Journal*, 1996; 312: 886.

139 *International Herald Tribune*, May 19, 1994.

140 *Current Opinion in Oncology*, 1995; 7 (4) 320–24.

141 *New England Journal of Medicine*, 1996; 334: 745–51.

142 *Journal of the National Cancer Institute*, 1996; 88: 270–78.

143 *New England Journal of Medicine*, 1989; 320: 69–75.

144 *Physicians' Desk Reference*, op cit.

145 Although a comprehensive discussion of alternatives for various illnesses is outside the scope of this book, a number of publications (including my newsletter *What Doctors Don't Tell You*) cover such alternatives in detail. For arthritis, consult John Mansfield, *Arthritis: Allergy, Nutrition and the Environment* (Thorsons, 1995). For asthma and eczema: Dr. Jonathan Brostoff and Linda Gamlin, *The Complete Guide to Food Allergy and Intolerance* (Bloomsbury, 1992). Also *What Doctors Don't Tell you*, 1991; 2 (12) and 1994; 5 (5). For proof of what works in all natural therapies, consult *Proof!: What Works in Alternative Medicine*, a monthly newsletter by the Wallace Press.

146 See *What Doctors Don't Tell You*, 1995; 6 (6) and Dr. Melvyn Werbach, *Healing Through Nutrition* (Thorsons, 1993), and his sourcebooks, *Nutritional Influences on Illness and Nutritional Influences on Mental Illness* (Tarzana, CA: Third Line Press, 1994 and 1991, respectively).

147 *Epilepsia*, 1992; 33 (6): 1132–36. See also *What Doctors Don't Tell You*, 1996; 6 (11): 12 and Werbach, op cit.

148 For discussion of the medical evidence of alternative cancer treatments, see Dr. Ralph Moss, *Cancer Therapy: The Independent Consumer's Guide to Non-Toxic Treatment & Prevention* (New York: Equinox Press, 1995), and Drs. Ross Pelton and Lee Overholser, *Alternatives in Cancer Therapy* (New York: Simon & Schuster, 1994).

Also *What Doctors Don't Tell You,* 1996; 7 (3) and 7 (4) and the *WDDTY Cancer Handbook* (The Wallace Press), 1997.

149 See Dr. Richard Evans, *Making the Right Choice* (Garden City Park, NY: Avery Publishing Group, 1995).

CHAPTER 9

1 For the history of amalgam, see Dr. Hal Huggins, *It's All in Your Head: The Link Between Mercury Amalgams and Illness* (Garden City Park, NY: Avery Publishing Group, 1993): 59–61.

2 Dr. Murray J. Vimy, symposium, 'Mercury from Dental Amalgam,' British Dental Society, April 14, 1992.

3 *Journal of the American Medical Association,* 1993; 269: 2491.

4 *Journal of the American Medical Association,* 1991; 265: 2934.

5 *The Lancet,* 1992; 339: 419.

6 *Bio-Probe Newsletter,* 1994; 10 (3): 3.

7 *Panorama,* 'Poison in the Mouth,' transmitted July 11, 1994.

8 Environmental Health Criteria 118: Inorganic Mercury (World Health Organization, Geneva, 1991).

9 *Panorama,* op cit.

10 M. Nylander, correspondence, *The Lancet,* 1986; i: 442; also *British Journal of Industrial Medicine,* 1991; 48: 729–34.

11 *Polsli Tygodnick Lekarski,* 1987; 42 (37): 1159–62; *International Archives of Occupational Environment Health,* 1987; 59: 551–57.

12 *Swedish Dental Journal,* 1989; 13: 235–43. *Adv. Dent. Res.* 1992; 6: 110–13.

13 *British Journal of Industrial Medicine,* 1992; 49: 782–90.

14 Dr. Diana Echeverria, as interviewed on *Panorama's* 'Poison in the Mouth,' op cit.

15 *British Medical Journal,* 1991; 302: 488, and *British Medical Journal,* 1994; 309: 621–22.

16 *Journal of Dental Research,* 1985; 64 (8): 1072–75.

17 Professor P. Soremark, Department of Prosthetic Dentistry, Karolinska Institute, Sweden, 'Mercury Release in Dentistry—I,' paper delivered July 15–16, 1985, 'Hazards in Dentistry: The Mercury Debate,' Kings College, Cambridge.

18 Prof. J. V. Masi, Ph.D., 'Corrosion of Restorative Materials: The Problem and the Promise.' Unpublished paper.

19 *FASEB Journal,* 1989; 3: 2641–46.

20 Ibid.

21 Dr. Murray J. Vimy, symposium, op cit.

22 Ibid.

23 Ibid.

24 Ibid.

25 *FASEB Journal,* 1992; 6: 2472–76; *Clinical Toxicology,* 1992; 30 (4): 505–28.

26 *American Journal of Physiology,* 1990; 258: R938–45.

27 Vimy, symposium, op cit.

28 *The Journal of Prosthetic Dentistry,* 1984; 51: 617–23.

29 Hal Huggins, personal interiew, April 1990.

30 Hal Huggins, *All in Your Head*: 126.

31 *The Journal of Epidemiology and Community Health,* 1978; 32: 155. *Swedish Journal of Biological Medicine,* January 1989: 6–7.

32 *International Journal of Risk and Safety Medicine,* 1994; 4: 229–36, as reported in *Bio-Probe Newsletter,* 1994; 10 (3): 6.

33 *American Journal of Physiology,* 1990; 258: R939–45.

34 *European Journal of Pediatrics,* 1994; 153: 607–10.

35 *Zentralbatt fur Gynäkologie,* 1992; 14, 593–602.

36 *Klinisches Labor,* 1992; 38: 469–76.

37 *International Journal of Risk and Safety Medicine,* 1994; 4: 229–36.

38 *Bio-Probe,* March 1993.

39 Huggins, interview, op cit.

40 *Annual Review of Microbiology,* 1986; 40: 607–34; *Antimicrobial Agents and Chemotherapy,* 1993; 37 (4): 825–34.

41 *Journal of Prosthetic Dentistry,* 1987; 58: 704–07.

42 P. Störtebecker, correspondence, *The Lancet,* 1989; i: 1207.

43 *Brain Research,* 1990; 553: 125–31.

44 Duhr *et al.,* FASEB 75th Annual Meeting, Atlanta, Georgia, April 21–25, 1991, Abstract 493.

45 *Journal of Neurochemistry,* 1994; 62: 2049–52.

46 *The Lancet,* 1994; 343: 993–97; 343: 989. See also studies reported in *What Doctors Don't Tell You,* 1995; 5 (12): 1–3.

47 Personal interview, Dr. M. Vimy, October 13, 1994.

48 For more information about the test, contact The British Society for Mercury-Free Dentistry (tel. 0171–486 3127). London naturopath Harald Gaier has adapted a simple test developed by Max Dauderer, in Munich, which your dentist can use to see if you are 'leaking' excessive amounts of mercury. All you need is a stick of sugarless chewing gum, some zinc-free wads of cotton, two syringes, and two sterile containers.

Make sure before you start the test that you haven't chewed anything for at least two hours. Then, take one of the two small wads of cotton and place them in your mouth for a short while, so that they are soaked with your saliva. Don't chew the cotton.

Take the plunger out of the syringe and insert the saliva-sodden cotton into it. Replace the plunger and squeeze the saliva out through the syringe into a sterile container marked 'Before.' Close it tightly.

Next, chew the stick of sugarless gum intensively (concentrating on those areas of your teeth covered with amalgam fillings). Discard the gum. Collect a second saliva sample the same way you did the first, with a second wad of cotton and the second syringe. Squeeze the saliva out into the second sterile container marked 'After.' Close it tightly.

Send both samples to a lab that can analyze each sample for its mercury content.

In Dr. Gaier's experience, people with large amounts of amalgam have far higher mercury content in the 'After' sample. For instance, in forty of his patients investigated for amalgam poisoning, the amount of mercury in their saliva went up by an average of 415 percent after chewing the gum. Thsoe patients with symptoms suggestive of mercury poisoning such as MS invariably had increased post-chewing mercury scores—often by as much as 1,800 percent.

Chapter 10

1   *British Medical Journal,* 1994; 309: 361–65.

2   E. A. Campling *et al.,* The Report of the National Confidential Enquiry into Perioperative Deaths, 1990 (National CEPOD, 1992). See also more recent editions of CEPOD.

3   *New England Journal of Medicine,* 1991; 325: 1002–07.

4   As cited in *Drugs and Therapeutic Bulletin,* 1980; 18: 7–8, as cited in Stephen Fulder, *How to Survive Medical Treatment* (Century Hutchinson, 1987): 90.

5   *Effective Health Care,* November 1992.

6   *GP,* August 6, 1993.

7   See studies mentioned in *The Lancet,* 1994; 344: 1652–53.

8   John G. F. Cleland, correspondence, *The Lancet,* 1994; 344: 1222–24.

9   *The Lancet,* 1994; 344: 563–70.

10 *New England Journal of Medicine,* 1992; 326: 10–16.

11 Gordon Waddell, 'A New Clinical Model for the Treatment of Low Back Pain,' in James Weinstein and Sam Wiesel (eds), *The Lumbar Spine* (Philadelphia: W.B. Saunders Co., 1990): 38–56.

12 See Henry La Rocca, 'Failed Lumbar Surgery: Principles of Management,' in Weinstein and Wiesel, *The Lumbar Spine*: 872–81.

13   *Spine*, 1980; 5: 87–94.

14   *Journal of the American Medical Association*, 1992; 268 (7): 907–11.

15   *The Mount Sinai Journal of Medicine*, 1991; 58 (2): 183–87.

16   Waddell, op cit.

17   La Rocca, op cit.

18   *Spine*, 1986; 11: 712–19.

19   *Journal of the American Medical Association*, 1991; 266: 1280–82.

20   *The Lancet*, 1994; 344: 1496–97.

21   *New England Journal of Medicine*, 1989; 320: 822–28.

22   *British Medical Journal*, 1994; 308: 809–10. *New England Journal of Medicine*, 1994; 330: 1460, and 330: 1448–50; *Lancet*, 1994; 343: 1049–50, and 343: 1496–97.

23   *New England Journal of Medicine*, 1995; 332 (14): 907–11.

24   *New England Journal of Medicine*, 1981; 305: 6–11; *European Journal of Cancer Clinical Oncology*, 1986; 22: 1085–89; *European Journal of Cancer*, 1990; 26: 668–70.

25   *British Medical Journal*, 1991; 303: 1431–35.

26   Ibid.

27   Both from *New England Journal of Medicine*, 1992; 326: 1102–07.

28   *Journal of the American Medical Association*, 1993; 268 (7): 869.

29   *British Medical Journal*, 1990; 301: 575–80.

30   Interview with surgeon Andrew Kingsnorth, October 1994; see also *British Journal Surgery*, 1992; 79: 1068–70.

31   *New England Journal of Medicine*, 1973; 289: 1224–29.

32   Kingsnorth, op cit.

33   *The Lancet*, 1994; 343: 251–54.

34   Cherald Chodak, *New England Journal of Medicine*, 1994; 330: 242–48.

35 *J. Pathol. Bacteriol.*, 1954; 68: 603–16, as reported in the *British Medical Journal*, 1993; 306: 407–08.

36 *The Lancet*, 1993; 341–91.

37 *Journal of the American Medical Association*, 1992; 267: 2191–96; *New England Journal of Medicine*, 1994; 330: 242–48.

38 *Journal of the American Medical Association*, 1993; 270: 948–54.

39 *Archives of Family Medicine*, 1993; 2: 487–93, as reported in *Journal of the American Medical Association*, 1993; 269 (20): 2676–77.

40 *Journal of the American Medical Association*, 1993; 269: 2633–36.

41 *National Cancer Institute Monogr.*, 1988; 7: 117–26.

42 *Journal of the American Medical Association*, 1995; 273 (2): 129–35.

43 Interview with Reginald Lloyd Davies, July 1995; see also *The Lancet*, 1994; 344: 700–01.

44 *New England Journal of Medicine*, 1994; 330: 242–48.

45 *Journal of the American Medical Association*, 1995; 274 (8): 626–31.

46 *The Lancet*, 1995; 346: 1528–30.

47 *The Lancet*, 1995; 346; 1334–35.

48 M. Baum, correspondence, *The Lancet*, 1996; 347: 260.

49 Hospital Episodes Statistics 1993–4 (HMSO) as cited in *What Doctors Don't Tell You*, 1996; 7 (1): 1–3.

50 *Obstetrics and Gynecology*, 1993; 82: 757–64. See also *The Hysterectomy Hoax* (New York: Doubleday, 1994).

51 *Fertility and Sterility*, 1984; 42: 510–14.

52 *New England Journal of Medicine*, 1993; 328: 856–60; *Cancer*, 1985; 56: 403–12.

53 *American Journal of Obstetrics and Gynecology*, 1982; 144: 841–48.

54 *The Pulse*, August 14, 1993.

55 *British Journal of Urology*, 1989; 64: 594–99.

56 *British Journal of Obstetrics and Gynaecology*, 1994; 101: 468–70.

57   *American Journal of Obstetrics and Gynecology*, 1981; 140: 725–29.

58   *American Journal of Obstetrics and Gynecology*, 1993; 168: 765–71.

59   *Fertility and Sterility*, 1987; 47: 94–100.

60   For specific alternatives to hysterectomy, see *What Doctors Don't Tell You*, 1996; 7 (1): 3.

61   *The Lancet*, 1991; 337: 1074–78.

62   Ruditer Pittrof *et al.*, *The Lancet*, 1991; 338: 197–98.

63   *Journal of the American Medical Association*, 1993; 270 (10): 1230–32.

64   Angela Coulter, correspondence, *The Lancet*, 1994; 344: 1367.

65   *British Journal of Obstetrics and Gynaecology*, 1996; 103: 142–49.

66   *World Journal of Surgery*, 1987; 11: 82–83.

67   Blood Technologies, Services and Issues, U.S. Office of Technology Assessment Task Force, U.S. Congress, 1988; 22/23: 121–29.

68   *Vox Sanguinis: The International Journal of Transfusion Medicine*, 1987; 52: 60–62.

69   Ibid.

70   *Transfusion Medical Reviews*, 1989; 3 (1): 39–54.

71   Ibid.

72   *British Medical Journal*, 1994; 308: 1205–06; also 308: 1180–81.

73   Ibid.

74   See Luc Montagnier, *AIDS: The Safety of Blood and Blood Products* (John Wiley & Sons, 1987).

75   *Gastroenterology*, 1988; 95: 530–31.

76   *Monitor Weekly*, April 7, 1988.

77   *British Medical Journal*, 1994; 308: 695–96.

78   N. Hallam *et al.*, correspondence, *British Medical Journal*, 1994; 308: 856.

79   *New England Journal of Medicine*, 1989; 320: 1172–75.

80   *Annals Otology, Rhinology & Laryngology*, 1989; 98: 171–73.

81 *Annals of Thoracic Surgery,* 1989; 47: 346–49.

82 *British Medical Journal,* 1986; 293: 530–32.

83 *Transfusion,* 1989; 29: 456–58. *British Journal of Surgery,* 1988; 75: 789–91.

84 *Annals of Surgery,* 1986; 203: 275–79.

85 *Vox Sanguinis,* 1989; 57 (1): 63–65.

86 *Journal of the American Medical Association,* 1986; 256: 2242–43.

87 *Journal of Bloodless Medicine and Surgery,* Spring 1986: 15–17.

88 *Journal of the American Medical Association,* 1973; 226: 1230. See also *Journal of the American Medical Association,* 1977; 238: 1256–58.

CHAPTER 11

1 *Times,* February 11, 1990.

2 Ajay K. Singh *et al.,* correspondence, *New England Journal of Medicine,* 1994; 331 (26): 1777–78; *New England Journal of Medicine,* 1994; 331 (17): 1110–15.

3 Dr. David Lomax, correspondence, *The Lancet,* 1993; 342: 1247.

4 *Times,* September 21, 1993.

5 *The Lancet,* 1996; 347: 527.

6 *American Journal of Surgery,* 1993; 165: 9–14.

7 *Journal of Gynecological Surgery,* 1989; 5: 131–32.

8 *The Lancet,* 1994; 344: 596–97.

9 *The Lancet,* 1993; 342: 674.

10 *Australian and New Zealand Journal of Obstetrics and Gynecology,* 1993; 31: 171–73.

11 *The Lancet,* 1993; 342: 633–37.

12 *The Lancet,* 1995; 345: 36–40.

13 *The Lancet,* 1994; 344: 596–97.

14   Ibid.

15   David Lomax, correspondence, *The Lancet*, 1993; 342: 1247.

16   *Journal of the American Medical Association*, 1995; 273 (20): 1581–85.

17   *The Lancet*, 1993; 341: 1057–58.

18   *Journal of the American Medical Association*, 1994; 271 (17): 1349–57.

19   R. Treacy *et al.*, correpsondence, *British Medical Journal*, 1992; 304: 317.

20   *The Guardian*, February 23, 1993.

21   *Journal of Bone and Joint Surgery*, July 1991.

22   *Acta Orthopaedica Scandinavica* (Supplement), 1990; 61: 1–26.

23   *Journal of Bone and Joint Surgery*, 1994; 76A: 959–64, as reported in Minerva, *British Medical Journal*, 1994; 309: 888.

24   *The Guardian*, op cit.

25   *British Medical Journal*, 1992; 303: 1431–35.

26   *Journal of the American Medical Association*, 1994; 271 (17): 1349–57.

27   *The Lancet*, 1993; 341: 1057–58.

28   *British Medical Journal*, 1994; 309: 880.

29   Interview with Chris Bulstrode, orthopedic surgeon at John Radcliffe Hospital in Oxford, *The Guardian*, op cit.

30   *The Journal of Bone and Joint Surgery*, 1994; 76B (5): 701–12.

31   Ibid.

32   *Journal of Bone and Joint Surgery*, 1992; 76B: 539–42; *Journal of Biomedical Materials Research*, 1977; 11: 157–64, as reported in *Journal of Bone and Joint Surgery*, 1994; 76B (5): 701–12.

33   *Fundamental and Applied Toxicology*, 1989; 13: 205–16.

34   *Science*, 1994; 266: 726–27, as reported in Minerva, *British Medical Journal*, 1994; 309: 1382.

35   *New England Journal of Medicine*, 1992; 326 (1): 57–58.

36   *Journal of the American Medical Association*, 1992; 268 (21): 3092–97.

37 *The Lancet*, 1992; 340: 1202–05.

38 *New England Journal of Medicine*, 1992; 327: 1329–35.

39 *Journal of the American College of Cardiologists*, 1992; 19: 946–47; *New England Journal of Medicine*, 1991; 326: 1053–57.

40 *New England Journal of Medicine*, 1992; 326 (1): 10–16.

41 *Chest*, 1992; 102: 375–79.

42 *New England Journal of Medicine*, 1991; 325: 556–62.

43 *Journal of the American Medical Association*, 1992; 268: 2537–40.

44 *The Lancet*, 1993; 341: 573–80 and 341: 599–600.

45 *New England Journal of Medicine*, 1994; 331 (16): 1044–49.

46 *New England Journal of Medicine*, 1994; 331 (16): 1037–43; *The Lancet*, 1995; 346: 1179–84.

47 *New England Journal of Medicine*, 1993; 329: 221–27.

48 Ibid.

49 *Physicians' Desk Reference* (Montvale, NJ: Medical Economics Data Production Company, 1995): 2340.

50 *New England Journal of Medicine*, 1994; 331: 771–76.

51 *The Lancet*, 1993; 341: 234.

52 Report of the Interim Licencing Authority, sponsored by the Medical Research Council and the British Royal College of Obstetricians and Gynaecologists, 1990.

53 *The Lancet*, August 13, 1994; *Teratology*, 1990; 42: 467; Les White *et al.*, correspondence, *The Lancet*, 1990, 386: 1577; Lyn Chitty *et al.*, correspondence, *British Medical Journal*, 1990; 300: 1726.

54 *British Medical Journal*, 1993; 307: 1239–43.

55 P. Boulot, correspondence, *The Lancet*, 1990; 335: 1156–56.

56 *What Doctors Don't Tell You*, 1994; 5·(6): 7.

57 Robert H. Heptinstall, *Pathology of the Kidney* (Boston: Little, Brown and Company, 1992): 1592.

58 *Nephron*, 1993; 63 (2): 242–43.

59 *Journal of Endourology*, 1994; 8 (1): 15–19.

60 *Journal of Urology*, 1993; 150 (6): 1765–67.

61 *Polskie Archiwum Medycyny Wewnetrznej*, 1993; 89 (5): 394–99.

62 *British Journal of Urology*, 1991; 68 (6): 657–58.

63 Japanese Journal of Clinical Radiology, 1990; 35 (9): 1015–20.

64 *Nephrologie*, 1993; 14 (6): 305–07.

65 *Rofo Fortschr Geb Rontgenstr Neuen Bildgeb Verfahr*, 1993; 158 (2): 121–26.

66 *Acta Urologica Japonica*, 1993; 39 (12): 1119–24.

67 *Acta Urologica Japonica*, 1992; 38 (9): 999–1003.

68 *Urologica Internationalist*, 1993; 51 (3): 152–57.

69 *Journal of Urology*, 1993; 150: 481–82.

70 *Journal of Urology*, 1991; 145 (5): 942–48.

71 *Journal of Pediatrics*, 1994; 125 (1): 149–51.

72 *Journal of the Association of Physicians of India*, 1993; 41 (11): 748–49.

73 *Journal of Urology*, 1990; 144 (6): 1339–40.

74 *Scandinavian Journal of Urology and Nephrology*, 1993; 27 (2): 267–69.

75 *Nephrology, Dialysis, Transplantation*, 1990; 5 (11): 974–76.

76 *Acta Urologica Belgica*, 1994; 62 (2): 25–29.

77 *Journal of Urology*, 1994; 151 (6): 1605–06.

78 E.S. Searle, correspondence, *British Medical Journal*, 1994; 309: 270.

79 *The Independent*, July 3, 1996.

80 Interview with Paul Balen, solicitor for U.K. cases, October 1994.

81 *Drugs and Therapeutics Bulletin*, 1994; 32 (3): 17–19.

82 Ibid.

83 *The Independent*, July 3, 1996.

CHAPTER 12

1   *The Netherlands 1986 Monthly Bulletin of Population of Health Statistics.*

2   Norman Cousins, Deepak Chopra and Andrew Weil are just a few of the authors who have popularized the mind-body connection. See also *The Lancet*, 1995; 345: 99–103 and *The Lancet*, 1994; 344: 995–98.

3   *The Lancet*, 1994; 344: 1319–22.

4   *The Lancet*, 1994; 344: 973–75.

5   *British Medical Journal*, 1992; 305: 341–46.

6   *What Doctors Don't Tell You*, 1995; 6 (4): 8–10.

7   *British Medical Journal*, 1991; 303; 1105–09; also 303: 1109–10.

8   Ibid. See also *British Medical Journal*, 1991; 303: 1105–09.

9   *British Medical Journal*, 1995; 310: 489–91.

10 *American Journal of Public Health*, 1993; 83: 1321–25, as reported in the *Journal of the American Medical Association*, 1993; 270 (18): 2170.

11 Leon Eisenberg, M.D., Special Communication, *Journal of the American Medical Association*, 1995; 274 (4): 331–34.

12 *Journal of the National Cancer Institute*, 1993; 85 (15): 1483–92.

13 *Journal of the American Medical Association*, 1994; 272 (18): 1413–20.

14 *New England Journal of Medicine*, 1994; 331: 141–47.

15 *The Lancet*, 1994; 343: 1454–59.

16 *Journal of the American Medical Association*, 1995; 273 (20): 1563.

17 Interview with Dr. Jonathan Wright, May 1996.

18 See Melvyn Werbach, *Nutritional Influences on Illness* (Tarzana, CA: Third Line Press, 1993) and *Nutritional Influences on Mental Illness* (Third Line Press, 1991), for an extensive review of the medical literature and scientific studies that exist on the role of nutrition in causing or treating illness. Also see the *Journal of Nutritional and Environmental Medicine*, a monthly scientific review of the United

States, and the *American Journal of Clinical Nutrition,* two excellent sources of scientific papers on the subject.

19 *The Lancet,* 1992; 340: 439–43.

20 Natural Resources Defense Council, 'Intolerance Risk: Pesticides in our Children's Food' (Washington, D.C.: NRDC, 1989). See also *What Doctors Don't Tell You,* 1995; 6 (3): 1–3.

21 Dr. John Mansfield, 'Chemical Crippling,' *What Doctors Don't Tell You,* 1995; 6 (7): 12. See also the work of Professor William Rea, head of the Environmental Health Center in Dallas, Texas.

22 *Journal of the American Medical Association,* 1995; 273: 1179–84.

23 *Times,* March 28, 1995.

24 *British Medical Journal,* 1995; 310: 1122–25.

25 *Times,* November 1, 1994.

26 See Melvyn Werbach and Michael T. Murray, *Botanical Influences on Illness* (Tarzana, CA: Third Line Press, 1994), and the 'Alternatives' column in *What Doctors Don't Tell You* and Proof! (both from The Wallace Press), which contain copious scientific evidence that alternative medicine works.

27 *Medical Biology,* 1977; 55: 88–94, as quoted in *New England Journal of Medicine,* 1995; 333 (4): 263.

28 See B. Pomeranz and G. Stu, *Scientific Bases of Acupuncture* (New York: Springer-Verlag, 1989), as quoted in *New England Journal of Medicine,* 1995; 333 (4): 263.

29 *New England Journal of Medicine,* 1995; 333 (4): 263.

30 *New England Journal of Medicine,* 1994; 330 (3): 223.

31 C. Hewlett, correspondence, *The Lancet,* 1994; 344: 695. See also *What Doctors Don't Tell You,* 1996; 7 (3): 5.

INDEX

Alternative Healing Approaches

KAVA
NATURE'S STRESS RELIEF
by Kathryn M. Connor, M.D. and Donald S. Vaughan
80641-X/$5.99 US/$7.99 Can

ST. JOHN'S WORT
NATURE'S MOOD BOOSTER
*Everything You Need to Know about This
Natural Antidepressant*
by Michael E. Thase, M.D. and Elizabeth E. Loredo
80288-0/$5.99 US/$7.99 Can

GINKGO
NATURE'S BRAIN BOOSTER
by Alan H. Pressman, D.C., Ph.D., C.C.N.
with Helen Tracy
80640-1/$5.99 US/$7.99 Can

A HANDBOOK OF NATURAL FOLK REMEDIES
by Elena Oumano, Ph.D.
78448-3/$5.99 US/$7.99 Can

A COMPLETE LINE OF
WOMEN'S HEALTH INFORMATION

THE WHOLE WOMAN
Take Charge of Your Health in
Every Phase of Your Life
by Lila A. Wallis, M.D., M.A.C.P. with Marian Betancourt
78081-X/$17.50 US/$25.50 Can

HELP YOUR MAN GET HEALTHY
An Essential Guide for Every Caring Woman
by Maria Kassberg Regan and Steve Jonas, M.D.
89769-0/$12.50 US/$18.50 Can

THE ATHLETIC WOMAN'S SOURCEBOOK
How To Stay Healthy and Competitive in Any Sport
by Janis Graham
79667-8/$12.50 US/$18.50 Can

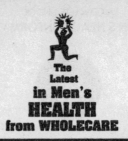